Physick
and the family

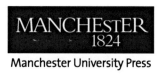

To Andy
A long overdue gift with
grateful thanks as always.
Alun.

MANCHESTER
1824

Manchester University Press

Physick and the family

HEALTH, MEDICINE AND CARE IN WALES, 1600-1750

Alun Withey

MANCHESTER UNIVERSITY PRESS

Manchester and New York

distributed in the United States exclusively by Palgrave Macmillan

Published by Manchester University Press
Oxford Road, Manchester M13 9NR, UK
and Room 400, 175 Fifth Avenue, New York, NY 10010, USA
www.manchesteruniversitypress.co.uk

Distributed in the United States exclusively by
Palgrave Macmillan, 175 Fifth Avenue,
New York, NY 10010, USA

Distributed in Canada exclusively by
UBC Press, University of British Columbia, 2029 West Mall,
Vancouver, BC, Canada V6T 1Z2

British Library Cataloguing-in-Publication Data is available

Library of Congress Cataloging-in-Publication Data is available

ISBN 978 0 7190 9125 4 paperback

First published by Manchester University Press in hardback 2011

This paperback edition first published 2013

Printed by Lightning Source

This book is dedicated to the memory of my sister, Susan Withey (1965–88)

Contents

Preface

This book is a new history of medicine in early modern Wales. It is also a new history of the medical knowledge, beliefs and practice of a distinct region of the British Isles – one that was largely rural and also far away from medical centres of licensing and training. More broadly, it is a work of social history, exploring the influences of a range of factors upon the everyday lives of 'ordinary' people.

This is not, however, a narrative story; such an approach in this case would prove unsatisfactory. The reader would soon conclude that humoral medicine was unsurprisingly dominant in Wales; that a range of healers practised; that a vast array of substances found their way into medical remedies and so on until the point of even studying it in medical terms might seem questionable. Instead, it uses evidence from Welsh sources to address a number of key themes in the history of medicine, including domestic medicine, the dissemination of knowledge, the market for medicines, medical language and literacy and the family. Much of what has already been written about Welsh medicine concentrates upon folklore and magic, both of which were undoubtedly important components in the medical worldview of the people of seventeenth- and eighteenth-century Wales. But they were not the only components.

Throughout the book it will become clear that Welsh people (and, it must be remembered, these were mostly Welsh-speaking people) belonged to a very broad medical culture which drew not only from elsewhere in Britain, but from continental Europe and far beyond. Welsh people were obviously aware of wider medical developments, not only through the strong Welsh oral culture of knowledge dissemination, but also through the increasing impact of English published texts. They could buy a range of materia medica from local shops, including exotic foreign ingredients. They could see foreign quacks and mountebanks in action in market towns, and also consult practitioners with strong links to urban medical centres. For a small, relatively sparsely populated and reputedly insular country, Wales was remarkably open for business.

But in other ways, Welsh sources allow us to ask broader questions about the sickness experience. How did sufferers understand, articulate and deploy sickness narratives? Who cared for the sick in both domestic and wider community contexts, and what can this reveal about social relations? How well equipped was the early modern household to deal with sickness? Evidence from Wales allows us to shed light on all of these issues.

A good regional medical history should not simply explore its subject in isolation, but instead use it as a means to open up new debates and pose new questions. These are the aims to which this book aspires.

Acknowledgements

The creation of this book owes much to the generosity, guidance and support of many academic colleagues, friends and family, which I should here like to acknowledge. I firstly owe a great debt of gratitude to my PhD supervisor, Dr David M. Turner. His patience, insight and expertise have guided me through the challenges of academic research and writing since undergraduate days. I also wish to thank my second supervisor, Professor Anne Borsay, for her support and valuable advice throughout my research. To study under two such excellent mentors has been a pleasure and a privilege. Professor Steve Hindle and Dr Adam Mosley provided thoughtful and useful feedback and comments on my work, as did the anonymous readers from Manchester University Press. Thanks also must go to the Wellcome Trust who supported the research for this work through a PhD studentship, and to the staff of the History departments at Swansea University and the University of Glamorgan, who have provided such fruitful and stimulating environments for my work.

Secondly, I would like to thank the staff of all the record offices and repositories whose help in locating sources has often been invaluable. These include The National Library of Wales (and especially Beryl Evans and her team), Bodleian Library, British Library, Wellcome Library, Cardiff Central Library, Carmarthenshire Record Office, Chester and Cheshire Archives, Flintshire Record Office, Glamorgan Record Office, Pembrokeshire Record Office, Powys County Archives. My most grateful thanks here are reserved for Tony Hopkins of the Gwent Record Office whose recommendation, in 2004, that I take a look at a certain Monmouthshire commonplace book serendipitously introduced me to Welsh medical history.

A number of academic colleagues have generously helped in locating and providing source material, suggesting new lines of enquiry and through numerous fruitful conversations. In this, I would especially like to thank Richard Allen, Peter Bowen, Mary Fissell, Robin Gwyndaf, David Haycock, Ralph Houlbrooke, Sharon Howard, Geraint H. Jenkins, J. Gwynfor Jones, Elaine Leong, Diana

Acknowledgements

Luft, Ross McFarlane, Morfydd Owen, Margaret Pelling, Sara Pennell, Lisa Smith, Anne Stobart, Jon Stobart, Lisa Tallis, Patrick Wallis, Jane Whittle and Nick Woodward. From the genesis of this book, many others have helped in a variety of ways, and probably more than they know. I would like to offer my sincere thanks and gratitude to Andy Mardell, Andy Croll, Chris Evans, Jane Finucane, Fiona Reid, Andy Bosson and Martyn Pease.

Finally, I have been blessed with a family who have shown unstinting support, encouragement and forbearance in their indulgence of a 'mature' (and doubtless seemingly eternal) student. To my parents, Pat and Colwyn, Rob and Alison, my parents-in-law Iris and Bill, and especially my mother Pat, I offer my grateful thanks for their love and constant support through the ups and downs of my work. My son Morgan came along as this book was in preparation, and has changed the life of his 'dadda' immeasurably for the better. But perhaps most importantly, I thank my wife Suzanne. Without her eternal patience, indulgence, selflessness and love, this book could never have been written.

Figures

Introduction

In 1739, Robert Lloyd, rector of the parish of Aber in Caernarvonshire, was unusually thorough in compiling his parish registers. Recording his parishioners' burials, Lloyd also noted their afflictions. 'Out of ye 9 yt were buried were infants no. 6, died of ye asthma and dropsy no. 1, consumption no. 1, feminine obstructions and dropsy no. 1'.[1] A range of other conditions afflicted his flock, from 'pleuritic fever' to 'decay', 'mortification in the bowels' to 'canker in the jaw' and the list goes on.[2] Sometimes we can put names to the sufferers, and even glean some basic information about their ages, where they lived, who their families were. But Lloyd's list makes a useful metaphor for our understanding of the medical history of Wales; we have the bare facts, but lack the wider understanding to complete the picture. How did early modern people, such as the parishioners of Aber, experience illness, and how well equipped were they, their homes and families to tackle it? To whom did they turn for advice and treatment? What were the sources of their medical knowledge and who, if anyone, supported and cared for them during their last days? In addressing each of these questions with reference to early modern Wales, this book will make an important contribution not only to Welsh medical history, but to the historiography of British and European medicine in the seventeenth and eighteenth centuries.

The medical history of any country goes straight to the heart of the culture and beliefs of its people. Medicine, sickness and death, all form the backdrop for the everyday beliefs, experiences and struggles of our ancestors as they lived out their lives. Sickness affected people's existence at the most basic level; it coloured how they approached their daily lives and interacted with others; it crossed boundaries of religion and magic and served to reinforce or question their beliefs of mortality and an afterlife. Medicine and illness, as Roy Porter noted, are therefore languages, as much social as biological, through which we can understand and reconnect with our past.[3] Medical history in the past three decades or so has indeed undergone at the very least a transformation and, at best, a complete rejuvenation. The rise of the Social History of Medicine, now virtually a discipline of its own, has provided much of the impetus for this change. Old Whig notions of 'Great Men' doctors, miraculous discoveries and linear teleological progress have been largely abandoned in favour of more nuanced explorations of the many side alleys and dead ends of medical history; of the continuities as well as the changes.[4] The influence of social-constructionism, to give one example, can be seen in the increasingly firm location of medical history, illness, disease and medicine within wider economic, political and cultural, as well as social and religious trends, demonstrating the close relationship between medicine and contemporary culture.[5] This has also served to address accusations that medical history lacked its own conceptual framework by providing ways of understanding medicine as being both reflective and formative of society as a whole.[6]

The early modern period, in particular, has benefited greatly from the works of a vanguard of social historians of medicine. Roy Porter initially did much to shift the emphasis away from doctors and back to the actual sickness sufferer, demonstrating also the extent of patient agency and power.[7] Porter's work also highlighted the multiplicity of treatment options open to sufferers, citing the 'catch-all' approach to healing and the many different forms which the growing body of medical healers could take.[8] Where traditional medical histories were practitioner-centred, they were also often male-dominated. It is therefore pleasing to note the growing body of recent works on gender and medicine, and especially an appreciation of the multifarious roles of women, drawing on a new range of sources such as domestic remedy collections. Much still remains to be done though, in order to move away from a general over-concentration on obstetrics, especially midwifery.[9]

Likewise, an increasing recognition of the importance of 'place' and regionalism in medicine has led to a number of smaller-scale studies of individual towns as well as wider demographics of disease, highlighting the possibilities of reconstructing local medical conditions where sufficient source materials survive.[10] Cross pollination with other historical disciplines has borne fruit in the exploration of previously marginalised subjects, such as death and disability, while the value of quantitative methodologies, highlighted first by Wrigley and Schofield, has done much to stimulate interest in disease demography.[11] A growing body of work on the economics of medicine has also done much to locate medical retail and retailers within wider patterns of consumption and notions of the marketplace for medicines.[12] On balance, medical history seems well on its way towards shaking off any perceptions of a 'plague-doctors and leeches' image. What, though, of the medical historiography of Wales?[13]

The relative lack of attention paid to Welsh medical history in recent historiography, and especially so for the early modern period, seems to reflect some deeply entrenched shibboleths about how to approach it. Overall, it seems that historians have not really known what to 'do' with the history of medicine in Wales, and this is certainly reflected in the existing secondary literature. Welsh medical historiography can generally be compartmentalised into two neat categories: nineteenth-century industrial health, and an enduring medical folklore. In many ways, the former seems perfectly logical and legitimate, and many such works emerged from 1980s' labour history, providing new studies on such themes as life in industrial towns like Merthyr Tydfil, with a 'second wave' of interest in social and national histories of Wales emerging in the 1990s as Wales began to come to terms with its newly devolved status.[14] In terms of medical histories, this has engendered some excellent works, such as Anne Borsay's 2003 collection of essays, exploring such matters as the rise of public health provision in Wales, and health and medicine in the industrial coalfields, with further welcome evidence of the influence of more recent trends towards previously marginalised subjects such as suicide.[15] Another recent and diverse collection of essays on such topics as maternal mortality, urbanisation and port health in twentieth-century Wales has served to highlight the relevance of medicine in both a Welsh and a wider context, while its editor, Pamela Michael, also highlights the need to understand Wales in terms of its own unique and indigenous characteristics.[16]

For the period between 1600 and 1800, however, the situation is markedly different. In the 1950s and 1960s, the Welsh historian Glyn Penrhyn Jones published variously on Welsh medical history, although only within Welsh local journals and, in the case of his book, only in the Welsh language, severely limiting the audience, and thus the impact, of his research.[17] In fact, at the time of writing, only one relevant book, *Wales and Medicine*, edited by John Cule, explores the topic at all, doing so in synchronic snapshots from pre-history through to the modern age, and this is now over thirty years old.[18] Despite its useful insights into some aspects of medicine in Wales, its emphasis on doctors and practice is showing its age in today's environment of 'history from below'.

Analysis of the sorts of academic articles published over the years reveals a wide assortment of varying quality ranging from antiquarian delight at the seemingly bizarre contents of early remedies to a multiplicity of works on magical and 'folkloric' medical practices and the colourful band of healers who undertook to use them.[19] But, importantly, some works have attempted to step outside the boundaries and use Welsh medical sources to make wider comparisons. In the 1970s, Morfydd Owen analysed the medieval medical manuscripts of Wales, including those of the Physicians of Myddfai, and set them in context of wider English and European medical books, concluding that Wales could boast a coherent tradition of medical writings.[20] More recently, Lisa Tallis has analysed the uniqueness of folkloric healing in Wales and its relationship with 'orthodox' healing, while Owen Davies has explored the role of cunning folk, examining such often ignored facets as gender roles and social status, stressing the importance of such figures in local communities, as well as their specific skills.[21] Colleen M. Seguin has even infused Foucauldian notions of power to Welsh medical history, by analysing governmental attempts to control or discredit the drawing power of healing wells in Wales.[22] In fairness, then, the problem lies not necessarily with the subject matter itself, since the case for an especially strong Welsh background of magical and lay healing within the wider context of a somewhat peculiar religious background has, in the main, been well made. Rather, it is the almost total lack of attention paid to alternatives to folklore in early modern Wales that corrals Welsh medical historiography into little more than a fringe subject category. While, over the years, many historians have made brief forays into the subject, their calls and conclusions have remained largely unheeded and atrophy into silence, leaving a trail of unanswered questions and dead ends. Metaphorically, Welsh medical historiography might neatly be summed up as so many acorns, but no oak trees.

What is needed, then, is a new direction and, accordingly, this book has three main aims. The first, and most important, is to provide a complete reappraisal of Welsh medical history in the early modern period. In doing so, it challenges current and prevailing depictions of pre-industrial medical culture, beliefs and practice as being dominated by magic and folklore. Given current trends towards exploring the geographical margins of the early modern medical world, Wales has been notably absent in existing studies of early modern Britain, and beyond. Bringing the Welsh experience to this corpus of existing knowledge can greatly enhance our understanding of the important confluences and divergences within distinct regions, as well as bridge a significant gap in the medical historiography of early modern Wales.

Secondly, this book will provide an important addition to the wider social history of Wales by using medicine as a way of revising and shaping our understanding of early modern Welsh culture and society. In Parts II and III of this book, such factors as medical economies, both of material goods and knowledge, into and within Wales are extremely important in highlighting its participation in social and economic networks. These sections question the extent to which the country really was insular or remote. Studies of medicine within the context of the family and domestic environment in Chapters 6 and 7 do much to shed light on issues such as social structures and networks of care in Wales, but also explore wider questions of gender and particularly male patriarchal roles within the Welsh household. Likewise, a detailed analysis of poor relief has wider utility in shedding light on the operations of the Old Poor Law in rural Wales, another area sparsely served by historians.

But the third, and vitally important, aim is to use the example of Wales as a means to address much wider issues of social and medical history. To fully explore the potentially unique or nuanced elements of medicine in (and of) Wales, it *must* be located far more firmly within the wider context of its relationship with other regions of early modern Britain and, indeed, Europe. The issue of the spread of medical knowledge raises important questions about the complex economic and cultural relationships between centres and peripheries, and is by no means limited, for example, to the relationship between London and Wales. As evidence in the book will demonstrate, even relatively small Welsh ports handled medical goods from all over the globe. Another essential question concerns cultural reciprocity and emulation. To what extent could regional and provincial medicine in England and Wales be seen as emulative of form and structure within large English towns and cities? Much evidence certainly indicates that Welsh patients and practitioners could be at least normatively aware of developments in London, through books, pamphlets and the availability of London goods through local dealers. Further issues such as the assimilation of English-language disease terms and nomenclature in Wales, the dissemination and consumption of medical texts, the networks of trade and supply, all dovetail with broader questions of the cultural hegemony of English urban centres over 'remote' regions. At a time when the boundaries between 'folkloric' and 'orthodox' medicine are being continually eroded, how too might indigenous 'popular culture' and 'folklore' be reconciled with the increasing influence of 'modern' medical provision, even in rural areas? Equally, understanding the important influences of factors such as religion, literacy, power, language and dialect in Wales can greatly enhance our understanding of the diversity of early modern sickness experiences, and especially away from urban centres.

This study is prescient in other ways. The form and structure of the family has been undergoing a reappraisal in recent times, and an understanding of the ways in which familial and wider community structures addressed illness crosses disciplinary boundaries.[23] The role of power in medical relationships is also timely, as Roger Cooter points out, at a time when shifts in medical power and authority in today's society continue to make headlines such as those concerning the increasing intrusion of the private sector into public healthcare.[24] On a wider level, the study of medical power and authority in Wales is interesting bearing in mind its peculiar position as a partially devolved region of the United Kingdom, while questions of the existence of indigenous elements to Welsh medical beliefs echo underlying questions of national identity. Here, then, the book seeks to move beyond its stated and immediate aims of a new medical history of Wales, by also providing a fresh and valuable study of life and health during the seventeenth and eighteenth centuries. In undertaking a new study of early modern medicine in Wales, we are in fact presented with the increasingly rare opportunity of mapping uncharted historiographical waters. It has recently been argued that much medical historiography relies upon the creation of a juxta-position to traditional, or else Whiggish, medical history – in essence, the setting up of a straw man against which the 'new social history' can be matched.[25] In Wales, however, there is little 'traditional' historiography against which to argue. Whilst this is in one way frustrating, it also paves the way for a new study, quite separate from what has gone before, but also able to be infused with the inherited theoretical, conceptual and structural net gains of the past thirty or so years of medical historiography. This means that, for the first time in more than a quarter of a century, Welsh medical history has the chance to lead by example. Rather than being a narrow or limited study, therefore, it is hoped that the analyses and studies within will appeal to a wide range of historians, and far beyond the Welsh borders.

Structure

The book is divided thematically into three parts which can be broadly catego-rised as disease, knowledge and care. In the first section, Chapter 1 establishes the contextual background for the book, investigating some of the factors affecting the types and spread of disease in Wales. In doing so, it explores something of the importance of geography and regional variation in affecting the sickness experience.

In Part II, themes of bodily concepts and the spread of medical information are developed. Chapter 2 investigates the ways in which Welsh people conceptu-alised their bodies and how this information was assimilated and disseminated. Studies of disease and the body in popular cultural sources, such as poetry and vernacular verse, contribute to a wider assessment of a 'Welsh' bodily concept. This is further brought out by analysis of the Welsh body in English literature, where it is argued that external depictions of Wales and the Welsh were surpris-ingly positive in comparison with those of other regions of the British Isles. The importance of religion in Wales in shaping attitudes to health and the body is also explored in detail. Much Welsh historiography concentrates on the con-servatism of Welsh religion and its role in preserving traditional, or else folkloric medicine. Here, a different approach is adopted and the ways in which Welsh religion could effect changes in medical approaches are explored. Chapters 3 and 4 examine the pathways through which medical information travelled in Wales, through detailed analyses of both oral and literate cultures in early modern Wales. Here, the study draws attention to the growing importance of medical texts, and highlights an inherent paradox that the strong Welsh-language oral culture of knowledge sharing was responsible for widespread dispersal of information from English-language printed texts.

The third and final section turns to the Welsh disease sufferer and questions of care. More broadly, it points to the ways in which Wales participated in a global medical economy. Chapter 5 utilises a comprehensive study of over 3000 probate inventories to investigate medical material culture within the home in early modern Wales. This is an important study since it investigates the propensity of 'ordinary' people to manufacture medicines within their own homes, and weighs up the increasing importance of consumption of medical goods and materials. This is accompanied by a further study of the probate inventories of apothecaries and other medical retailers, which finds much evidence for the widespread availability of medicines and medical equipment, even in deeply rural areas of Wales. Chapter 6 critically analyses the 'sick role' and the ways in which sufferers both experienced and described their symptoms, foregrounding the growing impact of literacy and letters in sickness self-fashioning. Chapters 7 and 8 look in more detail at the availability of medical care in the early modern community, arguing that sickness served to create a temporary medical family drawn from friends, neighbours and the wider community, who provided a comprehensive structure of support from visiting to the provision of physical care. Whilst the historiography of poor law provision in Wales often downplays the extent of support, studies of parish records here are used to argue against this view, and demonstrate that Welsh parishes often provided comprehensive, flexible and adaptable structures of support. In terms of medical practice, Chapter 7 provides evidence pointing to a large number of Welsh practitioners in both towns and rural areas, who provided a range of medical services to the communities they served. Addressing questions of emulation, this chapter argues that their desire to adopt English medical nomenclature points to a growing wish to be seen as 'legitimate' practitioners, a view backed up by the increasing numbers of medical licences granted to Welsh physicians in the eighteenth century. It is important to note at this point that, in focusing specifically on questions and depictions of illness, its physical and social effects on the sufferer, their families and those in their social networks, more specialised areas of medical treatment such as surgery and midwifery have deliberately not been included.

Throughout the book are several recurring themes: the relationship between England and Wales; the linguistic duality of medical knowledge in Wales; the relationship between 'traditional' and 'modern'; the importance and dynamics of social relations; the importance of regions; and the pathways of medical knowledge. In recent years too, medical historians have focused upon issues of power, a notable example being Mary Fissell's work on eighteenth-century Bristol, charting state control through the rise of institutions.[26] The situation is different in

Wales, however, where there simply were no medical institutions until much later than this period. Instead, therefore, we examine something of the issues surrounding the power of the ownership and exercise of medical knowledge. Medical knowledge was transacted freely through a culture of sharing and this sharing provides a unique lens through which to view social interaction since it transcended usual boundaries of social status. The conclusion proposes a new 'story' of Welsh medical history – that of the inherent tension of a country simultaneously drawn strongly to the traditions of its past, but also towards the growing influence, both consciously and unconsciously, of its near neighbour and of the wider world beyond.

There is also a wider question to address. On a broad scale, what has so far been lacking in Welsh medical history is a conceptual understanding not only of the ways in which medical knowledge and practice in Wales contained unique or indigenous elements, but also of how they were reconciled with wider medical culture. Is it possible, for example, to talk of 'Welsh Medicine' or should we think more in terms of 'medicine in Wales'?[27] The latter makes more sense, since it is questionable whether an autonomous 'Welsh medicine' can be discerned or inferred after the medieval period. For Scotland, Helen Dingwall defines 'Scottish Medicine' as that taught *by* Scots *to* Scots, placing the 'Scottishness' within the realm of practice and training.[28] Even on this reading, the lack of Welsh medical training and treatment infrastructure would not see the dawn of 'Welsh Medicine' until well into the nineteenth century. On a deeper level too, it is not realistic to expect to find a uniquely Welsh system of bodily concepts away from those of the humoral body. Local and regional sickness experiences did contain social or linguistic factors which fostered an experience unique to a given area, but, given the limited geographical scope of such experiences, it is difficult to consider these as 'Welsh'. Searching for 'medicine in Wales', on the other hand, allows a freer exploration of the Welsh experience and the ways in which being in Wales (and 'being Welsh'), contributed to the sickness experience, but without inferring that it was separate.

This raises a second, deeper, question: that of how the geographical entity of 'Wales' can be approached and indeed whether it is even possible to encapsulate the medical experiences of any particular country or region as a totality. Appreciation of the potential importance of regionalism and localism in history, and not just medical history, has borne fruit in recent years in the form of a 'New British History'. This has encouraged a shift away from previously Anglocentric historiography and towards a more inclusive understanding of the ways in which constituent and distinct regions, amongst them Wales, Scotland, Ireland and Cornwall, fitted into a wider 'nation' of the British Isles.[29] Although the 'New British History' originated in the late 1980s and early 1990s, it is still comparatively underused, especially in terms of medical history. The implicit assimilation of the various constituent regions of the British Isles into a wider English nation surely has implications for medical history and for Welsh history. The opportunity now exists to fully question Wales's role in this wider structure, taking into account its own history and indigenous elements. Dingwall notes the problems for Scotland, equally relevant to Wales, of assuming homogeneity to the whole region, and notes the ways in which local regional distinctions – such as upland and lowland, urban and rural – could bring their own nuances to medical beliefs.[30] Whilst Wales will be treated here as a distinct geographical country, with its own defining and unifying language, this book will also explore Wales inclusively in terms of its role within the wider medical economy. Through case studies from a variety of sources, and from a variety of themes, it will also seek to draw out the nuances of localism and regionalism, and their effects upon sickness experiences and medical knowledge.

The question of change is also one salient for Wales. 'Change over time' has been a central concern of historians, but the importance of continuity should also not be overlooked or downplayed. In Wales, and in the early modern period, there were many areas where change came slowly, if at all. Humoral conceptions of the body remained constant throughout this period, and changes in monarch, government and religion made relatively little impact overall. The lack of a Welsh print-trade meant that no Welsh medical books were available until 1733, while medical licensing in Wales did not really start to increase markedly until the latter years of the scope of this book. Alternatively, potentially far-reaching changes did occur in the ways in which Wales increasingly participated in much broader networks of medical trade and information. This is exemplified in aspects such as the assimilation of English-language medical print culture and disease terminology, and more subtle changes in sickness self-representation such as the increasing import of literacy in shaping depictions and narratives of sickness.

But, in stressing the inclusivity of medicine in Wales, and the fresh approaches within this book, it should be noted that this study does not attempt a complete rupture with what has gone before. 'Irregular' or 'magical' medicine, however defined, was a vitally important aspect of Welsh history, and has been amply and ably served by historians. In this sense, further investigation of these aspects might simply be seen as rehashing old ideas, and would contribute little to existing knowledge. What it does do, however, is question the extent to which 'folk-lore' was the only medical reality. Throughout the book it is argued that such depictions represent only a part of the Welsh experience while, in reality, Welsh people had access to a far greater 'bank' of knowledge, to far wider medical markets, and also participated in sophisticated socio-medical networks. This is an important point and one which invites further exploration. Whilst previous depictions of Welsh early modern medicine have tended to highlight the conservative elements of aspects such as religion and oral culture, countervailing influences from across the border were equally vital in stimulating the spread of medical knowledge, manifested most notably in the assimilation of English printed medical texts into Welsh vernacular, oral culture, and back again into manuscript. Likewise, whilst Welsh religion could certainly be seen as a conducive environment for superstition and magic to flourish, it could also provide the impetus for change, as seen in the introduction of Paracelsian and Helmontian medicine into Wales, and also again for the dissemination of medical knowledge in vernacular Welsh. Thus is found the inherent tension which lies at the heart of medicine in early modern Wales. It was a country pulled simultaneously by two different forces.

On the one hand, a traditional, conservative and, in some ways, insular country was drawn to 'superstitious' beliefs and practices through a combination of a strong oral culture and favourable religious background. Welsh traditions of manuscript copying throughout the early modern period served to preserve and promote early Welsh medical culture, and also to draw its people to the trusted knowledge of their forebears. At the same time, however, Wales was also being inexorably drawn towards 'modern' medicine through a variety of channels. In economic terms, the strong degree of interaction between Wales and England led to manifold areas of cultural permeation, from medical encounters and trade, to the increasing adoption of English-language medical terms. With no printing press in Wales until 1718, those wishing to read medical texts were compelled to buy English books, and these were available from a variety of sources. Conversely, a strong tradition of knowledge sharing in Welsh served to disseminate these ideas orally. Finally, medical goods, equipment and practitioners were available from a variety of sources across Wales, and these highlight the extent to which Wales participated in a global medical economy. Rural village shops sold a range of goods, including exotic spices and herbs, while a wide range of consumer goods passed through Welsh ports from all over the world. How far Wales was truly remote or cut off by either poor roads or topography should therefore be questioned. Moreover, the increasing desire of Welsh practitioners to achieve or assume legitimacy, noted above, whether by licensing or the adoption of English medical nomenclature, implies both a willingness to be seen as legitimate and sophisticated practitioners, and so shake off pejorative depictions, and an increasing willingness on the part of 'ordinary' Welsh people to patronise 'regular' practitioners as well as cunning folk.

In sum, therefore, the aim of this work is to provide not only a general history of medicine in Wales, but a number of histories, taking into account disease,

Introduction

sickness experience and medical treatment, as well as the influence of such important factors as geography, social status, social networks and religious beliefs on Welsh medical mores. It is not a progressive story of medical discoveries and enlightenment. Nor is it intended to be a national (or nationalist) history, of interest merely to Welsh historians. Rather, it is intended that studies of such issues as the rural sickness experience, the effects of medicine and disease on culture and vice versa and the effects of a vacuum of 'professional' medicine and medical practitioners, will provide the impetus for future studies not only of Wales, but of other similar areas, both geographically and socially.

Notes

1 T.J. Owen, 'The Records of the Parish of Aber', *Caernarvonshire Historical Society Transactions*, 14 (1953), p. 83.

2 Ibid., p. 83.

3 Roy Porter, *The Greatest Benefit to Mankind: A Medical History of Humanity from Antiquity to the Present* (London: Fontana, 1999 edition), pp. 35–36.

4 Ludmilla Jordanova, 'Has the Social History of Medicine Come of Age?', *Historical Journal*, 36:2 (1993), p. 438.

5 Ludmilla Jordanova, 'The Social Construction of Medical Knowledge', *Social History of Medicine*, 7:3 (1995), pp. 362–363, 365; for examples of such an approach, see Andrew Wear (ed.), *Health and Healing in Early Modern England: Studies in Social and Intellectual History* (Aldershot: Ashgate, 1998); Ralph Houlbrooke, *Death, Religion and the Family in England 1480–1750* (Oxford: Clarendon Press, 2000 edition).

6 David Harley, 'Rhetoric and the Social Construction of Sickness and Healing', *Social History of Medicine*, 12:3 (1999), pp. 407–408.

7 See Roy Porter (ed.), *Patients and Practitioners: Lay Perceptions of Medicine in Pre-Industrial Society* (Cambridge: Cambridge University Press, 2002 edition); Dorothy Porter and Roy Porter, *Patient's Progress: Doctors and Doctoring in Eighteenth Century England* (Stanford: Stanford University Press, 1989).

8 Roy Porter, *Quacks: Fakers and Charlatans in Medicine* (Stroud: Tempus, 2003 edition); Roy Porter, *Bodies Politic: Disease, Death and Doctors in Britain, 1650–1900* (London: Reaktion, 2001).

9 See Elaine Leong, 'Making Medicines in the Early Modern Household', *Bulletin of the History of Medicine*, 82:1 (2008), pp. 145–168; A.S. Weber, 'Women's Early Modern Medical Almanacs in Historical Context', *English Literary Renaissance*, 33:3 (2003), pp. 358–402; Jennifer K. Stine, 'Opening the Closets: The Discovery of Household Medicine in Early Modern England'(Stanford University: Unpublished PhD Thesis, May 1996); Wendy D. Churchill, 'The Medical Practice of the Sexed Body: Women, Men and Disease in Britain *circa* 1600 to 1740', *Social History of Medicine*, 18:1 (2005), pp. 3–22; for debates on the relative lack of studies of women and medicine see for example Nadja Durbach, 'The Social History of British Medicine: An Essay Review', *Journal of the History of Medicine and Allied Sciences*, 57:4 (2002), pp. 487–489.

10 Andrew Wear, *Knowledge and Practice in English Medicine, 1550–1680* (Cambridge: Cambridge University Press, 2000); Margaret Pelling, *The Common Lot: Sickness, Medical Occupations and the Urban Poor in Early Modern England* (London and New York: Longman, 1998); Charles Webster (ed.), *Health, Medicine and Mortality in the Sixteenth Century* (Cambridge: Cambridge University Press, 1979); Mary E. Fissell, *Patients, Power and the Poor in Eighteenth Century Bristol* (Cambridge: Cambridge University Press, 2002 edition); G. Melvyn Howe, *People, Environment, Disease and Death: A Medical Geography of Britain Throughout the Ages* (Cardiff: University of Wales Press, 1997); Helen M. Dingwall, '"General Practice" in Seventeenth Century Edinburgh: Evidence from the Burgh Court', *Social History of Medicine*, 6:1 (1993), pp. 125–142; Ian Mortimer, 'The Rural Medical Marketplace in Southern England, c. 1570–1720' in Mark S.R. Jenner and Patrick Wallis (eds, *Medicine and the Market in England and its Colonies, c. 1450 – c. 1850* (Basingstoke: Palgrave Macmillan, 2007), pp. 69–87.

11 See Margaret Pelling and Richard M. Smith (eds), *Life, Death and the Elderly: Historical Perspectives* (London and New York: Routledge, 1991); Mary J. Dobson, *Contours of Death and Disease in Early Modern England* (Cambridge: Cambridge University Press, 2002 edition); E.A. Wrigley and R.S. Schofield, *The Population History of England, 1541–1871* (Cambridge: Cambridge University Press, 1989).

12 See Jenner and Wallis (eds), *Medicine and the Market*; Sara Pennell, 'Consumption and Consumerism in Early Modern England, *Historical Journal*, 42:2 (1999), pp. 549–564; Steven King, 'Accessing Drugs in the Eighteenth-Century Regions' in Louise Hill Curth (ed.), *From Physick to Pharmacology: Five Hundred Years of British Drug Retailing* (Aldershot: Ashgate, 2006), pp. 49–78; Penelope J. Corfield, 'From Poison Peddlers to Civic Worthies: The Reputation of the Apothecaries in Georgian England', *Social History of Medicine*, 22:1 (2009), pp. 1–22; Patrick Wallis, 'Consumption, Retailing and Medicine in Early Modern London', *Economic History Review*, 61:1 (February 2008), pp. 26–53.

13 Some elements of the following discussion appear in an altered form in my review article, Alun Withey, 'Unhealthy Neglect? The Medicine and Medical Historiography of Early Modern Wales', *Social History of Medicine*, 21:1 (2008), pp. 163–174.

14 For example Kenneth O. Morgan, *Rebirth of a Nation: A History of Modern Wales* (Oxford: Oxford University Press, 1981); Gwyn A. Williams, *When Was Wales? A History of the Welsh* (Harmondsworth: Penguin, 1985); John Williams, *Was Wales Industrialised? Essays in Modern Welsh History* (Llandysul: Gomer, 1995); Andy Croll, *Civilising the Urban: Popular Culture and Public Space in Merthyr c.1870–1914* (Cardiff: University of Wales Press, 2000); Philip Jenkins, *A History of Modern Wales 1536–1990* (London and New York: Longman, 1992); Gareth Elwyn Jones and Dai Smith (eds), *The People of Wales* (Llandysul: Gomer Press, 2000 edition)

15 Anne Borsay (ed.), *Medicine in Wales c.1800–2000: Public Service or Private Commodity?* (Cardiff: University of Wales Press, 2003).

16 Pamela Michael and Charles Webster (eds), *Health and Society in Twentieth Century Wales* (Cardiff: University of Wales Press, 2006), p. 6.

17 Glyn Penrhyn Jones, *Newyn a Haint yng Nghymru* (Caernarfon: Llyfrfa'r Methodistiaid Calfinaidd, 1962); Jones, 'Some Aspects of the Medical History of Caernarvonshire',

Caernarvonshire Historical Society Transactions, 23 (1962), pp. 67–91; Jones, 'Some Aspects of the Medical History of Denbighshire', *Denbighshire Historical Society Transactions*, 8 (1959), pp. 40–66.

18   John Cule (ed.), *Wales and Medicine* (Llandysul: Gomer Press, 1975).

19   For some examples see Mary Vaughan, 'An Old Receipt Book', *Journal of the Merioneth Historical and Record Society*, 4 (1964), pp. 318–323; Geraint Jenkins, 'Popular Beliefs in Wales from Restoration to Methodism', *Bulletin of the Board of Celtic Studies*, 27:3 (1977), pp. 440–462; Richard C. Allen, 'Wizards or Charlatans? Doctors or Herbalists? An Appraisal of the "Cunning Men" of Cwrt-y-Cadno, Carmarthenshire', *North American Journal of Welsh Studies*, 1:2 (Summer 2001), pp. 68–85; Richard Suggett, *A History of Magic and Witchcraft in Wales* (Stroud: The History Press, 2008).

20   Morfydd E. Owen, 'MeddygonMyddfai: A Preliminary Survey of Some Medieval Medical Writing in Welsh', *Studia Celtica*, 10:11 (1975–76), pp. 210–233.

21   Lisa Tallis, 'The "Doctor Faustus" of Cwrt-Y-Cadno: A New Perspective on John Harries and Popular Medicine in Wales', *Welsh History Review*, 24:3 (2009), pp. 1–28; Lisa M. Tallis, 'The Conjuror, the Fairy, the Devil and the Preacher: Witchcraft, Popular Magic and Religion in Wales, 1700–1905' (University of Wales, Swansea: Unpublished PhD Thesis, 2007); Owen Davies, 'Cunning-Folk in England and Wales during the Eighteenth and Nineteenth Centuries', *Rural History*, 8:1 (1997), pp. 91–107.

22   Colleen M. Seguin, 'Cures and Controversy in Early Modern Wales: The Struggle to Control St. Winifred's Well', *North American Journal of Welsh Studies*, 3:2 (Summer 2003), pp. 1–17.

23   See, for example, Will Coster, *Family and Kinship in England 1450–1800* (London: Longman, 2001); Keith Wrightson, *English Society 1580–1680* (London and New York: Routledge, 2003 edition); Patricia Crawford, *Blood, Bodies and Families in Early Modern England* (Harlow: Pearson, 2004).

24   Roger Cooter, '"Framing" the End of the Social History of Medicine' in Frank Huisman and John Harley Warner (eds), *Locating Medical History: The Stories and Their Meanings* (Baltimore and London: Johns Hopkins University Press, 2004), p. 313.

25   Frank Huisman and John Harley Warner, 'Medical Histories' in Huisman and Harley Warner (eds), *Locating Medical History*, p. 2.

26   Fissell, *Patients, Power and the Poor.*

27   I am here paraphrasing a similar question asked recently of the medical history of Scotland. See Helen M. Dingwall, *A History of Scottish Medicine: Themes and Influences* (Edinburgh: Edinburgh University Press, 2003), p. 2.

28   Ibid., p. 2.

29   For the 'New British History' see John G.A. Pocock, 'British History: A Plea for a New Subject', *Journal of Modern History*, 47:4 (1975), pp. 601–621; Tony Claydon, 'Great Britain: Identities, Institutions and the Idea of Britishness', *Historical Journal*, 42:2 (1999), pp. 585–586; P.R. Coss, William Lamont and Neil Evans, 'British History: Past, Present – and Future?', *Past and Present*, 119 (May 1988), pp. 171–203; Philip Jenkins, 'A New History of Wales', *Historical Journal*, 32:2 (1989), p. 387.

30   Dingwall, *History of Scottish Medicine*, esp. pp. 3–5.

Part I

Disease and mortality in early modern Wales

Disease and Welsh society

'The gentry in general are pretty hearty in the Countrey [sic]. It's the common sort that drop off'.[1]

So wrote the Anglesey curate Owen Davies in March 1729 as an epidemic fever swept through his area. In many respects, however, his wry comment does represent something of the true situation in early modern Wales, since social status could have a strong influence on both susceptibility to disease and the chances of survival.

By the early eighteenth century, the population of Wales is estimated to have been around 400,000 following a pattern of growth which had begun in the Middle Ages and which continued through centuries afterward.[2] Large parts of Wales were given over to an agrarian economy and the majority of people lived in predominantly rural areas.[3] The lowest strata of Welsh society, the poor, was also the biggest, estimated by Glanmor Williams as being up to three-quarters of the population, while the biggest single occupation of the 'average' Welsh person as late as the nineteenth century was that of farm labourer.[4] The houses of the majority of the lowest orders of society were often dark, damp and uncomfortable, and offered scant shelter against the elements.[5] While writers extolled the healthy Cambrian landscape, they did not feel similarly well disposed towards Welsh houses. English visitors often spoke disparagingly of conditions in such houses and descriptions of 'hovels' and 'miserable huts' are characteristic. One notorious book about Wales and its people described a Welsh dwelling as 'a Dunghill modelled in the shape of a cottage, whose outward surface was so all to-be-negro'd with such swarthy plaister that it appear'd not unlike a great blot of Cow-Turd'.[6] Whilst clearly designed to be provocative, there is undoubtedly an element of truth behind the barbs. As late as the nineteenth century, an English writer, Walter Davies, wrote of labourers' cottages in North Wales that 'One smoky hearth, for it should not be styled a kitchen, and one damp litter cell, for it cannot be called a bedroom, are frequently all the space allotted' to six or seven people, adding that 'three fourths of the victims of the putrid fever perish in the mephitic air of these dwellings'.[7] Amongst the less fortunate, death rates rose in this period as the effects of a combination of epidemic diseases, poor harvests and rising grain prices tended to weed out the weak and vulnerable.[8] Conversely, wealthy gentry families living in better housing, and with presumably better living conditions, actually saw average life expectancy at age five improve by around five years for every quarter century between 1550 and 1750.[9]

Welsh travellers within the country were also aware of the sufferings of their fellow countrymen. Whilst accompanying the Duke of Beaufort on his 1684 tour of the Principality, Thomas Dineley wrote of one area in Cardiganshire that 'The vulgar here are most miserable and low as the rich are happy and high both to an extream'.[10] The tradition of will making, even amongst the less well off, also affords a glimpse into the types of conditions that the less fortunate endured. One 1630 will provides a rare mention of housing, listing 'a house or cottage' valued at one pound, together with only two other belongings, a bedsead and hutch, comprising the meagre acquisitions of a poor man.[11] Another frequent remark is the lack of space in such dwellings, where often large families shared a single room.[12] Such cramped and crowded living quarters afforded much opportunity for infections to spread within households and were compounded by the common practice of sharing living space with animals. Straw covered clay floors could become infested with fleas from animals, and stinking from urinal and faecal contamination.[13] Unwashed bodies, often infested with lice, provided further opportunity for the spread of disease from person to person, and lice were active at all seasons of the year, causing a range of symptoms from skin infections to fevers.[14] Moreover, the proximity of animals and poor construction of houses also provided a fertile breeding ground for flies, especially houseflies, blow flies and flesh flies, all capable of spreading deadly diseases such as bacillary and amoebic dysentery, typhoid and tuberculosis, all of which were widespread in Wales.[15] Lack of adequate heating made cold winters especially difficult and it was often the poorest and weakest who succumbed during prolonged periods of poor weather. We should note that this situation was not universally applicable however.

We should also not ignore towns and urban Welsh patterns of disease. Wales in the seventeenth and eighteenth centuries boasted no cities, relying instead on external 'regional capitals' of Bristol in the South, Chester in the North and Shrewsbury along the Welsh Marches.[16] There were few towns with more than 2,000 inhabitants – one notable exception being Wrexham – yet appreciation of the importance of such towns to Welsh economic, social and cultural history has grown markedly in recent years.[17] In the early modern period, contemporaries saw towns as unhealthy, noisome and pestiferous places where disease and poor

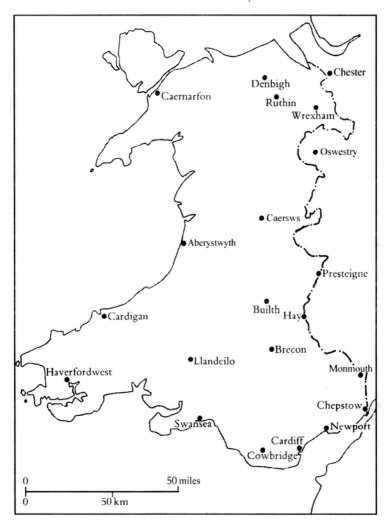

1 Map of Wales showing major towns

health were almost unavoidable companions to the urban dweller. Townsfolk were often derided as idle and prone to worry, which sapped their health and gave them poor digestion leading to more serious complaints.[18] The presence of large groups of people in close proximity proved a fertile breeding ground for all manner of epidemic and endemic diseases throughout the early modern period.

Water supplies were often contaminated as people empted their waste into the nearest available stream or river. Rich and poor lived cheek by jowl, sanitation was rudimentary and raw sewage and animal detritus frequently fouled the streets in which children played. In 1594, charges were brought against two bailiffs for 'suffrynge dy[ver]s abuses' in Cardiff, relating to the disposal of dunghills, and also for 'nott cawsynge ye highewayes'.[19] Clearly this problem bedevilled early modern towns since, even as late as 1740, the authorities of Aberystwyth were forced into legislation to prevent inhabitants from 'lay[ing] downe their dunghill opposite their doors'.[20] Anything from the unwashed bodies wearing filthy clothing, harbouring a multitude of vermin, to the immorality and drunkenness of the townspeople, to the foul and noxious odours of the urban environment could bring disease and spell disaster for the early modern town.[21]

Plague was certainly present during the sixteenth and early seventeenth centuries in Welsh towns, although it appears to have made less impact here than in some parts of England. Chester was one area that suffered greatly, with 650 people dying of the plague there in 1603 and 986 in 1604.[22] South and mid-Wales were hit badly in the late 1630s, with outbreaks in Llanidloes, Machynlleth and Newtown while north Wales, especially Wrexham, was hit in 1631. The years 1637–38 were apparently bad for plague across all parts of Wales and the diarist Walter Powell reported in 1639 that the disease was also 'very hot in diverse parts of Monmouthshire'.[23] One of the most prolonged outbreaks in Wales occurred in Presteigne in Powys, lasting from August 1636 until June the following year. Here, the authorities were forced into desperate measures to try and contain the epidemic by restricting public movements and even threatening to halt food supplies if people attempted to leave the town.[24] This outbreak seems to have provoked much popular fear in surrounding areas, and one man from the neighbouring parish of Upton on Severn was apparently even bound over for threatening to go to Presteigne in 1637 in order to deliberately bring the plague back upon his wife and children.[25] In general, plague visitations were more virulent in towns although not exclusively, as the outbreak in rural Bedwellty parish which killed 82 people in 1638 demonstrates.[26] The last reliable reports of an outbreak in Wales occurred in 1652 in Haverfordwest and Carmarthen, the disease wreaking havoc amongst populations and reportedly stretching resources in Haverfordwest almost to breaking point.[27] Wales, however, does appear to have escaped relatively unscathed in terms of the impact of bubonic plague, at least in comparison to some areas of England. The reasons for this may lie partly in the geography of the country. As Paul Slack's work on the effects of plague in Exeter has shown, the plague decreased at higher altitudes, and it is noticeable that Welsh outbreaks tended to occur most in lowland towns.[28] It is possible that the largely upland terrain of Wales was in some ways responsible for shielding its population from the worst of its ravages. In tandem with this, the lack of large towns, and distance between them may also have served to check the progress of the disease.

Smallpox too was an endemic disease which often became epidemic, and was certainly notorious throughout Wales during this period, killing around a quarter of those who contracted it.[29] Evidence of smallpox outbreaks can be found in sources throughout the country and across the time period and the disease was deeply embedded in Welsh popular culture as a deadly, or at the very least disfiguring, enemy. Indeed, by the end of the eighteenth century, few families in Wales were apparently left unaffected by the disease.[30] Although smallpox was endemic in many areas during the seventeenth century, the most severe epidemic outbreaks occurred in the eighteenth century and especially in 1722–23 in Carmarthen with over 71 deaths there, and again in 1729 and 1732, peaking in 1733 when it combined with an unusually virulent outbreak of measles. Later epidemics of smallpox in Wales in the mid-eighteenth century coincided with a more general outbreak across Britain.[31]

Urban areas tended to follow different patterns of mortality to those in the countryside. The density of population meant a constant supply of disease vectors, leading to a steadier mortality rate, without such marked seasonal variations as in the countryside parishes. Although winter still saw a peak in mortality, the presence of insects usually saw a second peak during the summer months, unlike in rural parishes where summer usually brought something of a respite in mortality.[32] Epidemic mortality often hit towns with greater virulence than in the countryside, and especially market towns and their surrounding parishes as those travelling in with their animals became exposed to epidemic disease. Other socio-economic constraints could entice impoverished country folk into towns looking for work, again exposing them to diseases to which they had not had chance to build up an immunity.[33] Housing, too, varied greatly from place to place. In Knighton and Presteigne in mid-Wales, the labouring poor suffered appalling conditions, dwelling in small alleys and courtyards away from the more affluent abodes of the better off. One woman complained to the authorities there in 1690 that her 'poor cot' had no roof, leaving her exposed to the elements.[34] Better built and ventilated housing, however, reduced the chances of infection from disease and there is evidence to show that some Welsh towns, such as Carmarthen and Hay-on-Wye, contained stone and slate housing which may have served to lessen the impact and prevalence of some diseases.[35]

Despite the apparently strong lines of demarcation, town and countryside should not necessarily be regarded as separate entities. Traditionally, the view of the early modern Welsh citizen has tended to be one of stasis, where people seldom left their own parish and lived their lives in relatively isolated communities.[36] In recent years, however, the relative mobility of the early modern population has begun to be appreciated, and this has implications for the spread of disease.[37] People moved around for various reasons. For farmers, visits to market towns were essential in order to sell their stock. Occupants of outlying hamlets required goods and services which a growing number of smaller towns and villages were gearing up to provide.[38] One consequence of this mobility was the potential for diseases to enter populations with no immunity as travellers acted as carriers. Thus, incoming traders from the Welsh hinterlands could introduce viruses which had little effect in areas of sparse population, but which could become epidemic in dense urban environments. In times of poor harvests and economic hardship, the poor often entered towns looking for work. Likewise, travelling traders and pedlars, as well as a steady stream of wandering vagrants and beggars, could all act as disease vectors.

Diet was another strong factor affecting susceptibility to disease. Malnutrition lowered immunity to disease, especially during harvest failures and poor weather when staple crops were in short supply. Many poor people were dependent on the most basic of foodstuffs such as barley and rye bread, and the Welsh diet was proverbially poor.[39] In Cardiganshire, 'The poorer sort for bread [eat] oaten cakes, and drink beer small made of oaten malt, some drink only water for necessity'.[40] As late as 1801, the majority of households in Wales were still dependent on oats and barley, a similar situation to that in rural Scotland, while some areas had their own more or less nutritious variations on the common oaten cakes and rye bread.[41] Barley bread was common in the eighteenth century in the hilly areas of west and north Wales and rye bread was more common in Cardiganshire and Radnorshire.[42] In pastoral areas, there was more access to milk, cheese and some meats although the lack of adequate storage meant that anything other than fresh meat was heavily salted. A diet heavy on rye was likely to bring other problems such as ergot poisoning or mycotoxicosis, both of which were caused by contaminated grain and which, it has been argued, may have been responsible for fever epidemics, such as those experienced in north Wales in the 1720s and 1730s.[43] Periods of dearth increased the chances of infection by lowering immunity and Wales was hit by several incidences of poor harvests, especially in 1667–69, 1678–83, 1694–1703 and 1708–9 and again during the 1720s and 1730s, the crop failures of the 1690s falling into a wider pattern of harvest failures which provoked mortality crises across Europe.[44] Uncooked meat could harbour intestinal worms which could be especially troublesome to children.[45] Less chronically, the monotonous diet of the majority of people could cause a variety of stomach complaints and gastro-intestinal complications. Parts of Wales, along with East Anglia, were reputedly amongst the worst in the country for incidences of urinary or bladder stone, caused by inadequate supplies of fresh water and vitamins.[46]

Constipation was an uncomfortable by-product of a bulky diet and might well have been the cause of the attack of 'stone and collick' noted by Walter Powell in 1651.[47] Given his earlier comments about the diet of the poor in Cardiganshire, it was not without a note of irony that Thomas Dineley recorded the epitaph of a man in Aberaeron who reputedly died of 'winde collick' – 'If his arse could have spoke, his heart had not brok[e]'.[48]

Notes

1 Leonard Owen, 'The Letters of an Anglesey Parson, 1712–1732', *Transactions of the Honourable Society of Cymmrodorion*, 1 (1961), p. 89.

2 Philip Jenkins, *A History of Modern Wales 1536–1990* (London and New York: Longman, 1992), p. 17.

3 Glyn Penrhyn Jones, 'A History of Medicine in Wales in the Eighteenth Century' (Liverpool University: Unpublished MA Thesis, 1957), p. 13.

4 Glanmor Williams, *Renewal and Reformation Wales, c. 1415–1642* (Oxford: Oxford University Press, 2002 edition), p. 418; David Howell, *The Rural Poor in Eighteenth Century Wales* (Cardiff: University of Wales Press, 2000), p. 66.

5 Howell, *The Rural Poor*, p. 89.

6 Jones, 'History of Medicine', p. 15; W. Richards, *Wallography* (1682) quoted in Iorweth Peate, *The Welsh House: A Study in Folk Culture* (Liverpool: Brython Press, 1944).

7 Quoted in Sir Leonard Twiston-Davies and Averyl Edwards, *Welsh Life in the Eighteenth Century* (London: Country Life, 1939), pp. 16–17.

8 Nick Woodward, 'Crisis Mortality in a Welsh Market Town: Carmarthen, 1675–1799', *Welsh History Review*, 22:3 (June 2005), p. 433.

9 Ralph Houlbrooke, *Death, Religion and the Family in England 1480–1750* (Oxford: Clarendon Press, 2000 edition), p. 8.

10 Thomas Dineley, *The Account of the Official Progress of His Grace Henry the First Duke of Beaufort . . . Through Wales in 1684.* (London: Blades, Facsimile edition 1888), p. 249.

11 Gerald Morgan, 'Bottom of the Heap: Identifying the Poor in West Wales Records', *Llafur*, 7:1 (1996), p. 20.

12 Peate, *The Welsh House*, p. 88.

13 Jones, 'History of Medicine', p. 16.

14 James C. Riley, 'Insects and the European Mortality Decline', *American Historical Review*, 91 (1986), p. 849.

15 Ibid., p. 845.

16 Jenkins, *History of Modern Wales*, p. 4.

17 Ibid., p. 34.

18 Andrew Wear, *Knowledge and Practice in English Medicine, 1550–1680* (Cambridge: Cambridge University Press, 2000), p. 160.

19 John Hobson Matthews (ed.), *Cardiff Records, Volume 2* (Cardiff: Cardiff Corporation, 1898), p. 146.

20 Jones, 'History of Medicine', p. 17.

21 Mary J. Dobson, *Contours of Death and Disease in Early Modern England* (Cambridge: Cambridge University Press, 2002 edition), pp. 16–17; See also Evan D. Jones, 'Gleanings from the Radnorshire Files of Great Sessions Papers. 1691–1699', *Radnorshire Society Transactions*, 13 (1943), pp. 28–31. For an excellent study of the early urban environment, see Emily Cockayne, *Hubbub: Noise, Filth and Stench in England* (Yale: Yale University Press, 2007).

22 Alun Withey, 'Medical Knowledge and Practice in Early Modern Wales' (Cardiff University: Unpublished MA Thesis, 2006), p. 11.

23 Ibid., p. 12; Joseph Alfred Bradney (ed.), *The Diary of Walter Powell of Llantilio Crossenny in the County of Monmouth, Gentleman, 1603–1654* (Bristol: John Wright & Co., 1907), p. 8; Glyn Penrhyn Jones, 'Some Aspects of the Medical History of Denbighshire', *Denbighshire Historical Society Transactions*, 8 (1959), p. 57.

24 Keith Parker, *A History of Presteigne* (Woonton Almeley, Herefordshire: Logaston Press, 1997), pp. 54, 58.

25 Ibid., p. 56.

26 R.W. McDonald, 'The Parish Registers of Wales', *National Library of Wales Journal*, 19:4 (1976), p. 422.

27 Geraint H. Jenkins, *The Foundations of Modern Wales, 1642–1780* (Oxford: Oxford University Press, 2002 edition), p. 89; Woodward, 'Crisis Mortality', p. 453.

28 Paul Slack, *The Impact of Plague in Tudor and Stuart England* (London: Routledge and Kegan Paul, 1985), p. 74.

29 Mary Lindemann, *Medicine and Society in Early Modern Europe* (Cambridge: Cambridge University Press, 1999), p. 48.

30 W.H. Howse, *Radnorshire* (Hereford: Radnorshire Society, 1973), p. 115.

31 Glyn Penrhyn Jones, *Newyn a Haint yng Nghymru* (Caernarfon: Llyfrfa'r Methodistiaid Calfinaidd, 1962), pp. 36–37.

32 Woodward, 'Crisis Mortality', p. 442.

33 Ibid., p. 434.

34 Keith Parker, *Radnorshire from Civil War to Restoration* (Woonton Almeley, Herefordshire: Logaston Press, 2000), p. 10.

35 Woodward, 'Crisis Mortality', p. 440; Geoffrey L. Fairs, *A History of the Hay: The Story of Hay-on-Wye* (Chichester: Phillimore, 1972), pp. 238–241.

36 See for example the arguments in Geraint H. Jenkins, 'Popular Beliefs in Wales from Restoration to Methodism', *Bulletin of the Board of Celtic Studies*, 27:3 (1977), pp. 440–462.

37 Keith Wrightson, *English Society 1580–1680* (London and New York: Routledge, 2003 edition), p. 49.

38 Peter Borsay et al., 'Introduction: Wales, a New Agenda for Urban History', *Urban History*, 32:1 (2005), p. 9.

39 Jenkins, *History of Modern Wales*, p. 89.

40 Dineley, *Official Progress*, p. 249.

41 Howell, *The Rural Poor*, p. 87.

42 Jones, 'History of Medicine', p. 18.

43 Dobson, *Contours of Death*, p. 476.

44 Jenkins, *Foundations*, p. 90.
45 Lindemann, *Medicine and Society*, p. 26.
46 Jones, 'History of Medicine', p. 23.
47 Bradney, *Diary of Walter Powell*, p. 43.
48 Dineley, *Official Progress*, p. 249.

Part II

Medical knowledge in early modern Wales

2

The Welsh body and popular medical culture

'Yn Mhob Clwyf mae Perygl'
In every disease lurks danger[1] (Welsh Proverb)

How did people in Wales conceptualise, reify or otherwise approach illness and their bodies? Indeed, for the early modern Welsh inhabitant, what *was* illness? In general terms, the early modern period is viewed as a period of transition. In England, a gradual move away from magical and superstitious medical forms has been noted, beginning in the seventeenth century, and accelerating through the secularising Georgian period. As people seemed to lose faith in spiritual causes and cures, more importance was attached to the tangible medical remedy. The doctor was to become a secondary figure to the patient in a society becoming more medically self-conscious.[2] In Wales, however, 'superstitious' views of medicine are generally shown as persisting for much longer, even into the twentieth century. If we take the view that much of Wales remained largely rural and conservative during this period, its people shielded by a combination of poor roads, difficult terrain and language differences from the wider intellectual changes, then it is easy to see how folklore (however defined) could be seen as the prevailing characteristic of Welsh medical history. There is indeed little doubt that the Welsh were inclined towards supernatural and spiritual conceptions of health, but this was only a part of the true picture. The other part is that of a country open and receptive to new ideas, far less cut off than is often assumed and also capable of keeping parity with wider English and European medical trends.

Individual concepts of illness and the body in Wales involved a range of dynamic and overlapping spheres, including lay referral networks, religious beliefs and affiliation, literacy, language, popular illness narratives and so on. Equally, individual concepts of illness could vary greatly according to factors such as location and social status in Wales, making it difficult to assume a universal experience. For these reasons, a straightforward narrative of medical approaches, merely identifying what people 'believed', would probably fail to encapsulate the fluidity and dynamism of the situation, since no single aspect can realistically be taken in isolation. It would be difficult to explore folkloric medical beliefs in Wales, without understanding the overlap and reciprocity between apparently magical rituals and charms and the unique religious situation in Wales. Likewise, in talking of orthodox printed medical literature, we must note that many such works stressed the role of God and prayer, as well as reinforcing the importance of medicine and regimen.[3] This study of medical beliefs in Wales proposes a fresh model, and one which shifts focus from the medical to the social. Medicine was a social currency – a means of knowledge exchange – which was freely shared across Welsh society, supported by the presence of certain favourable conditions. People's understandings of illness and the body were expressed and reinforced through a number of social frameworks. They included common understandings of the humoral body, location, religious concepts of the body, underpinned by the somewhat unique religious background in Wales, and cultural and linguistic representations of the body, reinforced and recycled through a strong oral tradition. In fact, linguistic changes over the course of the seventeenth and eighteenth centuries provide strong evidence for a growing Anglicisation in Welsh medicine, belying the image of a pastoral country cut off from wider developments which can sometimes be perpetuated by existing historiography. Before proceeding, the formal structure of medicine in Wales must be addressed.

The structure of 'official' medicine in Wales

During the early Middle Ages European medicine was, as Katherine Park notes, 'fluid and undifferentiated', with hazy boundaries between types of healers and a lack of formalised medical care.[4] After 1050, she argues, the rise of medical institutions created the beginnings of a medical profession and also of attempts to discourage lay practice.[5] Italian, French and eventually English universities began to offer formal medical training and by 1500 a structure of medical practitioners was well developed. In England, the London College of Physicians received its charter in 1518 and was the organ of the academically trained 'learneds.[6] Scotland had a tradition of medical training and guild structure amongst its physicians and surgeons, dating to the early sixteenth century. This was made manifest in the establishment of the Incorporation of Surgeons in 1505 and later the Royal College of Physicians in Edinburgh in 1681, and subsequent provision of medical training in Scotland.[7] Ireland, too, had the potential to train its own physicians and had, in Dublin, its own Royal College, chartered in 1667 as well as surgeons' guilds. Medical training had been available through Trinity College in Dublin since the early seventeenth century, although few licences were granted during the early to mid seventeenth century.[8] Likewise, the increasing translation of medical works from Latin into vernacular English contributed to a broadening of medical knowledge amongst the English laity.[9]

Until the nineteenth century, however, there were no Welsh universities to offer medical courses, meaning that those wishing to study medicine had to go elsewhere. With no indigenous, systematised medical training, there was no formal Welsh medical faculty able to research, contribute or publish in Wales or in Welsh. In fact, the lack of a vibrant Welsh print trade until the eighteenth century meant that there was little opportunity for Welsh doctors to publish, and certainly not in the vernacular until much later. One notable exception was the Tenby-born physician and lexicographer Robert Recorde, who was court practitioner to the English monarch Edward VI. Recorde, however, wrote in English from England, and was less than sympathetic to the general practices of his kinsmen.[10]

Nominally, Wales fell under the purview of the London institutions but in practice it was generally too remote and even, perhaps, culturally intractable to be fully subsumed in this way. There is little evidence for the seeking and granting of medical licences in Wales before the last quarter of the seventeenth century. This lack of institutional and public medicine, together with a favourable religious culture of tolerance for old practices and beliefs, seemingly served to create a vacuum of 'orthodox' practitioners in Wales, paving the way for the flourishing of traditional, alternative, lay and otherwise irregular forms of medical practice. Given this evidence, it is unsurprising that such themes have continued to prevail in Welsh medical history.

But in itself, this lack of 'official' infrastructure does not fully encapsulate the Welsh experience. Nor does the apparent paucity of licensed medical practitioners tell us much about the everyday medical attitudes of the Welsh population for whom official medicine was a small, and probably largely irrelevant, feature. Parts of rural England were equally remote from licensing and the centres of learning, and many people had a similarly poor access to 'learned' practitioners, even though they lived in a country where medical training was available. The Scottish Highlands provide a similar example during this period, as does Ireland which, despite having the Royal College in Dublin, issued few licences, leaving contemporaries to complain about the omnipresence of quacks and charlatans.[11] The crucial difference, and in fact the unique characteristic of Wales, was its language, which acted as a shield for older traditions, but also a field upon which was fought the battle for linguistic medical supremacy. Where 'official' medicine interacted with rural England, it did so in English. Literate farmers from areas as similarly remote as Wales from medical centres, say Cumbria, had no language barrier to cross when they purchased medical self-help works. For

English-language medical works to embed in Wales to any social depth, which they certainly did, therefore required a different process.

Neither does this lack of formal medicine mean that Wales was medically backward for the pull of its near neighbour was inexorable. Medical knowledge permeated Wales in many different ways throughout the early modern period. English medical texts were collected and absorbed by an eager and growing literate section of Welsh society, linked to the growing importance of even small Welsh towns as cosmopolitan cultural and economic centres. But it was the strong culture of oral transmission of ideas through storytelling, gossip and free-sharing of medical information which ensured that such knowledge spread beyond the literate. More than this, it became assimilated into the Welsh vernacular, meaning that up-to-date ideas could penetrate to surprising social depths. There was also, however, something of a tension caused by the very people who sought to appear most 'modern'. One notable feature of the Welsh literati was a desire to collect, copy and recycle old texts, such as those of the Meddygon Myddfai and other medieval manuscript collections. Thus, while simultaneously adopting English fashions and sensibilities, educated elites in Wales moved to protect and preserve traditional Welsh cultures. Such innately conservative tendencies also had an effect of pulling the Welsh people in two directions – to the past and their strong and ancient medical traditions, and also to a future more allied with the path of 'modern' medicine.

Overall, people in Wales in fact had access to a great deal of medical information, and were nowhere near as isolated as previous accounts have tended to imply. This was made possible by the paradox of a traditional, oral culture of storytelling and information spread, which perpetuated the wide dispersal of information from English-language printed medical texts to a broadly illiterate people. But, there was also a growing interest amongst some sections of society in acquiring and promoting literacy. This, and the increasing numbers of Welsh vernacular medical publications from the late seventeenth century, served to provide a more inclusive medical culture.

Concepts of the body

As elsewhere, ideas about the body in Wales were understood and articulated through a number of spheres. Across the scope of this book little changed in the basic ways that the Welsh people conceptualised the workings of their bodies. Essentially, the Welsh body was a humoral one derived, as in the rest of Europe, ultimately from the Hippocratic corpus, systematised by Galen of Pergamum in the second century.[12] There was little deviation from this model in Welsh culture, and health and illness were understood and described in humoral terms.

The Welsh body and popular medical culture

How was this model of the body assimilated? From around the fourth and fifth centuries AD, medical literature from a range of sources had begun to filter through the Western world in the form of Greek and Latin manuscripts. These were translated into Welsh at some stage between the ninth and eleventh centuries, and were followed from the twelfth century onwards by an influx of medical texts from Arabia through the medical school at Salerno in Italy.[13] From such works began a gradual process of embedment as Welsh writers began to copy and rework the originals into manuscript collections, augmenting them with their own empirical remedies and local herbal lore. The importance of early monasteries as healing sites probably did much to disseminate this information into the oral vernacular.

By the fifteenth century, several fully formed Welsh-language remedy collections had been created including the works of the Physicians of Myddfai, the collection of Bened Feddyg and the manuscript known by its library reference as Hafod 16.[14] Such early practitioners were probably, like Bened Feddyg and the Myddfai physicians, members of families who passed their compilations down through generations, each making their own additions.[15] Moreover, increasingly during the sixteenth century, literate Welshmen were beginning to translate English medical texts into vernacular Welsh. John ap Ifan, who translated Humphrey Llwyd's edition of the *Treasury of Health*, addressed his fellow countrymen at the end of the work, stating that the translation was 'Howe thou shalt knowe to gyve the quantytye of mede-cynnes'.[16] Familiar figures such as astrological charts, bloodletting diagrams and 'dangerous days' of the year had appeared in early Welsh manuscripts.[17] Certainly by the sixteenth century, vernacular remedy collections were solidly humoral and parts of this learned literate culture had clearly made the transition into popular currency.[18]

It is probable, however, that the process of transmitting such remedies orally had begun long before this, giving the illiterate access to the ideas of the literati.[19] This is an important point since, although there was clearly much cultural inter-action with England and the wider world through trade links, it is likely that the Welsh people also assimilated humoral medicine through an internal process dating back to the original Latin texts, rather than translating the English versions into Welsh. In this sense, if indigenous language can be taken as a cultural marker, there may well have been a proto-'Welsh' medical culture at the beginning of the early modern period even if it did not persist far beyond that point. The fact that classical medical texts were ever translated into Welsh is also significant, both in demonstrating ready demand for such works in the native tongue, and in that there were practitioners suitably qualified to be able to understand the potentially esoteric applications of the remedies, and privileged knowledge of the workings of the body.

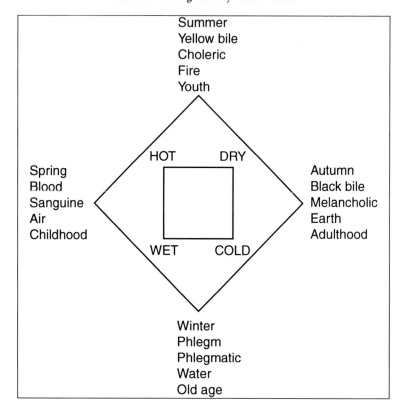

Summer
Yellow bile
Choleric
Fire
Youth

HOT   DRY

Spring   Autumn
Blood   Black bile
Sanguine   Melancholic
Air   Earth
Childhood   Adulthood

WET   COLD

Winter
Phlegm
Phlegmatic
Water
Old age

2   The humoral system

In Wales, therefore, and in general terms, disease was widely viewed as resulting from disequilibrium in the body caused by an excess of humours and, regardless of the type of practitioner, treatment usually involved evacuative procedures, such as bleeding, sweating and vomiting, to restore the body to its natural state.[20] As elsewhere, beliefs in the maintenance of a healthy body at all levels of Welsh society involved regular purges, enemas, vomits and any means to ensure that bad humours were evacuated and the body was able to renew itself. Purging was *the* basis of early modern treatment, often the first line of defence against illness and even a routine prophylactic. This was ultimately linked to Aristotelian notions of the four elements of earth, air, fire and water and the states of hot, cold, wet and dry, thus codifying the human body as a microcosm of the wider universe, susceptible to astrological and planetary activity as well as terrestrial environmental conditions.[21] In terms of everyday experience, however, it is important to remember that most people did not comprehend a systematic view of Galenic medicine and were probably not aware of its ultimate origins. Rather, what prevailed was a 'popular humoralism' where the body was widely understood in humoral terms alongside astrological and magical theories of sickness and recovery.[22] The largely agrarian context of Wales was certainly conducive to supernatural beliefs and it has been argued that the Welsh character, together with a propensity towards innate localism and conservatism, heightened their sensitivity to their surroundings.[23] Cycles of life and death mirrored the patterns of nature, and there were correlations between the cycles of the sun and the moon and those of the body, such as menstruation.[24]

Long before Galen systematised medicine, as Roy Porter noted, people had analogised their bodies with nature, interpreting bodily flows with the workings of the weather and the seasons, and adopting the suggestive power of a range of plants and animals as a means of palliating their symptoms.[25] The body might be also susceptible to infiltration through a range of other both temporal and supernatural means. The actions of malevolent or friendly spirits might be invoked as either cause or salvation and certain bodily signs could be interpreted as providential. Environmental factors likewise played a part in spreading illness, and the Welsh were deeply aware of the dangers lurking in bad airs and places.[26] Astrology too formed an important part of popular views of the body and people were ever mindful of the potential influence of the stars and planets upon their health. Many remedies stipulated that the substance should be taken 'at full and New Moon', as did 'Dr. Ratcliff's Receipt for Convulsion Fitts'.[27] Such information was readily available from the seventeenth century in popular almanacs, such as *Rider's British Merlin* and *Gallen's Almanack*, which provided detailed astrological predictions for the year ahead, and were eagerly collected in Wales.

Unsurprisingly, on an individual level, it is clear that Welsh people understood that each person had their own particular humoral balance. Here, one humour might be dominant, leading to states of body and mind, such as sanguine, melancholic, choleric and so on, while different ages of man, and also either sex, could harbour predominant humours. Youth was considered to be hotter and drier than old age, with an excess of yellow bile, leading to a fiery choleric temperament.[28] Disease, as well as being an external entity, dwelling in particular environments or in noxious airs or waters, might also be let in to the body by the particular humoral temperament of the individual.[29] Even within this schema, however, there was much scope for interpretation and also for local variations, given the relationship between the human body and its environment. Thus it could be possible for bodily beliefs and characteristics to emerge which were peculiar to a given geographical area. Was there though, in any sense, a readily identifiable 'Welsh body', or bodily conception?

Popular culture and the Welsh body

For the majority of people in Wales, oral culture was the main means of reception and transmission of ideas. Across early modern Europe, traditional songs and stories formed an important part of both domestic and social gatherings, and were a welcome and necessary means to pass long, winter nights. Indeed, fireside gatherings also performed a useful economic function in saving and spreading the cost of winter fuel.[30] The tradition in Wales of storytelling appears to have been particularly strong, bolstered by the bardic tradition and the ready presence of large numbers of balladeers and minstrels.[31] Although declining markedly during the centuries after the Reformation, patronage from the Welsh gentry continued to be important in recycling traditional Welsh poetical forms. Traditional Welsh poetry was designed with performance in mind; it was meant to be read out loud, in front of a public which might include both the patron and his employees or local people.[32] Typical subjects were local figures or landmarks, familiar to indigenous people.[33] In this sense it was not a high culture of poetry, but a uniquely Welsh vernacular tradition through which knowledge and ideas could disseminate.

The ageing body was a constant theme in Welsh poetry. Given the supposed hot temper of the Welsh, discussed below, much poetry is instead geared towards the ravages of old age, and its deleterious effects upon the body. The seventeenth-century Welsh poet Owen Gruffydd used repeated humoral metaphors of cold and dry in his poem 'The men that once were'.

> Old, old. To live on, wretched to behold, my hair is white, my smile is cold . . .
> Harsh stroke to the old when the cold weather broke,
> Longing, a dull ache in my side, for the kind chieftains that have died
> I'm cold for all those generous men . . .
> Unthieving givers are gone, and my ways are heavy, cold and long.[34]

Old age, for Gruffydd, was a state of wretchedness, stripping the body of its warmth. He presents himself as a person robbed of his virility by the rigours of disease and old age, in fact a regular theme in Welsh verse dating back to early times. In the ninth century, an anonymous Welsh poet wrote of the deterioration of his body:

> Four ills, of all my hates the chief, are met in me together
> Coughing: Old age: Sickness: Grief,

I'm senile, lonely, twisted and cold,
After the bed of desire I'm galled with misery
My back's thrice snarled,
No girl wants me, no friend haunts me.[35]

Here again, the emphasis lies firmly upon the loss of sexual potency and the impotency engendered by age and sickness. The deliberate separation of coughing from other forms of sickness emphasises its severity, rendering it synonymous with poor health and symbolic of a body in demise. Others used the popular humoral convention, although certainly not specific to Wales, of comparing the life of the body with seasons or months of the year. The medieval Welsh poet Dafydd ap Gwilym used the months of May and January to signify the marriage between a young girl and an old man, the girl being represented by the metaphorical warmth and burgeoning of May, with the old man marked out by the cold and harsh winter month.[36] This use of May as a metaphor for youth was utilised in another poem 'May Month' by Gwilym, and described as 'a fair and handsome youth who has enriched me . . . yesterday great God gave May'.[37] The 'January and May' marriage, i.e. that between couples with large disparities of age, was in fact a common idiom which sometimes attracted social disapproval, not least because of the potential for the younger partner to be forced onto parish charity on the death of their elderly spouse.[38]

Others, however, concentrated on the physical and social effects which disease could render upon the body and, of these, the most compelling relate to the physical ravages engendered by smallpox. It was indeed a disease to be feared. According to Geraint Jenkins, advertisements for servants in Wales commonly included the phrase 'must have had the smallpox', highlighting the deeply rooted fear that outsiders could introduce the disease into families and households.[39] This fear is also often explicit in verse. The Welsh poet Tudur Aled spoke of pockmarked shields which resembled the marks of variola.[40] Cadwaladr Roberts of Pennant Mellangell, Montgomeryshire wrote a satire about the disease, and bemoaned the ways in which the characteristic symptoms of *y frech wen* could have severe physical and even social ramifications for the sufferer.[41] Roberts wrote of 'a pox of pain, lifeless plague [that] blemished my whole skin'.[42] Unable now to attract a 'beautiful and unstained girl', he lamented that 'only . . . a keen witch' would now have him, arguing that people would mock his appearance, 'this grubby elf with perforated skin'.[43] But the fear culture of smallpox was by no means solely an adult phenomenon since even children's nursery rhymes played upon the social stigma of the smallpox. In one rhyme, 'cân nant y eira' (song of the snow brook) a Welsh boy wears a beaver hat low on the side of his head to hide his dimpled nose and smallpox scars.[44] For the sufferer, and even the child, the mark of smallpox was clearly represented as one of shame.[45]

At other times, sickness might sometimes appear in poetry as a device to insult or curse. Robin Clidro's 'Satire on a Stingy Parson' condemned the unfortunate curate to a noisy, flea ridden prison with mice in the bedsraw, but also 'ar cryd, ar ddanoedd am dano'n ymdynny' (with fever and toothache growing upon him). Apart from the potential power of the imagery, Clidro clearly considered the symptoms to be something occurring *upon* the body, rather than within it.[46] In fact, in terms of the symptomatic effects of disease, awareness of physical 'difference' was evidently an important aspect in Welsh popular mentalities, with deformity or disability, and especially blindness, often particularly remarked upon. In burial records, those with physical deformities or disabilities were often noted. In 1623, Rees ap John ap Ieuan was buried, 'an olde, blinde and beddered man'.[47] 'Oliver Lloid with one Eie' was likewise recorded, as was Margaret Verch Ellis, 'an old blind woman'.[48] Physical appearance could strongly affect even the ways in which people were referred to. Nicknames were often based on physical characteristics, and these could transmute into permanent surnames. In the parish register of Bedwellty in Monmouthshire in 1638 was the burial of Thomas William, known as 'vocatus y coch mud' (the red mute), while the presence of other striking physical characteristics might result in a nickname, such as that of David Powell 'penfelyn' (yellow head).[49] That these sobriquets were sufficiently well recognised to be recorded in burial entries, suggests that conceptions and representations of the body were widely recognised and used.

While, logically, Wales did not have its own unique set of biological diseases, cultural influences could still impinge upon beliefs about the origins and spread of disease. It is important to recognise that disease terminology was not static, and varied much depending on such issues as the status of the individual and location, and also over time. There were certainly instances of local Welsh idiosyncrasies in terms of names for particular diseases. In Cardiganshire, malaria was referred to by the name 'y Hen Wrach' (the old witch) due to a local legend telling of a witch who lived in marshlands, who would emerge from the mists and seize her unsuspecting victims in a vice-like grip, causing them to display the characteristic shivering malarial symptoms.[50] Richard Suggett has identified several references to Welsh disease terms connected with witchcraft and esoteric magical and supernatural medicine, which appear to have no corresponding form in English; the diseases themselves appeared to defy treatment by orthodox means.[51] One such condition was 'liveranartegro', a condition supposedly caused by witchcraft which caused the fusing of the heart and liver. Beliefs in this disease were apparently limited to south Pembrokeshire, while west and mid-Wales contained references to 'clwyf yr edau wlân' (the woollen-yarn disease), similar to consumption, and 'clefyd y galôn' (disease of the heart), but relating to depressive illness.[52] It is worth mentioning as a side note, however, that 'liveranartegro' appears to be bastardised from the English 'liver and heart to/do grow'. If so, this provides a useful example of the assimilation of English terminology into Welsh vernacular, explored in more detail later in the next chapter. Such diseases were so strongly linked to particular environments that they would not respond to anything other than a local healer who possessed specialist knowledge both of diagnosis of these conditions, and medical environment in which they dwelt.

The Welsh body in English literature

In English popular culture, there were certainly perceptions of a Welsh stereotype, and these included references to physical characteristics. One pamphlet viewed the Welsh as being possessed of 'a Hot Cholorick Temper [who] will, upon a word's speaking, run at you with their Knives full drive'.[53] The literary Welshman was often feisty and quick to take offence at any perceived slight upon himself or his country, and this made a useful angle for republican Civil War satirists, angry at Wales's royalist stance, to attack.[54] In one political pamphlet, adversaries of a fiery Welshman, Jenkin, mock his ebullience by observing that 'your Welch bloud is up'.[55] Clearly, this was a recognised literary trope which the intended audience would understand, but its deployment in popular literature does appear to differ from representations of other regional stereotypes – at least in medical terms.

In references to health in popular and literary depictions of Wales and the Welsh, little mention is made of specific maladies or conditions.[56] Indeed, compared to his Scottish and Irish counterparts, the stage and literary Welshman fares comparatively well.[57] The literary Welshman was poor, sometimes beggarly, had a predilection for toasted cheese and metheglin, and was mildly ridiculed for his rustic ignorance. He does not, however, seem to have been viewed as unhealthy or physically repellent. Compare this to the Welshman James Howell's mid-seventeenth-century depiction of the Scots who, 'naturally abhor cleanliness . . . their breath commonly stinks of pottage, their linen of piss, their hands of pigs turds, their body of sweat'.[58] Later, in a 1701 publication, the Scots are further described as dirty, verminous and possessed of unsanitary personal habits.[59] Popular depictions of the Irish centred around their apparently unusual appearance and, like the Welsh, quick tempers.[60] Moreover, the Irish, according to the Dublin-based English physician Thomas Sydenham, were 'naturally lazy and content to feed hardly upon cheaper food which is plentifull among them and will therefore betake themselves to no industry'.[61] Sydenham noted the prevalence of fevers in Ireland, and especially Dublin, due to the moist airs and marshy country only remedied, he argued, by English settlers draining the bogs.[62] The most likely reason for these differences is political, and especially in the somewhat unique relationship between Wales and the centre of power. Wales was a nation without a state, and had no existence in law beyond that simply of a region of England.[63] During the Civil War, Welsh soldiers fought for the King at Edgehill, but their poor performance on the field underlined the fact that they posed no significant military threat to centres of power.[64] Unlike the Scots, and especially the Irish, who were viewed by pamphleteers with dislike, even overt apathy, the Welsh were portrayed more as ignorant and misguided, but essentially harmless and rustic, neighbours.[65] The presence of national stereotypes was a constant feature of early modern culture and historians have analysed such characters in order to access popular views of the countries depicted. Obviously stereotypes, by their nature, are intended as extreme caricatures – even grotesques, and must be used with caution. Nevertheless, they had also to be recognisable to audiences in order to work as a stereotype, and the contrast between Welsh and Scottish depictions of health and appearance, in particular, seems telling.

Such examples underline the fact that an entire social group, just as an individual, could be characterised by single or unique aspects of their humoral makeup. This, in turn, highlights the strong humoral link between body and environment. As a simultaneous inhabitant of Earth and the wider universe, the body was seen as most naturally suited to its native environment. Air, climate, earth and landscape all influenced the body, and a person's humoral balance was naturally attuned to the physical characteristics of their birthplace. Venturing outside one's home area invited illness.[66] While Wales did not have its own peculiar set of biological diseases (even if it possessed cultural and regional variations in disease nomenclature), the path and spread of disease was affected by landscape and topography. Thus, the landscape of Wales, its airs and waters, could render tangible effects on the bodies and minds of the early modern Welsh population, and this could also have an impact on perceptions of health and illness.

Given its overwhelmingly rural context, the landscape of Wales should have made for a healthy population since the countryside, in the early modern period, was lauded by writers as a place of robust health. The hard, physical labour of agricultural work reputedly hardened the bodies and immune systems of country dwellers. Thus, even though the rural population were often poorer than their urban counterparts, their cast-iron constitutions were viewed as better able to digest a range of foods, in turn expelling noxious humours from the body through their naturally hotter constitutions.[67] This bucolic depiction of health was reinforced by beliefs in the healthiness (and otherwise) of different types of landscape, ranging from the mephitic low-lying marshes where fevers and agues dwelt, to the healthier airs of upland, pastoral regions.[68] Was Wales viewed from the outside as a healthy place to dwell? One late seventeenth-century pamphlet may serve to shed light on this question.

In 1695 an English writer, probably Nathaniel Crouch (writing under his pseudonym of R.B.) printed an account of his journey throughout Wales. Crouch assessed the features of all Welsh counties but, importantly, also remarked upon the physical characteristics of the people within.[69] The Welsh people as a whole he saw as 'generally healthy, strong, swift and witty, which is imputed to the clear and wholesome Air of the mountains, the cleanly and moderate Diet of the people and the hardship to which they are inured from their childhood'.[70] The reference here to the healthiness of their moderate diet seems unusual given that the usual Welsh diet of barley bread and toasted cheese, depicted elsewhere, was proverbially poor. Likewise remarked upon is the natural robustness of the Welsh people developed through their hardships. It is difficult to say why, where many others were dismissive of the landscape of Wales, Crouch chose a different tack, although it is not inconceivable that his writings were a deliberate attempt to juxtapose a healthy, rural life against life in the city of London where the pamphlet was printed and which, in 1695, was still fearful of the return of the plague.

Moving on to specific counties, it was generally those upland regions with their sharper and colder air which seemed healthiest to Crouch. In Breconshire, 'the mountains of Talgar and Ewias in the east seem to defend it from the excessive heat of the sun, which makes a wholesome and temperate air' while in Caernarvonshire 'the air is sharp and piercing by reason of the high mountains'.[71] The hilly terrain of Monmouthshire contained 'temperate, clear and healthful' air and was 'fruitful of cattel [sic], corn and all other accommodations of life'. Glamorganshire, with its abundance of 'Cattel, pleasant springs and fruits' was the 'Garden of Wales' for its inhabitants.[72] Flintshire was a particular favourite, with its 'healthful [air] and the soil plentiful of corn'.[73] Other counties fare less well, and often those regarded as poorest and least populous. Denbighshire was 'mountainous, cold and barren' although Crouch conceded that it is 'yet not without some fruitful valleys'.[74] Poor Merionethshire was 'like a Welsh harp although it yields but dull musick to the inhabitants, being the roughest and most barren shires of all Wales'.[75] Here, the rough and stony soil meant that 'the plow cannot go, nor the Corn thrive' although, as Crouch notes, 'some have causelessly imputed the scarcity of grain to the sloth of the people'.[76] In general, however, the picture given is of a healthy land, whose people are generally hardy. The importance of individual environments is also thrown into sharp relief. While the intended audience or readership must be considered, Crouch provides a useful potential glimpse into outsiders' views of the Principality, and of the Welsh body, during this period.

Religion and medical knowledge in Wales

Certainly one of the strongest contributory factors in concepts of health and sickness in Wales was religion. God was a healer, but He also sent sickness as punishment for sin or as a test of faith. Christianity provided an explanatory framework for the body, and stressed the duty of each individual to look after their bodies as the vehicle for their immortal souls.[77] Divine providence was seen as being at work regardless of religious affiliation – it was just a matter of degree as to how it was interpreted and addressed. For Welsh Anglicans and Catholics alike, the healing power of God was reinforced through rituals such as prayer and pilgrimage to holy sites. Protestants were equally as likely as Catholics to respond to their maladies through prayer. Likewise, despite opposing the symbolism of Catholic rituals, Welsh Protestants still visited holy wells, and journeyed to London to be touched by the monarch for the 'King's Evil'.[78]

As is so often the case, it is those who left the least in terms of tangible historical record who represent the majority of 'ordinary' people. For most Welsh people, though, Anglicanism certainly provided familiar and comforting links with the past. Wales was sheltered from repeated waves of reformers and divines by the combined action of several factors – the often unforgiving landscape; an impoverished clergy who were unable or unwilling to fully carry out their duties; a relative lack of Welsh-language vernacular religious literature during the Reformation; and a gentry by and large unwilling to persecute recusants.[79] Old trusts in the power of saints, spirits and the supernatural were so deeply embedded that, although they may have lost their pre-Reformation connections, they existed still in the popular imagination.[80] The strong tradition of storytelling in Wales, together with the potential for the spread of information orally through other means, such as fairs, markets and village gossip, served further to perpetuate shared cultural mores.[81] Thus, although most Welsh people accepted the imposition of Protestantism upon them (it has been argued that nine out of ten considered themselves Anglicans even if they did not regularly attend services), they had no great theoretical understanding or love of it in the same way that they did the older pre-Reformation church.[82] In some ways, the church certainly served to preserve such traditions since views of the power of spiritual and supernatural healing reinforced the practices of faith healers and cunning folk.[83] The church was the epicentre of Welsh community life, and the source of many public social events and celebrations, often based around time honoured public rituals.[84] The impoverished Welsh clergy were not up to the task of reform and sometimes were not above superstitious practices themselves.[85] As Helen Dingwall also reminds us, beliefs in a Christian God and beliefs in the power of superstitions and charms were not mutually exclusive, and such beliefs were not an alternative to any medical 'orthodoxy' but rather a part of it.[86] There was therefore, in essence, a very hazy boundary between religion and 'superstition'.[87]

The problem with assessing the impact of religion upon medical beliefs and practices in Wales, however, is that it is too easy to concentrate on the conservative aspects of religion and miss the extent to which it also fostered change. In medical terms, this retention of the 'old ways' has tended to be viewed as simultaneously preserving, and even promoting, magical and folkloric medicine. Whilst this is true to a certain extent, we also need to recognise the extent to which religion could also act as a driver for change. Rather than simply serving to promote a particular 'type' of medical belief, this somewhat unique Welsh religious background in fact fostered a duality of beliefs, giving effective licence to the retention of pre-Reformation symbolism on one hand, and the development of a more pragmatic Protestant realism on the other.

Religion certainly performed a strong didactic function in terms of disseminating medical knowledge and, crucially, one which was transmitted in vernacular Welsh. At every service, Welsh congregations would have listened to Biblical passages which hammered home the correlations between physical and spiritual health. Disease was a common theme in the Bible, with everything from Christ's healing of the lame and disfigured to the Egyptian plagues. Crucially, this information was imparted in Welsh. Since the sixteenth century, the Welsh had had their own Bible translated by William Salesbury, also usefully translating disease terms into Welsh. Often fulfilling roles as healers in the community, the Welsh clergy were well placed to be able to minister to both the spiritual and physical needs of their flocks, and could also act as conduits for the spread of medical knowledge. Popular religious sayings intertwined with concepts of health and illness. Collecting medical manuscripts was also becoming more popular amongst the clergy, supporting their role as healers, and also emphasising their own worldliness and learning.

Regarding the everyday medical experience of the majority of Welsh people, what existed was a combination of secular and religious notions of the body and illness enmeshed in, and articulated through, the framework of popular humoralism. Christianity provided both an explanation for illness and a potential source of relief. Humoral medicine meshed easily with these religious concepts of sickness and also made sense as a worldview, involving observations of nature and the ways in which the natural world tied in with the human body. Since rural life, such as that experienced by much of the Welsh population in this period, was so closely tied in with the seasons, it was not hard to find metaphors amongst nature for the workings of the body. The notion of God as both sender and healer of illness was common across early modern society. But for certain groups, such as Non-conformists and dissenters in particular, ill health was most readily attributed to divine providence, and sickness could be construed as a punishment upon the ungodly or those pursuing a 'false' faith.[88] By attributing disease and sickness to the will of God, people could in some ways shield themselves against the otherwise harsh realities of daily life since this provided a means of explaining the otherwise unfathomable. Prayer was cheap physic. For those unable to afford the services of a 'regular' doctor, the power of faith should not be underestimated. Of the importance of religion in certain aspects of popular healing there can be no doubt since a variety of cures and rituals held special significance through their religious connotations. Neither did supernatural healing exist in a separate sphere to 'regular' or 'orthodox' medicine, such as they existed in Wales, as there were strong points of crossover. Even though 'folkloric' medicine contained many aspects of what could be construed as magical or spiritual, the influence of Christianity was never far away in terms of providing reference points or imbuing objects or practices with religious symbolism. Indeed, as Lucinda McCray Beier has argued, belief in the healing power of magic was crucial since it allowed people to espouse the esoteric remedies of cunning folk and white witches whilst still condemning the practice of black magic.[89]

Healing charms provide a useful case in point. Charms had a long history in Wales and are found in many sources across the country, demonstrating the coexistence of religious imagery with other types of symbolism and ritual. Charms dovetailed easily with humoral notions of illness as a foreign matter which needed to be driven out, often involving a large degree of symbolism. They crossed oral and literate boundaries being either spoken aloud verbatim or written down and carried as a protection. They might also be secreted around the home as protection against evil forces.[90] Sometimes, charms were symbolic practices reinforced by the verbatim recitation of Biblical passages. One charm for jaundice involved the placing of a gold coin into a mug of clear mead. The sufferer was then required to look into the glass without drinking any of the contents, while repeating the Lord's Prayer nine times without error.[91] Another, for 'St Antony's Fire', called upon 'Saint Telphin' to 'send this man whole hand and foot in the name Father son Holy gost [sic] Amen'.[92] In most cases, the core factor was the alliance of cure and Christianity in the belief that this provided extra cachet. In fact, the conscious development of a close relationship between religion and medical remedies in particular is noteworthy. This could be manifest in many forms including the collection of remedies and charms within religious texts. In one Welsh-language notebook, medical remedies are scattered within pages of Biblical verse, perhaps in the belief that they would benefit from an increased efficacy through this association.[93] Purloined church record paper came in useful for David Williams of Bodeulwen, Anglesey in the early eighteenth century, who recorded medical remedies alongside ballads, poems and prayers.[94]

Likewise, in a more formal use of church paper, William Harris, the incumbent of Llantilio Pertholey church in Monmouthshire, noted down a remedy for the 'biting of a mad dog' on the back page of the parish register, which he obviously felt might come in useful for his flock.[95] Given their role as community healers, it made sense for the clergy to keep a store of remedies, and their notebooks often served a dual role containing sermons and medical remedies together.[96] Such associations also extended to other practices connected with healing and the warding off of illness. The use of genuflection and religious symbolism has also been noted as an apparently common practice amongst the Welsh poor. According to one eighteenth-century observer, Welsh women habitually 'flourish[ed] a little with their thumb to their jaws, something like making a figure of the cross' especially when first entering church and also when taking communion.[97]

Dissent and medical beliefs

The impact of Non-conformity on medical ideas in Wales should not be downplayed. Puritanism, a section of Christianity for whom superstition and symbolism were anathema, had begun to spread in pockets in Wales during the early seventeenth century, and amongst certain social groups such as the newly prosperous middle orders of yeoman and merchants.[98] During the Interregnum, Puritan ministers, such as Walter Cradock and Vavasor Powell, toured Wales attempting to propagate the word and cure people of their allegedly godless ways, but Puritanism faded rapidly in the years following the Restoration of the monarchy, and arguably impacted little upon wider popular structures of belief. Dissenters and evangelists proved more dogged in their determination to rid the Welsh of superstition and symbolism. In the later seventeenth century, reforming societies came and went, such as the 'Welsh Trust', and the Society for the Propagation of Christian Knowledge (SPCK), which launched in 1699 with the intention of increasing popular literacy.[99] In national terms, dissent was not a widespread phenomenon and during this period accounted for no more than around 5% or 6% of the Welsh population.[100] Nevertheless, Protestantism, Puritanism and Methodism all played a part in both introducing and disseminating medical ideas in Wales, as well as colouring the personal views of those who followed them. Some of the best records of Puritan and Methodist approaches to sickness are those of ministers. Although such figures represent the most distilled form of religious influence, they demonstrate well the ways in which religious beliefs impinged upon views of sickness and the body. Here, sickness and death could be a direct result of individual conduct on earth, and believers looked to their own lifestyles to explain their own afflictions. As such, illnesses, injuries and even deaths of others could appear as either a just retribution or miraculous salvation.

For the Puritan minister Philip Henry of Broad Oak, Flintshire, like his English contemporary Ralph Josselin, illness in himself and his family was a straightforward matter of personal sinfulness.[101] In 1657, Henry recorded that 'the lord in this month shook his rod over me, 1. in a violent distemper upon mys[elf] 2. in much danger of life to Sister Mary'.[102] Henry went on to list what he saw as the offending faults which included 'pride', 'much forwardnesse' and 'my owne iniquity'.[103] For Henry, sickness was a test of his character, a signpost from God for him to mend his ways. Suffering from a 'cold and tooth-ake caught at Chester', he commented that 'sickness doth not, as it should, make mee more fervent & earnest, but rather more remiss'.[104] Where recovery followed, this was almost always attributed to God's mercy, just one example from many being that of his injury with an iron maul which, he wrote, 'was the great mercy of God it was not much worse, blessed be his name'.[105] Protestantism, and especially Puritanism, also emphasised the need to be constantly prepared for death, and Philip Henry was clearly keen not to be found wanting. On several occasions, he reasoned that his end must be nigh. In 1657, 'I was ill, I thought unto death' while in 1661 'I was not well in the evening of this day & thought, it may bee tis death'.[106] This could even occur in apparently minor conditions, as in 1665, 'through pain in my limbs like a cramp [I] made my will, not knowing but it may be a summons to death'.[107] Henry appeared keen to anticipate situations of potential mortality in order that he be properly prepared for his soul to be judged. For the devout Puritan, death provided the opportunity for rebirth, and the chance to know if the soul had been chosen for redemption.[108]

But for Puritans, there were clear correlations between medicine and faith, with spiritual cleansing being analogous with the workings of physic. Philip Henry, in another diary entry, implored Jesus to 'wash mee in thy Bloud, purge mee, cleanse mee, take away all my defilement'.[109] Here, humoral terminology was interwoven with the concept of Jesus as a healer, emphasising the close relationship between spiritual and physical health. At other times, he was even more explicit in his comparison, more than once quoting the Biblical passage of Matthew 9. 12. 'They that are whole need not a physician but they [th]at are sick. Sin is the sickness of the soule and sin-sick soules stand in great need of a Physician, and that Physician is no other but Jesus Xt'.[110] If sin was indeed a sickness of the soul, it was not hard to draw the further parallel between physical illness and sin, requiring prayer and repentance to regain health.

Welsh Methodists too were encouraged to be introspective and humble in the face of illness. In the 1730s, the Methodist minister John Harries of Mynydd Bach and Abergorlech in Carmarthenshire, kept an unusually detailed log of the lives and behaviour of those parishioners whom he buried. Harries was particularly concerned with the Christian conduct of the sick, believing that only the pious would gain salvation in the afterlife. Of one Mary William John William (sic), he commented that 'shee relied wholly on Jesus X for her soul [and] behaved herself very patient in ye time of her long sickness', while Joyce Evan, 'troubled with ye asthma or shortness of breath long time before shee died . . . was very cheerful, expected but to live but hop'd to be saved'.[111] Gwenllian Jones, who died in 1741, was noted for her 'Christian like' behaviour and for the fact that she 'distributed much of her substance to the poor'.[112] Her charitable nature reassured Harries that she 'ended [this] life and went to another'.[113] Those who were not always resolute in their faith, however, were playing a dangerous game. In July 1742 died Mary Richard who, according to Harries, 'was very wavering and inconstant in her profession [of faith], sometimes in and sometimes out'.[114] Harries wrote pointedly that she had called for the sacrament on her deathbed, implying that her apparent call to faith was only a last act of desperation. 'God grant we may be constant steadfast and immovable, always abounding the work of the Lord, knowing that our labour shall not be in vain' was his final comment on the matter.[115] How far Harries's views translate to his parishioners is unclear, since their conduct is only available through his eyes. Nevertheless, the fleeting glimpses of such people in his diary show the great extent to which sickness conduct could be affected by religious affiliation.

Personal religious beliefs, too, could actually exert a direct influence upon an individual's health by rendering some people more susceptible to certain conditions. Glyn Penrhyn Jones noted the prevalency for depressive illnesses amongst eighteenth-century Welsh Methodists, due to their intensive introspection and concentration upon personal weaknesses and failings.[116] Griffith Jones of Llanddowror, the founder of SPCK schools in Wales certainly suffered from depression, while Hywel Harris, the Breconshire Methodist revivalist suffered extremely low self-esteem and depression as a direct result of his self-image as a 'depraved sinner'.[117] It is unwise to assume this was a blanket experience, since the effects of other causes than religion cannot be ruled out. Many other denominations included similar patterns of self-recrimination and introspection, and it seems unlikely that one in particular could be adjudged especially prone. But some Welsh ministers certainly suffered under their duty of care to the sick and especially the dying. Philip Henry made several references to his uneasiness about having to attend the dying, and certain visits in particular seem to have played on his mind. In January 1651, he attended three dying parishioners within the short space of a few days, and fretted that such frequent exposure to death was leaving him with a diminished sense of his own spirituality.[118] John Harries too was affected by constantly keeping company with the terminally ill. In 1737, after spending several long hours with a dying parishioner, he glumly considered his own mortality, noting that 'I see both young and old are carried away to another world unobserved'.[119] This phenomenon has certainly been noted elsewhere. In 1652, the young Presbyterian minister Henry Newcome, newly arrived in Manchester from a rural parish, found that the continual round of deathbed sittings and funerals deeply affected his own state of mind.[120] Exposure to the many faces of death was commonplace during the early modern period, and people were somewhat inured to the reality of death and dying. Religion taught that mortal life was short in contrast to the afterlife which was eternal, making death a beginning rather than an end.[121] Nevertheless, it is not hard to see how exposure to the physical manifestations of death upon the human frame could affect those who witnessed it repeatedly.

In other ways, religion could also stimulate the spread of medicines and medical knowledge. It is possible, for example, to see the introduction of Paracelsian chemical medicine into Wales as being a direct result of the interests of Protestant reformers.[122] Paracelsian and Helmontian remedies were alternatives to Galenic cures, although there was still much continuity in terms of their underlying theories of therapeutic practices. Helmontian physicians, however, railed against the invasive techniques of orthodox Galenism, and especially against its painful and dangerous procedures, believing instead in the power of chemical remedies.[123] For advocates of this type of medicine, the physician was directly endowed by God with healing powers. This especially appealed to Protestant reformers, and to some of the more radical religious sects, since it divested the priest of any especial healing powers and removed some of the ritualistic elements of medicine.[124] Helmontianism was often championed by apothecaries who, in turn, were often patronised by the middle levels of society.[125] The Monmouthshire yeoman John Gwin was typical of the audience for Helmontian literature, and owned several works by the New England practitioner George Starkey, as well as others by Nicholas Culpeper.[126] Related by marriage to the Puritan divine Walter Cradock, Gwin was also a fairly well-to-do yeoman farmer, regularly travelling back and forth to Bristol to conduct business as well as buy his books. Other examples of 'chymical' medicine seem to appear in areas with strong Protestant or Puritan sympathies. Sir Owen Wynn of Gwydir owned an entire library of chemical books.[127] Wynn lived in Flintshire which, although not itself an especially strong Puritan area, was near to other areas such as Chester and Denbighshire, which were more sympathetic to Puritanism; these areas had a broad base of literate elites, receptive to alternative ideas.[128]

As well as influencing alternative medical regimes, religion could also stimulate attacks on popular healing practices. In 1721, Erasmus Saunders wrote complainingly of the Welsh vulgar who habitually invoked saints in their prayers and put their faith in the power of holy objects to heal themselves.[129] Later in 1745, Griffith Jones of Llanddowror condemned the 'abominable relics of Popery', while other writers such as Simon Thomas and William Wynne noted the various customs and practices of the Welsh lower orders which seemed grounded more in ancient than contemporary times.[130] Such men certainly had a spiritual axe to grind. Erasmus Saunders and Griffith Jones were members of the SPCK, with a vested interest in trying to divest the populace of papist practices, while Thomas was likewise an evangelist minister. Exaggerating the extent of popular healing practices could be a useful means of reinforcing their own message.

But care should be taken not to overstate the role of religion in everyday sickness experiences since in many written records of personal illness there is little evidence of either religious causation or cure. The 1630–36 diary of Robert Bulkeley of Dronwy, Anglesey contains many examples of his illnesses, but little to support views of his afflictions in religious terms. Bulkeley was also a regular visitor to the sickbedsof his friends and neighbours but exhortations to God to intervene are notably absent.[131] The fact that he does not make reference to religion clearly does not indicate that he did not regard it as important, but the lack of any reference whatsoever is notable. Perhaps Bulkeley was a pragmatist who simply did not 'believe' in supernatural healing, preferring to rely on the skills of flesh and blood, rather than spiritual healers. He certainly enjoyed many leisure pursuits which were actively discouraged by the church, such as gambling and attending blood sports. Another source, the Monmouthshire Civil War diarist Walter Powell, provides a further example of entirely secular approaches to illness, noting his many maladies but never referring to accidents or cures in religious terms.[132] Once again, Powell was one of the up-and-coming 'middling sort', a yeoman farmer and man of business. Even religious figures were not always so quick to look to their faiths in times of illness, and this seems increasingly noticeable during the eighteenth century. The 1720s diary of the Quaker, John Kelsall contains scant evidence that he equated illness with faith, and in fact little mention of health at all, unusual for a denomination so concerned with introspection and conduct.[133] The letters of the Anglesey parson Owen Davies, covering the years 1712–32, are also curiously devoid of direct connections of illness and religion. Occasionally, Davies thanks God for the recovery of local children, as in December 1724 when he wrote 'About a fortnight ago the measles seised [sic] upon most of the children but, God be praised, they are pretty well recruited'.[134] The reference to God here, though, appears almost as a convention, rather than a genuine expression of piety.

Religion and magic, then, certainly played an important part in the ways that people conceptualised illness throughout this period, although they were by no means the only framework. Individual conceptions of sickness causality were mutable and adaptable, and could be greatly affected by the religious affiliation or denomination of the individual sufferer. Religion might be an overt or explicit influence on personal sickness, or instead be little more than background 'noise'; in either case, though, it was there. It would therefore be a mistake to assume, as others seem tacitly to have done, that Welsh religion was responsible for somehow limiting or fixing medicine in Wales to a single, and conservative, category.

Having now dealt in some detail with Welsh concepts of illness and the body, and the effects of a range of different social, cultural and geographical factors upon these concepts, we now turn to the question of the spread of medical information in Wales. How did Welsh people obtain their medical knowledge, remedies, and so on? Up until now, little work has been done to try to ascertain the movement of medical knowledge both into and within Wales, and the extent of outside influence upon the types of medicines to which people had access. It is to such questions that the next chapters in this book will turn.

Notes

1 Henry Halford Vaughan, *Welsh Proverbs with English Translations* (London: Kegan Paul and Trench, 1889), p. 149.

2 Roy Porter, 'The Patient in England c. 1660 – c. 1800' in Andrew Wear (ed.), *Medicine in Society: Historical Essays* (Cambridge: Cambridge University Press, 1998 edition), pp. 101, 108; Jonathan Barry, 'Piety and the Patient: Medicine and Religion in Eighteenth Century Bristol' in Roy Porter (ed.), *Patients and Practitioners: Lay Perceptions of Medicine in Pre-Industrial Society* (Cambridge: Cambridge University Press, 2002 edition), pp. 145–147.

3 Lucinda McCray Beier, *Sufferers and Healers: The Experience of Illness in Seventeenth Century England* (London and New York: Routledge and Kegan Paul, 1987), pp. 156–157.

4 Katherine Park, 'Medicine and Society in Medieval Europe, 500–1500' in Wear (ed.), *Medicine in Society*, p. 75.

5 Ibid., pp. 75–76.

6 Mary Lindemann, *Medicine and Society in Early Modern Europe* (Cambridge: Cambridge University Press, 1999), p. 175.

7 Helen M. Dingwall, *A History of Scottish Medicine: Themes and Influences* (Edinburgh: Edinburgh University Press, 2003), pp. 4, 88–89.

8 James Kelly, 'The Emergence of Scientific and Institutional Medical Practice in Ireland, 1650–1800' in Greta Jones and Elizabeth Malcolm (eds), *Medicine, Disease and the State in Ireland, 1650–1940* (Cork: Cork University Press, 1999), pp. 21–22.

9 Park, 'Medicine and Society', p. 81.

10 See Robert Recorde, *The Urinal of Physick* (London: Printed by Reynold Wolfe, 1548).

11 Dingwall, *History of Scottish Medicine*, p. 99; Kelly, 'Emergence', p. 22.

12 See, for example, Beier, *Sufferers and Healers*, p. 31.

13 Morfydd E. Owen, 'The Medical Books of Medieval Wales and the Physicians of Myddfai', *Carmarthenshire Antiquary*, 31 (1995), p. 37.

14 See Ida B. Jones, 'Hafod 16: A Mediaeval Welsh Medical Treatise', *Études Celtiques*, 8 (1958–59), pp. 346–393.

15 W. Gerallt Harries, 'Bened Feddyg: A Welsh Medical Practitioner in the Late Medieval Period' in John Cule (ed.), *Wales and Medicine* (Llandysul: Gomer Press, 1975), p. 170.

16 British Library, BM Add. MS 15078, John ap Ifan, Welsh translation of Humfrey Llwyd's English version of the treatise by Petrus Hispanus entitled 'The Treasury of Health', unknown date.

17 Owen, 'Medical Books', pp. 39–40.

18 See for example National Library of Wales (hereafter NLW) MS 572D, Anon., Medical Herbal and Remedy Collection, 16th century.

19 Ibid., pp. 37–38.

20 Ibid., p. 31.

21 Lindemann, *Medicine and Society*, pp. 9–10.

22 Ibid., p. 164.

23 Geraint H. Jenkins, 'Popular Beliefs in Wales from Restoration to Methodism', *Bulletin of the Board of Celtic Studies*, 27:3 (1977), p. 442; David Howell, *The Rural Poor in Eighteenth Century Wales* (Cardiff: University of Wales Press, 2000), pp. 154–155.

24 Roy Porter, *The Greatest Benefit to Mankind: A Medical History of Humanity from Antiquity to the Present* (London: Fontana, 1999 edition), p. 38.

25 Ibid., p. 38.

26 See John Hobson Matthews (ed.), *Cardiff Records, Volume 1* (Cardiff: Cardiff Corporation, 1898), p. 199, for an account of death from the 'damps'.

27 Mary Vaughan, 'An Old Receipt Book', *Journal of the Merioneth Historical and Record Society*, 4 (1964), p. 319.

28 Andrew Wear, *Knowledge and Practice in English Medicine, 1550–1680* (Cambridge: Cambridge University Press, 2000), p. 38.

29 Ibid., p. 106.

30 Howell, *The Rural Poor*, p. 139.

31 For Welsh minstrels see Richard Suggett, 'Vagabonds and Minstrels in Sixteenth-Century Wales' in Adam Fox and Daniel Woolf (eds), *The Spoken Word: Oral Culture in Britain, 1500–1850* (Manchester: Manchester University Press, 2002), pp. 138–172.

32 Philip Jenkins, *A History of Modern Wales 1536–1990* (London and New York: Longman, 1992), p. 61.

33 Ibid., p. 64.

34 Quoted in Gwyn Jones, *The Oxford Book of Welsh Verse in English* (Oxford: Oxford University Press, 1977), pp. 110–111. The poems quoted here were translated from the original Welsh by Jones.

35 Ibid., p. 10.

36 Rachel Bromwich, *Dafydd ap Gwilym: A Selection of Poems* (Llandysul: Gomer Press, 1982), pp. 2, 18.

37 Ibid., p. 4.

38 For discussions of 'January-May' marriages see Martin Ingram, *Church Courts, Sex and Marriage in England, 1570–1640* (Cambridge: Cambridge University Press, 1994 edition), pp. 140–141 and E.A. Wrigley, *English Population History from Family Reconstitution* (Cambridge: Cambridge University Press, 1997), pp. 151–153; see also discussions of remarriage in E.A. Wrigley and R.S. Schofield, *The Population History of England 1541–1871* (Cambridge: Cambridge University Press, 1989), pp. 28–29, 190–191 and 258–259 and Jeremy Boulton, 'London Widowhood Revisited: the Decline of Female Remarriage in the Seventeenth and Early Eighteenth Centuries', *Continuity and Change*, 5 (1990), pp. 323–355.

39 Geraint H. Jenkins, *The Foundations of Modern Wales, 1642–1780* (Oxford: Oxford University Press, 2002 edition), p. 89.

40 Quoted in Glyn Penrhyn Jones, *Newyn a Haint yng Nghymru* (Caernarfon: Llyfrfa'r Methodistiaid Calfinaidd, 1962), p. 34.

41 Ibid., p. 35; 'y frech wen' – the Welsh name for smallpox, literally the white pox/rash.

42 Ibid., p. 35.

43 Ibid., p. 35.

44 Ibid., p. 36.

45 Detailed discussions of the physical, social and cultural impact of smallpox can be found in David Shuttleton, *Smallpox and the Literary Imagination, 1660–1820* (Cambridge: Cambridge University Press, 2007).

46 Gwyn Williams, *An Introduction to Welsh Poetry* (London: Faber and Faber, 1964), p. 221.

47 D.R. Thomas, *Y Cwtta Cyfarwydd: 'The Chronicle' written by the famous clarke Peter Roberts, Notary Public, From the Years 1607–1646* (London: Whiting and Co., 1883), p. 99.

48 Ibid., pp. 53, 85.

49 R.W. McDonald, 'The Parish Registers of Wales', *National Library of Wales Journal*, 19:4 (1976), p. 35.

50 Glyn Penrhyn Jones, 'A History of Medicine in Wales in the Eighteenth Century' (Liverpool University: Unpublished MA Thesis, 1957), pp. 203–220.

51 Richard Suggett, *A History of Magic and Witchcraft in Wales* (Stroud: The History Press, 2008), p. 105.

52 Ibid., pp. 105–106.

53 E.B., *A Trip to North Wales: Being a Description of That Country and People* (London: 1701), p. 6.

54 See Lloyd Bowen, 'Representations of Wales and the Welsh during the Civil Wars and Interregnum', *Historical Research*, 77:197 (2004), pp. 358–376.

55 Quoted in Mark Stoyle, 'Caricaturing Cymru: Images of the Welsh in the London Press 1642–46' in Diana Dunn (ed.), *War and Society in Medieval and Early Modern Britain* (Liverpool: Liverpool University Press, 2000), p. 170.

56 One pamphlet does suggest that Poor Taff suffered from flatulence due to his leek and cheese diet! See Alexander Brome, *Rump or an exact collection of the choycest poems and*

songs relayting to the late times by the most eminent wits from 1639 to anno 1661 (London: Printed for Henry Brome, 1662), p. 261.

57 J.O. Bartley, *Teague, Shenkin and Sawney, Being an Historical Study of the Earliest Irish, Welsh and Scottish Characters in English Plays* (Cork: Cork University Press, 1954), pp. 63–65; for examples of Welsh in English pamphlets see Anon., *The Welch Man's Inventory* (London: Printed for Thomas Lambert Dwelling in Smithfield, 1641); Anon., *The Welch-Mans complements* (London: S.B., 1643); Morgan ap Shinkin, *The Welch Doctor or The Welch Man Turned Physician being a New Way to Cure all diseases in these times* (London: 1643).

58 Quoted in Bartley, *Teague, Shenkin and Sawney*, p. 158.

59 Ibid., p. 158.

60 Ibid., p. 39.

61 Bodleian Library, MS Rawl.C.406, Notebook of Thomas Sydenham, 1683, p. 72.

62 Ibid., p. 73.

63 Stephen Roberts, 'Religion, Politics and Welshness, 1649–1660' in Ivan Roots (ed.), '*Into Another Mould*': *Aspects of the Interregnum* (Exeter: University of Exeter Press, 1998 edition), p. 30.

64 Bowen, 'Representations', p. 365.

65 Ibid., pp. 367–368.

66 Wear, *Knowledge and Practice*, p. 186.

67 Ibid., p. 161.

68 Mary J. Dobson, *Contours of Death and Disease in Early Modern England* (Cambridge: Cambridge University Press, 2002 edition), pp. 502–503.

69 R.B., *A Natural History of the Principality of Wales* . . . (London: Printed for Nath. Crouch at the Bell, Cheapside, 1695). See entry on Nathaniel Crouch in the Oxford Dictionary of National Biography.

70 Ibid., p. 123.

71 Ibid., pp. 131, 148.

72 Ibid., pp. 165, 171.

73 Ibid., p. 154.

74 Ibid., p. 151.

75 Ibid., p. 169.

76 Ibid., p. 169.

77 Wear, *Knowledge and Practice*, p. 30.

78 Protestant visitors to holy wells are discussed at length in Colleen M. Seguin, 'Cures and Controversy in Early Modern Wales: The Struggle to Control St. Winifred's Well', *North American Journal of Welsh Studies*, 3:2 (Summer 2003), p. 7; for visits relating to the King's Evil see NLW, Wigfair (2) MS 12402E, Letter from John Lloyde of Wigfair, undated, c. 1664.

79 Glanmor Williams, *Renewal and Reformation Wales c. 1415–1642* (Oxford: Oxford University Press, 2002 edition), pp. 279–280; Jenkins, *History of Modern Wales*, pp. 102, 114.

80 Jenkins, 'Popular Beliefs', p. 442.

81 Howell, *The Rural Poor*, p. 139.
82 Jenkins, *Foundations*, p. 181.
83 Doreen G. Nagy, *Popular Medicine in Seventeenth Century England* (Bowling Green, OH: Bowling Green State University Popular Press, 1988), p. 37.
84 Ibid., p. 181.
85 W.S.K. Thomas, *Stuart Wales* (Llandysul: Gomer Press, 1988), p. 58.
86 Dingwall, *History of Scottish Medicine*, p. 42.
87 Beier, *Sufferers and Healers*, p. 161.
88 Wear, *Knowledge and Practice*, p. 30.
89 Beier, *Sufferers and Healers*, p. 163.
90 Keith Thomas, *Religion and the Decline of Magic* (London: Penguin, 1991 edition), p. 215.
91 Wellcome Library, MS 8968, Notes and Drafts for Unfinished Volume 'The History and Lore of Cymric Medicine' by David Fraser-Harris, c. 1928, p. 12.
92 British Medical Association, *Catalogue of the Manuscripts, Charms, Remedies and Various Objects Illustrating the History of Medicine in Wales, Exhibited in the National Museum of Wales* (Aberystwyth: National Library of Wales, 1928), p. 10.
93 NLW MS 5932A, Anon., Medical Remedies and Miscellany, c. 1635; Alun Withey, 'Medical Knowledge and Practice in Early Modern Wales' (Cardiff University: Unpublished MA Thesis, 2006), p. 32.
94 NLW MS 836D, 'Piser Alice Uch Rees' Miscellany, 1718–42, pp. 130–131.
95 Gwent Record Office, MS D/Pa. 140.24, Parish Register of Llantilio Pertholey, remedy c. 1730.
96 For example see NLW MS 1023B, Sermons and Medical Remedies of Ellis Owen, 1712, pp. 11, 13, 24, 50, 52; NLW MS 5932A, Anon., Medical Remedies and Miscellany, c. 1635; British Library, BM Add. MS 14900, Anon., 'Llyfr Byr Llangadwaladr', Miscellaneous sermons and remedies, 18th century.
97 NLW MS 2576B, Letter giving account of medical superstitions in Wales, relating to Thomas Pennant's tour, July 1755, p. 77.
98 Thomas, *Stuart Wales*, p. 59.
99 Jenkins, *Foundations*, pp. 199–200, 202–203.
100 Jenkins, *History of Modern Wales*, p. 146.
101 For Josselin see Alan Macfarlane (ed.), *The Diary of Ralph Josselin, 1616–1683* (London: Oxford University Press printed for the Royal Academy, 1976); Alan Macfarlane, *The Family Life of Ralph Josselin, a Seventeenth Century Clergyman: An Essay in Historical Anthropology* (London: Cambridge University Press, 1970).
102 Matthew Henry Lee (ed.), *The Diaries and Letters of Philip Henry, M.A. of Broad Oak, Flintshire A.D. 1631–1696* (London: Kegan Paul, Trench and Co., 1882), p. 41; for other discussions of the Henry diaries see David Harley, 'The Theology of Affliction and the Experience of Sickness in the Godly Family, 1650–1714: The Henrys and the Newcomes' in Ole Peter Grell and Andrew Cunningham (eds), *Religio Medici: Medicine and Religion in Seventeenth-Century England* (Aldershot: Scolar Press, 1996), pp. 273–292.
103 Lee (ed.), *Diaries of Philip Henry*, p. 41.
104 Ibid., p. 96.

105 Ibid., p. 56.
106 Ibid., pp. 41, 98.
107 Ibid., p. 168.
108 For some discussions of the 'good death' see Ralph Houlbrooke, *Death, Religion and the Family in England 1480–1750* (Oxford: Clarendon Press, 2000 edition); Clare Gittings, *Death, Burial and the Individual in Early Modern England* (London: Routledge, 1988); David Cressy, *Birth, Marriage and Death* (Oxford: Oxford University Press, 1997); Richard Wunderli and Gerald Broce, 'The Final Moment before Death in Early Modern England' *Sixteenth Century Journal*, 20:2 (1989), pp. 259–275; Philippe Ariés, *Western Attitudes Toward Death from the Middle Ages to the Present*, trans. Patricia M. Ranum (London: Marion Boyars, 1976 edition); J.A Sharpe, '"Last Dying Speeches": Religion, Ideology and Public Execution in Seventeenth Century England', *Past and Present*, 107:1 (1985), pp. 144–167.
109 Lee (ed.), *Diaries of Philip Henry*, p. 45.
110 Ibid., pp. 62–63.
111 NLW MS 371B, Register of Mynydd Bach Chapel, c. 1715–50, pp. 59, 61.
112 Ibid., p. 62.
113 Ibid., p. 62.
114 Ibid., p. 64.
115 Ibid., p. 64.
116 Jones, 'History of Medicine', p. 47.
117 Geraint Tudur, *Hywel Harris: From Conversion to Separation 1735–1750* (Cardiff: University of Wales Press, 2000), p. 9.
118 Lee (ed.), *Diaries of Philip Henry*, p. 166.
119 NLW MS 371B, Register of Mynydd Bach Chapel, c. 1715–50, p. 60.
120 Houlbrooke, *Death, Religion and the Family*, p. 14.
121 Ibid., p. 28.
122 Paracelsus (Phillipus von Hohenheim, 1493–1541) was a Swiss physician, astrologer and philosopher who proposed an alternative, chemical-based physiology to Galen's humoralism. Johannes Baptista Van Helmont (1579–1644) was a Flemish nobleman-physician who also advocated chemical processes in the body, and moved away from astrological and magical associations with healing.
123 Wear, *Knowledge and Practice*, p. 353.
124 Ibid., p. 354.
125 Ibid., p. 355.
126 Gwent Record Office, MS D43:4216, Commonplace Book of John Gwin of Llangwm, 17th century, pp. 62, 65. For a more detailed discussion of Gwin see Alun Withey, 'Medicine and Mortality in Early Modern Monmouthshire: The Commonplace Book of John Gwin of Llangwm', *Welsh History Review*, 23:1 (June 2006), pp. 48–73.
127 Owen Morris, *The 'CHYMICK BOOKES' of Sir Owen Wynne of Gwydir: An Annotated Catalogue* (Cambridge: LP Publications, 1997).
128 Jenkins, *Foundations*, pp. 43, 51.
129 From passage quoted in Jenkins, *History of Modern Wales*, p. 112.

130 Jenkins, 'Popular Beliefs', p. 441.

131 Ibid., pp. 91, 96, 106, 133–135.

132 Christabel Powell, *Walter Powell's Gwent: An Architectural Biography of a 17th Century Diarist* (Risca: Starling Press, 1985), pp. 15, 17.

133 NLW MS 2699B, Quaker Diary of John Kelsall of Dolybran, 1722–34.

134 Leonard Owen, 'The Letters of an Anglesey Parson, 1712–1732', *Transactions of the Honourable Society of Cymmrodorion*, 1 (1961), p. 88.

3

The spread of medical information: medicine, and oral and print culture

How did medical knowledge move into and around early modern Wales? What sorts of factors influenced the availability of medical knowledge, and how did information cross boundaries of literacy and orality? The question of the portability of information is important since it raises wider questions of cultural hegemony and informational relations and networks between centres and peripheries. We have already explored the ways in which 'being' Welsh could nuance bodily approaches and conceptions. The other side of this concerns the nature of information entering Wales from outside and how far Wales was affected by wider medical cultures. Further, how far were contemporary Welsh conceptions of medicine formed and informed by developments in England, and what can this reveal of the extent of 'trickle-down' from cultural centres to the provinces?

During the mid-eighteenth century, and like many of his contemporaries, John Morgan of Palleg, near Ystradgynlais, Glamorganshire, kept an ad hoc notebook in which he recorded information of interest. Morgan appears to have been a fairly wealthy yeoman farmer, and may have belonged to a large family who owned estates in Monmouthshire and Glamorganshire.[1] In amongst family records, such as accounts and farming information, Morgan frequently recorded potentially useful medical remedies and, valuably for our purposes, often noted the sources of these remedies. Within his book are details of remedies from local people given verbally, often containing elements of 'magical' or folkloric medicine, receipts from consultations with medical practitioners, and passages copied from published books and texts.[2] It is apparent from his records that John Morgan regularly sought a range of different opinions in order to try and palliate his symptoms. In one entry, Morgan noted that he was suffering from pain in his knees, apparently exacerbated by walking. Possibly unwilling to leave nature to run its course, he consulted a local doctor in Cardigan, who duly prescribed a poultice made of feverfew and camomile, boiled in human urine.[3] On other occasions, it seems that he was happy to accept the advice of lay healers, as well as family friends and neighbours. A receipt for sciatica was 'directed by the woman of the Kengkod near Carmarthen', perhaps a cunning woman, while others were attributed to local people.[4] But, as well as these informal sources, Morgan also either owned or borrowed medical texts and copied out long passages from these printed works into his notebooks. Entries on the virtues and medical uses of herbs in one section bear strong resemblance to corresponding parts of *The English Physician* by Nicholas Culpeper, a widely available English medical text.[5] Elsewhere, an account by 'Simon Head, Surgeon of His Majesty's Ship Success' of reviving a girl afflicted with worms, appears to originate from a newspaper or pamphlet.[6] The types of remedies and ingredients indicate that Morgan was prepared to utilise virtually any type of remedy if he thought it would be beneficial. Thus, as well as a range of more traditional herbal and animal ingredients can be found evidence of chemical alternatives such as 'half an ounce of Paracelsus', 'Chymical oil of aniseed' and 'opeldeldock oil', all of which are linked to Paracelsian and Helmontian medicine of the mid-seventeenth century, but seem to have survived in remedy collections long afterwards.[7]

Morgan's book is just one example, but illustrates a key point in this study: information, and especially medical information, spread through a variety of channels. It crossed boundaries of orality and literacy, social status, geography and gender. Morgan clearly partook in several socio-medical networks. He was, it seems, as likely to consult a member of his immediate domestic circle as he was an 'orthodox' practitioner. He derived medical information from a range of people in his immediate locality and beyond, but also shared his information by lending his books to others. He sometimes took remedies verbally, but transferred them back into literate form in his own book. He wrote largely in English but sometimes recorded the Welsh names for ingredients, as well as where they might be obtained. Within this source, therefore, is effectively the entire compass of early modern Welsh medical knowledge and, importantly, something of the actual processes of knowledge transmission. It not only highlights the individual practices of an early modern disease sufferer, but also draws attention to the many overlapping spheres – social, cultural, verbal, literate, lay and orthodox – which together formed and informed Welsh medical approaches.

Medicine and the Welsh oral tradition

As Adam Fox has noted, there was constant reciprocity between oral and literate cultures, to the extent that it is questionable whether they should even be considered as being monolithic.[8] In his magisterial study of oral and literate culture in early modern England, Fox argues that the ability to absorb, retain and transmit information orally was far more keenly developed in our early modern counterparts.[9] For many people, such as those involved in working the land and in rural communities, literacy was simply unnecessary in their day-to-day activities. Instead, they developed a range of alternative techniques including rhymes, mnemonics and symbols in order to commit important information to memory.[10] Traditional histories of Wales have often stressed the orality of Welsh culture, and not without reason. The vast majority of people spoke Welsh and, by 1700, the number of monoglot Welsh speakers was still as high as 90%.[11] Gauging literacy levels is difficult due to variations of demography, social status and gender, but they were low in comparison with other areas. By the mid seventeenth century, only around 15% to 20% of the Welsh population could read, compared to an estimated 30% in England.[12] By the eighteenth century, although having risen to something in the order of between 30% and 45%, this was still lower than the English levels of between 40% and 60%.[13] As in many other European agrarian societies, Wales had a rich tradition of popular tales and legends which were continually reinforced and recycled through popular gatherings and public recitations and performances, as well as fireside tales and gossip.[14] This verbal sharing of ideas was also reinforced through work patterns. Markets and fairs brought people into contact with those from other areas, and the normal conduct of business was interspersed with news and gossip.[15]

Health was undoubtedly a central popular concern, and a regular topic of conversation in correspondence amongst friends and acquaintances.[16] But where did popular medical knowledge come from and how did it travel? As Adam Fox notes, we must understand the capacity of early modern people to commit information to memory.[17] Given the high levels of illiteracy in Wales, this ability was almost essential. People routinely called upon a large number of opinions in times of sickness and, with no way of putting remedies to paper, the only option was therefore to learn verbatim. Much medicine and herbal knowledge was based around local conditions and thus fixed within a community's consciousness. Medical knowledge was also part of the wider currency of knowledge sharing and interaction within communities. People simply 'knew' what herbs to use for particular conditions, or where they might find healing waters. In the parish of Caerwedros in Ceredigion, 'the old people knew all the herbal plants by name . . . as they were certain cure for many diseases'.[18] A nearby pool in the river Dewi 'was regarded as cure with the old inhabitants' as well as 'the waters of the Marllyn at Cwmtdu'.[19] Here, again, is the strong link between body and environment. This information was not part of any literate tradition, but survived because of constant reinforcement through verbal traditions, only finding its way onto paper through the observations of a visiting traveller. The emphasis too is clearly on the 'old people', passing down this local knowledge since time out of mind. This information had to be learned, and was often learned simply by following the example of others, with people having little comprehension of the ultimate source of this remedy or that compound.[20]

But a wealth of information was available to the illiterate through a variety of other channels, and these demonstrate the permeability of Wales to outside influences. It is easy to forget, for example, that Wales was part of the 'official' medical networks of the centre. Public proclamations were just one means through which specific medical information or instruction from London could be conveyed. In 1637, Charles I issued a proclamation requiring public prayer for the retreat of the plague 'in all other parts of the kingdom, on the 2nd of August'.[21] In the case of the 'King's Evil', proclamations were regularly sent out across Britain to inform the public of the allotted dates upon which it might be possible to gain access to the monarch and be ritually touched. One such proclamation was painted on a board and displayed at the church of St Gwydd in Disserth, Radnorshire in 1683.[22] From this official notice, people were able to not only discern basic information about the disease itself and its potential cure, but also derive extra information about the threat of contagion, since the practice of touching was suspended during the summer months for fear of disease spreading in warm conditions and in large crowds.[23] Importantly, this information would have been read out in local communities, and presumably translated into Welsh, bringing it from the literate to the verbal by one remove.

During the early modern period, there was in fact much interaction between Wales and England. Welsh cattle drovers often made their way to London to trade their livestock, doubtless encountering a range of potentially useful sources of knowledge along the way.[24] Despite poor roads and transport, the Welsh people were able to keep pace with wider trends and fashions although the degree to which this occurred varied greatly with location. Welsh towns, too, were medical marketplaces where people came into contact with a variety of goods, services and sellers. The presence of itinerant practitioners is especially noticeable in north Wales. The so-called 'Water Poet', John Taylor, for example, referred to his consulting a 'reverend Italian physition', 'Vincent Lancelles', referred to by locals as a 'mountebank' whilst journeying around Flintshire in 1652.[25] Lancelles was a Venetian who evidently travelled round Britain in the mid-seventeenth century, another record placing him in Oxford during this period.[26] Such practitioners sometimes advertised their services in ad hoc posters, especially in and around towns, and one such record survives for Lancelles' services in curing a broad spectrum of conditions in Derbyshire. Given his presence in north Wales, it is not inconceivable that a version of this same poster may have found its way onto noticeboards in Welsh towns. But Lancelles was by no means an exceptional visitor. In Wrexham in 1663, Philip Henry noted the presence of an Italian quack doctor who sold his wares upon a stage in the town centre.[27] Indeed, it was an incident involving the servant of this 'Giovanni, an Italian Mountebank' which prompted Henry's entry, since the man died of blows from a scuffle on the stage with one of the crowd, perhaps angered by an over-zealous pitch.[28] Little attention has been paid to the fact that Wales was in fact an active participant in the 'medical marketplace'. Indeed, the presence of medical entrepreneurs highlights the extent to which early modern Wales was open for business. This is backed up by other sources. Eighteenth-century Carmarthen certainly had trading connections with Bath and London, likely to have involved quacks and pedlars eager to push their goods into a fresh market.[29] Strong links with the large town of Bristol brought large numbers of travelling salesmen into Glamorgan and the southern counties of Wales. Itinerant 'Scotchmen' also made their way into remoter areas, although their presence was not always welcomed by the 'wild welch'.[30] Such figures as the travelling 'vagabond' who undertook to cure William Bulkeley of Anglesey of his toothache for a penny in 1632, were doubtless common across Wales throughout the early modern period, their mobility highlighting their potential utility both for the dissemination of information, and the introduction of compound or proprietary medicines into Wales.[31]

But much common-sense lore and bodily references were also available through other means, such as proverbs and aphorisms, with the early modern period being described as a 'golden age of proverbial expression'.[32] Proverbs were conveyors of essential knowledge, deployed by the church to underpin norms of moral behaviour as well as in schools as teaching aids.[33] From proverbs, people could glean a variety of useful information from general rules for health to specific ailments. How far they reflected actual beliefs or practices, though, is open to question A dry cough, for example, attracted several sayings. In one proverb, 'Peswch sych diwedd pob nych' ('A dry cough is the end of every weakness') or, as another had it, a dry cough was the 'trumpet of death'.[34] Others laid emphasis on the need to maintain a healthy body. The Welsh saying 'A fyno iechyd, bid lawen' asserted that health will come from being cheerful, while another, 'Deuparth iechyd, ymrwysiaw' stressed the importance of exercise in maintaining health.[35] One popular saying, 'Neb y dynno nyth a dryw, Ni cheiff iechyd yn y fyw' even entreated those who desired good health never to disturb a wren's nest.[36]

Especially for the old and sick, other sayings stressed the need to trust in God and highlighted the special role of God as a healer. 'Lles pawb pan feddyger' ('Everyone benefits when one is healed') and 'Goreu meddyg, meddyg enaid' ('The best physician is the physician of the soul') are a couple of examples which might fall into this category.[37] Here, too, was another strong crossover between religion and medicine. During the second half of the seventeenth century, one collection of the religious aphorisms of an elderly Puritan minister, John Dod, was apparently popular in Wales and was translated and published into Welsh.[38] Dod's work reinforced notions of the role of God in both sending and preventing illness, his belief being that 'There can be no afflictions or miseries befall us but by God's appointment, and canne hurt us, but must needsdo us good'.[39] The published sayings of Rees Pridderch of Llandovery, otherwise known as 'Vicar Prichard' provide another case in point. Prichard's proverbs and popular verses were extremely popular in Wales from the first editions of 1658 and onwards as late as the nineteenth century.[40] Deeply rooted in oral traditions, and also written using dialects local to Carmarthenshire and Glamorgan, the brevity of Prichard's verses made them easy to commit to memory and equally easily disseminated verbally.[41]

Many elements of oral culture also drew strongly from the printed word. Through oral channels such as minstrelsy and public recitation of ballads, even the unlettered poor could access a far greater range of ideas than might be expected.[42] In medical terms, much vernacular oral information, including medicine and medical remedies, was derived from print or manuscript.[43] This was certainly true of Galenic and Hippocratic texts, which often found their way into domestic remedy collections through published vernacular medical works, but were comprehended and referred to by people who had never seen the original printed forms.[44] Likewise, print culture could be informed by the vast database of popular and proverbial knowledge. Collections of popular wisdom, such as anthologies of proverbs which were amongst the first publications in Welsh, joined the burgeoning early modern print trade, and included *Oll Synnwyr pen Kembero Ygyd (All the Wisdom in a Welshman's Head Gathered Together)* (1547) by William Salesbury, the creator of the first Welsh dictionary.[45] In terms of medical information, tying these two groups together were manuscript remedy collections, of which a fuller discussion will follow later and which were a point of crossover. Here, remedies were recorded from both verbal and printed sources. They almost always contained tried and trusted remedies gleaned from networks of family, friends and kin.[46] They also contained book knowledge which may have come directly from the original publications, or instead may have entered the work through verbal transmission.

Corralling Welsh culture firmly within this fictive and monolithic category of 'oral culture', however, downplays the undoubted impact of printed literature upon Welsh medical mores during the early modern period. Traditional histories of Wales have often tended to emphasise both the geographical and cultural 'otherness' of the country. Under this schema, Wales is portrayed solely as a land of superstitions, magic and omens; a place where orthodox medicine failed to penetrate. Poor communications and transport meant that people were generally tied to their parishes, fostering an insular and conservative worldview.[47]

Generally unable to read English, most Welsh people could therefore not comprehend wider medical developments and this reinforced their need for local and
magical medicine. Such were broadly the views of David Fraser-Harris, the first
author who attempted a medical history of Wales in the early twentieth century, and so they have largely remained since.[48] But there is another, untold, side
to this story. Far from being isolated and conservative, Welsh medical culture
was increasingly shaped and informed by medical literature and, in particular,
English language medical literature. On their own, English medical texts can
clearly have made little practical difference to the majority of people who spoke
mainly Welsh and could not read anyway. What happened instead was a process
of permeation and assimilation. What was literate eventually found its way into
oral and vice versa. This is crucial to our understanding of the spread of medical
knowledge in Wales, since it highlights the fact that even the illiterate could have
access to knowledge perhaps originally intended for a literate, and potentially
higher socially located, audience.

In England, this process of literate knowledge embedding through several
'removes', each of which might add or subtract from the original form, has been
well noted.[49] In Wales, however, there was an extra 'remove' – that of the jump
from the English language into the Welsh before assimilation could even begin.
Here, then, we arrive at the dichotomy at the heart of Welsh medicine in the
early modern period: print culture from England was growing in importance and
had effects not only on the types of medical remedies available and their uses, but
even on the very language used to describe illnesses in Wales. This was effectively
a 'modernising' trend running counter to the natural conservatism of the Welsh
people. By contrast, though, it was only through the strong, traditional, Welsh
oral culture that such information was able to disseminate so widely. In medical
terms, then, Wales was a country effectively pulling in two different directions.
Its traditional culture of magical medicine hearkened back, but the growing influence of English language medical print kept it in step with 'modern' medical
developments.

The impact of medical print in Wales

The mid-seventeenth century saw what is often referred to as an 'explosion' of
print, as publishing became easier and cheaper, and the market for small and
cheap volumes increased.[50] Publications of chapbooks and almanacs could run
into the hundredsof thousands and there was an increasing demand for the
printed word across early modern society, although this was not necessarily uniform.[51] Lay medical works fitted into this increasing print culture and catered for
the needsof a literate public increasingly distrustful of the medical profession. In

England, between 1641 and 1800, Mary Fissell has identified over 2,700 editions of vernacular medical texts, or books containing medical information, intended for self-help and lay use.[52] However, the number of titles published was not high, something in the order of fifteen to eighteen per year in the seventeenth century, and a better indicator is the number of repeat editions, and also the longevity of books in circulation. Fissell proposes a rough average of one book per four households for the first half of the eighteenth century.[53] A brief glance at the publishing situation in Wales, however, reveals why medical books have been largely overlooked as potential sources. Four-fifths of people in Wales were illiterate, and there was no printing press located in Wales until 1718. As in Scotland, literacy varied markedly in Welsh rural and urban areas, and even in upland and lowland regions.[54] Scotland, however, had had its own printing press since 1507 and, although few books were printed in Gaelic, this reflected the fact that Gaelic was far more prevalent in the Highlands than in other areas, as opposed to Wales where the vast majority spoke their native tongue.[55]

Relatively few books were printed in Welsh (only ten between 1660 and 1669) and these were largely religious and devotional instructions, with some volumes of literature and poetry.[56] Numbers grew steadily and in fact increased five-fold during the eighteenth century through the growing Welsh print industry and book trade, and increasing output of presses at Shrewsbury, Trehedfyn and Carmarthen.[57] Nevertheless, in Wales, and in Welsh, the number of specifically medical books printed in the period 1600–1733 is somewhat easier to gauge precisely than for England; there were none. Some Welsh religious books did contain medical references, often reminding the sick of the need for piety, while almanacs or volumes of miscellanea also often included some medical information. Works like *Meddyginiaeth a Chyssur* (Medicine and Relief) (1722) by Edward Lloyd, contained passages from the scriptures from which sick people could draw comfort.[58] Thomas Richards's *Cyngor Difrifol i un ar ol bod yn glaf* (Serious Advice to a Patient) (1730) was a morality tract to give people spiritual guidance in plague-ridden years.[59] The first fully Welsh medical text to be published was *Llyfr Meddyginiaeth, ir anafys ar chlwfus* (a book of medicine for the wounded and sick) by William Bevan in 1733 (see Figure 3).[60] This was an important text, not least since it was designed with local distribution in mind. It was apparently distributed from the author's own home and was priced cheaply to appeal to a mass market. A subtitle also states that the contents were derived from a work by Robert Shiffery of Llanberis, near Caernarvon. This was probably an earlier, similar work, but one which unfortunately cannot be traced. By the time this book was published, literacy in Welsh was actually declining as the language was becoming increasingly stigmatised, not least given the attempts to eradicate it from all official institutions.[61] This fact alone may partially explain the lack of

LJyfyr Medd'giniaeth, ir a- nafy,s ar chlwfus.

Yr

Hwn fydd yn cynwns amryw gyng-
horion byddiol i ddyn ac Anifail,
yr hwn a gymerwyd allan o hen
Lyfur o fcrifen Law yr hwn a fafe
Lyfur ei *Thomas Ab Robert Shiffery*
o blwy *Llanberis* yn Sir *Gaernarvon*.

Gaŝ *William Bevan,* blwŷs *Llaafaes,* yn Sir fon
ac ar Werth gan yr Unrhŷw.

Yr hwn a.

Argraffwyd Yng'aerlleon gan ROGER ADAMS,
Printiwr, 1733.

3 Title page of *Llyfr Meddyginiaeth, ir anafys ar chlwfus,* 1733,
by William Bevan

printed medical sources in Welsh during this period, since many authors were probably deterred by the limited audience for Welsh language texts. There were undoubtedly some efforts to cater for a Welsh audience by English publishers. Andrew Wear states that John Gerard's 1633 edition of *The herball or Generall historie of plantes* included Welsh plant names in its indices.[62] Where Welsh authors did attempt to make forays into medical publishing, therefore, most chose to target the more lucrative English market. To name a few, Robert Recorde's sixteenth-century works, *Judgement of Urines* and *The Urinal of Physick*, were both still in print during the late seventeenth century, the latter going through multiple editions.[63] One Edward Edwards wrote a series of manuals based on surgical knowledge, printed during the 1630s, but these were intended for a learned, rather than a lay readership.[64] John Jones, the chancellor of Llandaff during the later seventeenth century, wrote a number of books in English and Latin, including treatises on the plague in Ireland.[65] None of these authors, however, made any play on their Welsh nationality in these books, or pretended to belong to anything other than an English medical faculty.

Based on these points, it is tempting to draw the conclusion that Wales was simply divorced from wider medical print culture and, until eighteenth-century industrialisation brought about fundamental changes, simply retained its traditional, folkloric ways. Recently, however, Welsh historians have begun to explore the extent to which the Welsh people were, as Richard Suggett has put it, 'surrounded by expressions of print culture'.[66] We need to look beyond mere literacy levels in order to assess the impact of print, and examine such issues as the portability of printed material, and its value and longevity in terms of gift exchange. The actual audience for books could be different from, and much wider than, its intended readership, as books were gifted, bequeathed and sold on.[67] Welsh people in fact had access to a wide variety of knowledge, of which the printed word was an important source.

The first printed translations of popular self-help books into Welsh did not occur until the nineteenth century. Nicholas Culpeper's *British Herbal* was not published in Welsh until 1816, over two centuries after its initial publication.[68] William Buchan's *Domestic Medicine*, first published in England in 1769, did not find its way into Welsh translation for another forty-seven years.[69] This is not to say, however, that such works were entirely unavailable in Welsh before this period, since there were a growing number of manuscript translations of English and Latin works into Welsh by literate scholars. Manuscripts were an extremely important form of transmission of literate knowledge, and there was a very strong tradition of both collecting and copying manuscripts in Wales which continued well into the eighteenth century. People like John Jones of Gellilyfdy, Flintshire, made a virtual cottage industry out of copying manuscripts, doing so in prodigious quantities whilst serving several prison sentences.[70] Thomas ap Ifan of Hendreforfydd likewise copied medical manuscripts originally belonging to Thomas Wiliems of Trefriw.[71] Medical manuscripts fell solidly into this tradition with collections such as those of the Physicians of Myddfai and Bened Feddyg being continually copied and recycled down the centuries. In the early modern period, men like the Tudor chronicler and administrator Elis Gruffydd compiled medical herbals; Gruffydd also translated Elyot's *Castell of Health* into Welsh.[72] Gruffydd was a collector of manuscripts and also regularly borrowed French manuscripts to translate, introducing a European element to Welsh medicine. Welsh scholars such as William Salesbury and, later, Moses Williams also compiled medical herbals in Welsh, although there is little evidence of their dissemination at the time.[73] British Library Add. MS 15078 is a manuscript Welsh translation of *The Treasury of Health*, originally by Petrus Hispanus but translated into English by the Welsh antiquary, Humfrey Llwyd.[74] Although this MS is difficult to date precisely, the handwriting style is consonant with a date during the late sixteenth or early seventeenth centuries. Given the 1559 publication of Llwyd's English-language version, the Welsh translation was probably done fairly soon afterwards, suggesting that such works were at least beginning to find their way into Wales by then. Another document, in the possession of Thomas ap Hugh of Llanweroedd, also in Welsh, appears to contain direct translation from a medical text given as 'Most exelent and aprved medicines and remedies for divers diseases and maladies'.[75] A trawl of the titles of published medical works brings forth the most likely candidate, Alexander Read's *Most Excellent and Approved Medicines and Remedies for Most Diseases and Maladies Incident to Man's Body*, which would place the translation no earlier than 1651.[76]

The very act of translating these books indicates that they were intended for the use of others who could not read English. In each case, the translator was obviously bilingual, so why go to the trouble of translating the works at all if only for their own use? It seems plausible that the manuscripts were intended for use by people other than the translators themselves which further hints at a market for such works in Welsh. Copied manuscripts, as Harold Love noted, should not necessarily be seen as separate to printed works, in the sense that they were both 'published' for an intended audience.[77] There is little evidence, however, for such translations beyond the late seventeenth century, leaving a gap of many decades before medical information transferred back from manuscript to print in Welsh. Obviously, this assertion is reliant upon limited source material, which may be due to several reasons. Firstly, it may simply be the case that no manuscript translations have survived for the eighteenth century, but that the practice continued. Secondly, though, information from these medical texts was increasingly subsumed into oral culture. This meant that the process of translation had already occurred by the time the information was disseminated, and thus sidestepped the need to commit the information to paper in Welsh. Finally, it is also possible that the increasing importance and availability of English language books, together with an increasing literacy in English, rendered translation superfluous since, as noted above, literacy in Welsh was declining. Despite these points, translations from the late seventeenth century and before highlight the increasing availability of medical texts in Wales during the early modern period.

The book trade in Wales

If there were no printed Welsh-language medical texts available until relatively late on in the early modern period, there was certainly a ready demand for English-language medical books. The book trade in Wales grew steadily during the early modern period, and there were a number of means through which English books could be obtained. The growth of Welsh towns brought with it a burgeoning demand for consumer goods, including books. Urban traders began to supply books alongside other goods, and the presence of publishers' agents in many Welsh towns meant that this could prove a lucrative sideline to their businesses.[78] Some, such as Thomas Durston of Shrewsbury, sold medicines as well, providing the complete means for self-treatment.[79] It seems that Durston was also a publisher, his output including several chapbooks containing medical information.[80] Gauging the exact extent to which medical books were available is difficult since there is little source material from shops to shed light on this issue. One 1639 probate inventory of a mercer's shop in Llanidloes contains a list of 133 books. Most are in English, many are religious or literary works, including collections of fables and Psalters as well as Latin and grammatical dictionaries. But some 40 books are unnamed, and it is not unreasonable to assume that medical texts were amongst these anonymous volumes.[81] Shops selling books could be found in towns throughout Wales, with extant evidence for such trade in Pembrokeshire, Cardiganshire, Carmarthenshire and also along the Marches.[82] Welsh apothecaries certainly used English medical texts in the course of their business, with some owning several different volumes. Market towns attracted customers from the hinterlands to participate in popular cultural activities, as well as to purchase goods and services. Indeed, towns depended on the trade of their rural peripheries for their prosperity.[83] This burgeoning book trade was therefore not simply an urban phenomenon, although the availability of particular types of books depended greatly upon the geographical location of the seller. Marcher towns were in close proximity to the printing presses at Shrewsbury, giving them potential access to a wide range of titles. Towns in Flintshire and Monmouthshire were close to the larger urban centres of Chester and Bristol and it should be no surprise to find evidence that inhabitants of such regions took the opportunity for cross-border shopping to purchase medical books.[84] Aside from shops, there was also a range of other sources through which books could be circulated around Wales. Richard Suggett has found some limited evidence for the sale of books by itinerant traders and pedlars, their transience and mobility giving them much opportunity to trade across the border.[85] Once again, though, it is difficult without direct evidence to assume that medical texts were necessarily a part of the pedlar's pack.

If the means of acquiring books are not always clear, we can be more assertive regarding the actual ownership of medical books in Wales. Clearly, wealthy elites and gentry were in the vanguard of literacy. The Welsh gentry faced something of a battle for legitimacy as they fought to shake off pejorative English carica-tures of the Welsh. Literacy and booklearning evinced sophistication, and the Welsh gentry were keen to accumulate personal libraries to rival those of their English counterparts. Medicine fitted in with the intellectual pursuits expected of a gentleman, and the library of Sir Owen Wynn of Gwydir contained over a hundred medical books, most of which concerned the esoteric chemical medicine of the Helmontians and Paracelsians.[86] But medical books were also increasingly to be found amongst the possessions of those lower down the social scale. A copy of George Hartman's *A Collection of Choice Approved and Experienced Remedies* was owned by Pryce Hughes, and signed 1707. Hughes was an agent on the estate of Lord Powis in Montgomeryshire, and probably a comfortably off, but not necessarily wealthy man.[87] An English-language edition of Culpeper's *The English Physician Enlarged* passed through several hands in Carmarthenshire during the early eighteenth century. The first attributed owner is one Lewis Walters in 1730, but the book later passed to Benjamin Simon of Abergwili and finally to William Bona of Llanpumpsaint, a well-known manuscript copyist, demonstrating both the longevity and the portability of books.[88] Bona made his own annotations to the book, noting which of the herbs he recognised and also marked with a 'BG' (denoting Bona's garden) those which were growing in his own beds[89]

One of the fullest records of the ownership of medical books comes from the Monmouthshire yeoman John Gwin, who referred to and paraphrased several passages from printed works in his commonplace book. Amongst the Paracelsian and Helmontian titles referenced by Gwin are *Natures Explication and Helmonts Vindication* by George Starkey and Richard Matthews's *The Unlearned Alchymist* from 1657 and 1662 respectively.[90] Other passages were paraphrased from Nicholas Culpeper. Gwin wrote that 'for physitians, sayes culpeper, first know or learne, what hower, and what daie a p[ar]ty falls sick. For everie hower and daie there is a planet raynes and governes'.[91] It is not clear whether Gwin actually owned these books, or whether he had merely seen and copied from them. The fact that he twice uses the phrase 'sayes Culpeper' implies that his passage is a précis from the original, rather than a direct quotation. But why copy passages from a book that you already own? Clearly, it may be the case that such passages reflect the reduction of weighty texts into a more useable form. Gwin also noted, for example, the name of a London apothecary recommended by Culpeper, perhaps as an *aide-mémoire* for a future visit to the city. The other strong possibility is that Gwin borrowed the books, and this highlights another important means by which book knowledge could spread.

The records of John Morgan of Palleg, noted earlier, demonstrate that books were routinely lent and borrowed. In 1747, Morgan kept accounts of his books, noting that '3 Wylch Bibles [were] lent to Thos Phillips' and 'A help to Magistrates, lent to Morgan' and that they had been duly returned.[92] Although no specific medical texts were amongst them, John Morgan's book list included 'dy[v]ers Cyfoethir Cymru', a collection of Welsh sayings, and 'Vicar Prichards Welsh poems', both of which might include medical aphorisms.[93] Some of the medical remedies written in his book appear to have come from an untraced text called 'Physical Observations' which does not appear in his inventory. It seems fair to conclude that he copied the passages from a borrowed book. This practice is important because it hints at what might be the first stage in the dissemination of book knowledge, that of print to manuscript.

Some Welsh sources are direct and deliberate copies of printed works, but which survive through use as manuscript remedy collections. One such is the purported remedy book of a 'Dr Samson Jones' of Bettws in Monmouthshire, which appears to be at least a partial copy of an untraced sixteenth-century book by 'Alexander Spraggot', titled *The Noblest Teaching of Urine*.[94] Other sources, however, show direct evidence of selectivity in the types of information recorded. One Welsh miscellany attributed to Humphrey Owen, and later to a blacksmith, John Morgan, but unfortunately undated, contains a passage which is clearly derived from a printed work. Under the heading, 'Severall secrets of Great Excellency in Phisik Surgery', Owen noted a publication date of 1660.[95] The book from which the quotes are taken appears to be *Eighteen Books of the Secrets of Art and Nature Being the Sum and Substance of Naturall Philosophy*, indeed printed in 1660 and authored by the sixteenth-century Swiss chemist and physician, Johannes Jacob Wecker. This work contains some unusual remedies even by early modern standards, such as the swallowing of a (still-beating) lapwing or weasel's heart to improve memory.[96] Owen included several remedies from the work but his comment that 'tis a book in folio of the work of some hundredsof the best Philosophers', together with his different version of the title, suggests that it was not necessarily his own possession and that he was instead quickly recording basic details from a borrowed copy.[97] This process is supported elsewhere in Welsh sources. An anonymous medical remedy collection in Pembrokeshire Record Office provides further evidence of copying, since it contains many remedies which are directly taken from the copy of George Hartman's book belonging to Pryce Hughes, mentioned above. Under the heading of '1698 Receipts' this collection lists many of the same remedies, and largely in the same order, as the printed version although it also contains some remedies not from the printed book.[98] Although coincidence cannot be ruled out, the survival of both documents within the same collection makes it plausible that they originated from the same area, and thus that the owners were connected. The borrowing of books certainly made financial sense in that it was mutually beneficial in widening the pool of knowledge available to the literate. To copy down medical remedies into manuscript sources also allowed for the 'cherry picking' of potentially useful information, spreading it from household to household and ensuring that extraneous detail could be omitted. Such passages are, for the most part, transcriptions and not translations. Unlike Thomas ap Ifan's translation of Humfrey Llwyd's book, which deliberately sought to preserve the whole document in the Welsh language, those who selected information from borrowed texts usually did so in English, without bothering to translate it. This probably reflects a desire to record the information quickly, and also the status of information recorded in notebooks and commonplace books as rough notes or *aides-mémoire*. It does, however, also demonstrate that the language of the vernacular written word in Wales was often English.

It was not only from books, however, that medical information could be obtained. Almanacs and chapbooks were becoming increasingly popular in Wales and were an important part of a literate culture intended for a mass, lay readership. Especially from the later seventeenth century, literacy levels began to increase amongst the lower levels of society, probably at least partly due to the work of the SPCK and the religious schools of Griffith Jones from the 1730s onwards.[99] Again, neither was this a purely urban phenomenon, and rural farmers and shepherds were amongst this newly literate audience. Reading was a popular pastime amongst craftsmen whose work kept them indoors, and Geraint Jenkins has noted that rural Welsh craftsmen, such as weavers and carpenters, were often well read.[100] Almanacs catered for popular tastes, and routinely contained a variety of information which might be useful to a broad section of society. This might include anything from weather and astrological information, market days and locations, to medical remedies and also adverts for proprietary medicines and the services of quacks.

By the end of the seventeenth century almanacs were available in Welsh, greatly increasing their potential readership in Wales. When Thomas Jones, from Tre'r-ddôl, Merioneddshire, published the first edition of his almanac, *Newyddion oddi wrth y Sêr* in 1680, Welsh people had access to a range of information including advertisements for products such as false teeth, glass eyes and patent medicines which Jones claimed, probably with tongue firmly in cheek, to be 'as infallible as the pope'.[101] Jones's almanacs were clearly intended for a wide audience. Priced at twopence, they were deliberately aimed at the lower end of the market, and intended to provide cheap entertainment and distraction from the hard living of ordinary people.[102] Elsewhere, Jones provided useful snippets of medical information based on his own experiences. In his almanac for 1681, he referred to an oil or ointment to treat worms, and also lists those herbs from Culpeper's herbals which he had personally found to be efficacious, bringing this English-language work to a Welsh audience.[103] In the edition for 1699, he even provided a list of all the ailments under which he had laboured since 1692, as well as the various cures he had used, and experiences he had had with doctors and apothecaries.[104] Other important inclusions in such works were elements such as the 'anatomical man', showing parts of the body with their corresponding planets, and also the bloodletting chart, which gave details for bloodletting and purging, including 'yr Arwŷddion ynghorph Dyn ac anifail' (dangerous/portentous days for the bodies of man and beast).[105] This is significant since, although such information was widespread in oral culture, it was possibly the first time that orthodox Galenic medical information had been available to the Welsh people in print in their own tongue. Between 1680 and 1712, Jones published thirty-four Welsh almanacs from London and Shrewsbury. From 1715 other authors had joined the almanac trade, with John Rhydderch authoring the first almanac to be printed on Welsh soil, from Carmarthen in 1734.[106] Somewhat frustratingly, however, there is little evidence to uncover levels of ownership of these Welsh publications, although the very fact that such information found its way into print in the first place hints at a ready, or at least potential, audience. We can, however, again be more confident about the possession of English-language almanacs and the broad popularity of such publications in Wales.

Griffith Wynn of Bodfaen, connected with the Nanney family of north Wales, owned a copy of *Gallen 1668: A New Almanack for the said year* which contained a variety of potentially useful information, including two receipts which Wynn particularly noted for 'a digestive powder for ye stomacke takin out of Riverkins [and] Another taken out of Wirklunge'.[107] Thomas Griffiths, a doctor from Mold, read *Parker's Ephemeris* for 1726, and indeed incorporated the whole publication into his diary, the variety of information found within it appearing to satisfy his apparent demand for collecting ephemera.[108] Other records of the Nanney family include a number of English almanacs including *Gallen*, *Rider's Merlin*, *Trigge* and the *Daily Journal*.[109] In many cases, almanacs were used as proxy notebooks by themselves, the reverse sides of pages providing a useful extra source of paper for handwritten additions, of which extra remedies could be a part.[110] Almanacs could be collected and retained over a long period of time, belying their usually brief temporal function. In 1724, Thomas Ffoulkes of Martyn, near Holywell, owned a collection of *Rider's British Merlin* almanacs dating back to 1693.[111] Given the time-limited aspect of much of the information within almanacs and chapbooks, the intact survival of this collection is all the more remarkable. It may simply be the case that the collection grew unintentionally as a result of repeated purchases, but the retention of useful information, of which medical remedies were certainly a part, seems an equally likely motive. Further, a note by Ffoulkes indicates that the collection was given to him by another man, John Evans, indicating that such items did have an especial value and were worthy of presenting as gifts.[112]

Not only the literate had access to the printed word, however. Much work has begun to recover the world of the illiterate, and the extent to which they were affected by print.[113] We must be somewhat cautious not to overestimate the extent to which books and printed literature were, in themselves, a *direct* influence upon medical views in Wales, since much medical knowledge was inherent. There is some evidence, but indeed still relatively little, to show that book ownership was growing and that medical books and publications were beginning to become more prominent in Wales, especially into the eighteenth century. But the vast majority of people, however, were still illiterate and so there must have been a further mechanism by which medical knowledge became as widespread as it apparently did. Literate knowledge was freely shared amongst fellow literates in the form of book lending. Thus, medical remedies were part of a currency of information exchange, as people used the opportunities provided by lending to increase their own personal store of knowledge.

At the most basic level, people who owned medical books were not proprietorial with their information, and instead shared their knowledge with others. The process of book lending, noted above, certainly did much to disseminate literate knowledge, but this was not merely the preserve of the literate. There were in fact many ways in which those who could not read could gain direct access to print culture. Literate individuals within communities, for example, often undertook reading and writing tasks for their illiterate neighbours. One such Welsh amanuensis was Robert Bulkeley MA of Dronwy in Anglesey. In the 1630s, Bulkeley regularly wrote letters for people in his village, and was certainly in a position to be able to pass on information from printed books.[114] Reading aloud was certainly popular in the early modern period, and much printed material was indeed designed to be read in this way.[115] Importantly, as Adam Fox notes, even those who could not read sometimes bought books on the basis that they could be read to them by others.[116] The practice of reading aloud ties in well with other performance-related aspects of Welsh culture, such as poetry.

Traditional Welsh poetry was designed with performance in mind; it was meant to be read verbatim, in front of a public which might include both the patron and his employees or local people.[117] In literate households, the practice of reading aloud to servants and other members of the household provided an ad hoc means of education, but also indirectly edified members of the lower orders, giving them access to otherwise exclusive information, which could then be passed on verbally. John Gwin, a literate yeoman farmer, wrote down Helmontian medical remedies from a practitioner, which he then passed on to his 'landladies boy'.[118] It is not inconceivable that the boy might have committed this remedy to memory, later passing it on verbally to others. In 1721, the Welsh writer Erasmus Saunders asserted that many of the common people took occasion to disseminate whatever book knowledge they had accumulated, by reading to one another.[119] Likewise, some Welsh books even included directions on how to use a pen, and charts to help promote reading skills.[120]

How, though, can we chart the potential impact of print, and especially English-language texts at a more basic level? Thus far, the discussion has centred upon the impact of the printed word, and the crossover between oral and literate cultures. We have seen the ways in which the lack of a literate Welsh medical culture pushed the literate towards English texts, which became disseminated and translated more widely into vernacular Welsh. One of the most convincing arguments for the impact of Anglicisation, however, comes in the changes which are apparent in the medical language of Wales during the early modern period.

Literacy and language

The medical language of Wales was a complex mix of original, inherited and adopted forms. It was through language and communication that people discovered, shared and reinforced their medical beliefs. Throughout the early modern period, Welsh medical language underwent some profound changes, most importantly through the influx and assimilation of English medical terminology. In linguistic terms, Anglicisation had a profound effect on the ways in which many people in early modern Wales referred to their own bodies and to their afflictions.

The assimilation of Latin medical texts in medieval Wales systematised Galenic medicine into Welsh and probably overlapped with existing indigenous disease terminology to expand the medical language of Wales.[121] The difficulty lies, however, in locating this original Welsh medical vocabulary. Mary Dobson has produced a list of conditions noted in sources for the south-east of England in the seventeenth and eighteenth centuries, using a wide range and large number of sources, and the number of disease terms exceeds200.[122] Andrew Wear has produced a similar list based on the causes of death noted in the London Bills of Mortality.[123] One feature of such lists is the level of interchangeability in disease nosology. People were confident in their own diagnoses and, as Lucinda McCray Beier puts it, '*knew* what they had', regardless of what the modern view of such descriptions may be, and meaning that some conditions may be repeated under other names.[124] It should come as no surprise that where Welsh sources are written in the English language, they employ the same range of terms to identify, presumably, the same conditions.[125]

Appendix A displays a small sample of Welsh language disease terms which belong to texts which largely predate the early modern period. Amongst such sources are terms which might be considered to be 'original' Welsh, inasmuch as they are derived from translations of Latin texts, and not from English translations. Here, we are interested not so much in what people were actually suffering from, since the presence of the signifier does not necessarily presuppose the existence of the condition, but rather in the terminology which they used to describe their symptoms.

Some evidence, for example, shows an apparent common derivation from the original Latin transcripts, such as in the Welsh terms surrounding the bodily humours, 'fleuma' (phlegm), 'malencolia' (melancholy), 'colera' (choler), demonstrating something of the common Latin origins of medical terminology in Europe.[126] There were important similarities too between English and Welsh terms. One example is 'haint dygwyd' (modernised to 'heint digwydd') for epilepsy. The word 'haint' means disease or sickness, while 'digwyd' is the Welsh term for 'fall'. The literal translation is therefore 'falling sickness' – the same terminology as that of seventeenth-century English for what is now called epilepsy. Another is 'haint y brenhinoedd', the 'King's Evil' or scrofula. The original Welsh term used for scrofula in medieval Welsh texts was 'manwyn'.[127] The first instance of 'haint y brenhinoedd' occurs in the late sixteenth century, coinciding with the burgeoning popularity of the royal touch under the late Tudors and Stuarts.[128] It seems possible that the Welsh language incorporated a corresponding change in English terminology, perhaps influenced by the fact that times of cures for the disease were regulated by proclamations issued and published in English. Although no direct evidence exists to support this, recognition of the change may have been a requisite of law. The likelihood of an 'official' change in the nomenclature of the disease is further strengthened by the inclusion of the ceremony for 'King's Evil' in the English Book of Common Prayer which was translated into Welsh, making this another possible source.[129]

As with English, many Welsh disease terms are descriptive of the symptoms of the particular disease, rather than possessing a distinct name. The noun 'brech' (mutated to 'frech') is the Welsh word for rash, and is commonly used in tandem with other descriptive nouns to connote diseases. Thus, smallpox becomes 'y frech wen' in Welsh, meaning 'the white pox' or 'white rash', and 'y frech goch' is the red pox or measles. The 'pla gwyn' ('white plague') refers to tuberculosis and indicates the pale and emaciated appearance of TB sufferers, hence also the English term 'consumption' referring to the body being literally wasted by the disease. The Welsh term 'wastio' may also be a bastardisation of the English term 'wasted', again connoting consumption. 'Gwaetlin' (haemorrhaging) is derived from the Welsh word 'gwaed' meaning blood, and the Welsh term means, literally, bleeding to death. Others are more general, such as 'clefyt o vwyn' which translates literally as 'internal disease' or sickness.

Sometime around the fourteenth century, though, Welsh bards began to adopt English-language terms in their writing. This process began slowly but rapidly increased to the point where English colloquialisms were beginning to find their way into vernacular Welsh in increasing numbers.[130] Some of the first of these loan-words occurred in fifteenth-century bardic works, with words such as 'balsam', 'cut', 'doctor', 'plastr' and 'physig' all making early appearances.[131] During the sixteenth century, the Welsh lexicographer William Salesbury included further terms in his Welsh dictionary, such as 'Medsn', 'meigryn' and 'pisso' indicating that they were already in common enough parlance to warrant inclusion.[132] By the seventeenth century vernacular remedy collections had begun to include such loan-words in numbers. Given the strong levels of crossover between oral and literate sources, such words were probably commonly used as part of colloquial speech in Wales, indicating a general shift away from older Welsh terms. Examples are Welsh terms such as 'pwygatione' (purge/purgation) and 'gonsympsion' (consumption). [133]This increasing usage of English loan-words was not merely a phenomenon of medical terminology, but also reflected wider changes in literacy and education. But a shift towards a more Anglicised medical language shows that the Welsh language was adopting and assimilating, rather than generating or regenerating its own medical terminologies. This is despite the fact that Welsh words do exist for each of the terms above.[134] The possible reasons for this are manifold. One is the lack of a professional medical faculty in Wales. This meant that there was no 'official' Welsh school of medical thought willing or able to contribute to wider debates, and is reinforced by the fact that the Welsh intelligentsia often eschewed their native tongue and wrote in English. The lack of a printing press in Wales during this period meant that no medical texts were produced in Wales until the eighteenth century, further limiting the printed medical word to English. Another possibility is that the strong Welsh traditions of oral transmission of ideas through ballads and storytelling brought English terms into the vernacular phonetically, explaining the often very slight changes seen in words such as 'gowt', 'cholick' and 'dropsi'.

It is also important to remember though that Welsh and English disease terms were used interchangeably, and this is especially noteworthy in the records of educated elites. Amongst such figures, there was a tension between wishing to be more Anglicised in education and language on the one hand, while not wishing to renounce Welsh culture and identity on the other. The medical manuscripts of Thomas Evans (Thomas ap Ifan) of Hendreforfydd, Merionethshire, contain evidence of this cross-lingual style with some remedies with English headings, such as 'to stoppe fluxe', continuing entirely in Welsh thereafter.[135] Elsewhere in this document, many of the Anglo-Welsh (we might refer to them as 'Cymricised') terms are present, such as 'melakolia', 'meigrin' and 'plasteire'.[136] Evans was a Welsh poet and transcriber of English documents, giving something of a clue as to the derivation of some of his terminology.[137] Over time, this tendency to write in English, whilst still retaining elements of the Welsh translation, seems to have increased. The Monmouthshire yeoman John Gwin made a point of noting the Welsh term 'lloy perthy' for the herb cleavers in his commonplace book.[138] In the book of John Morgan of Palleg, Carmarthenshire, some remedies, such as 'Gwaith y Llech' ('For the Rickets'), continue in English under the Welsh heading.[139] Further, whilst noting the inclusion of 'Ground Ivy' in a remedy for a 'fitt of the spleen', Morgan felt compelled to add that it was 'Llysiau'r Gorwm called in Welch'.[140] It is difficult to say exactly why men such as Gwin and Morgan were seemingly keen to record such Welsh names. It is likely that both were Welsh speakers, and keen to preserve the language. Such examples may also represent the earlier noted linguistic division between Welsh as a spoken language and English as that of the written word. Equally possible is that notes such as this were prompts for use when purchasing the items from a potentially monoglot Welsh apothecary. Nevertheless, the trend for using Welsh and English interchangeably is also particularly noticeable in the letters of the polymath Morris brothers of Anglesey, often in the same letter and sometimes even within a single paragraph or sentence. To give just one example from the many, a letter from Lewis Morris to his brother Richard in March 1740 describes the presence of much sickness in the locality from which he was writing. 'Mae ymma glefydon mawr, sef y bloody flux, neu glwy'r gwaed mewn rhai mannau, ar cryd poeth yn arteithio teuluoedd'(roughly translated, 'There is much disease here, namely bloody flux, or blood disease in some parts, and fever travels through families').[141] Here the English term 'bloody flux' is used within the same sentence as the Welsh 'cryd poeth' and 'glwy'r gwaed'. The Morris brothers were certainly well-travelled and spent much time in England. Their continued swapping between English and Welsh may reflect their status as educated literati, involved in business both within Wales and across the border. Eighteenth-century Anglesey, however, was not a particularly Anglicised area and it would be interesting to discover the extent to which English was employed in day-to-day speech there. It might be possible that, in some areas at least, these interchangeable terms were a phenomenon solely of the written word.

A second point is the potential relevance of the timing of these 'Cymricised' terms. Many terms emerged during and after the sixteenth century and it may be no coincidence that the 1588 Acts of Union were playing on the minds of the Welsh intelligentsia. English was now the language of the law, forcing a certain degree of interface. Despite exhortations by fellow countrymen to preserve the ancient language and publish in Welsh, the lack of institutional education in Wales sent many to Oxford and to London from where they began to move into the more lucrative English-language publishing market.[142] Equally, many of the gentry were keen to adopt English terminology in order to shake off the image of the stubborn and ignorant 'Taffy' with his guttural language, so lampooned by English satirists.[143] To begin to adopt and incorporate English styles of medical terminology was perhaps seen as a step towards achieving some sort of parity with the English medical community by bringing the Welsh language more closely in line. Contemporaries were certainly aware of this Anglicising trend and the writer of an Anglo-Welsh dictionary, John Rhydderch, noted in 1725 the appearance of a greater number of hybrids such as 'iwsio' (use) and 'mendio' (mend).[144]

Such points seemingly assume a somewhat negative and deterministic view of the adoption of English style terms but, alternatively, they could also demonstrate a straightforward conversion through vernacular spoken Welsh which then found its way into written sources and is still a feature of the Welsh language today. In this respect, a growing knowledge and assimilation of English materia medica again demonstrates the extent to which Welsh people were part of a wider medical milieu, and could adapt to new developments accordingly. Medicine fitted into a broad knowledge economy which crossed boundaries of class and literacy, and which highlights the potentially wide dispersal of such ideas across early modern Wales. To go further, then, we must look beyond the mere possession of texts and address the wider question of the importance of social networks in spreading medical information in early modern Wales.

Notes

1 See National Library of Wales (hereafter NLW), Aberpergwm MSS 2124–5, 2355.
2 West Glamorgan Archives, MS D/DZ/123/1, Notebook of John Morgan of Palleg, c. 1728–68, pp. 8, 9, 10, 18, 21, 32, 38.
3 Ibid., p. 8.
4 Ibid., pp. 21, 38, 53.
5 See for example the entries on the virtues of the Alder tree ibid., pp. 40–52 and

Nicholas Culpeper, *The English Physician: or an astrologo-physical discourse of the vulgar herbs of this nation* (London: Printed for Peter Cole, 1652), p. 4 and Nicholas Culpeper, *The Complete Herbal and English Physitian Enlarged* (London: Wordsworth, 1995 edition), p. 10.

6 West Glamorgan Archives, MS D/DZ/123/1, Notebook of John Morgan of Palleg, c. 1728–68, p. 53. The entry seems to correspond in both form and type with publications such as *The Gentleman's Magazine* or *Philosophical Transactions*, although searches of those particular publications failed to identify the exact source of this quote.

7 Ibid., pp. 18, 21, 53.

8 See Adam Fox, *Oral and Literate Culture in England 1500–1700* (Oxford: Oxford University Press, 2000); also, Keith Thomas, 'The Meaning of Literacy in Early Modern England' in Gerd Baumann (ed.), *The Written Word: Literacy in Transition* (Oxford: Clarendon Press, 1986), pp. 97–131.

9 Fox, *Oral and Literate Culture*, p. 19.

10 Ibid., pp. 20–21.

11 Adam Fox and Daniel Woolf, 'Introduction' in Fox and Woolf (eds), *The Spoken Word: Oral Culture in Britain, 1500–1850* (Manchester: Manchester University Press, 2002), p. 14.

12 RheinalltLlywd, 'Printing and Publishing in the Seventeenth Century' in Philip Henry Jones and Eiluned Rees (eds), *A Nation and its Books: A History of the Book in Wales* (Aberystwyth: National Library of Wales, 1998), p. 93; J.A. Sharpe, *Early Modern England: A Social History 1550–1760* (London: Arnold, 2006 edition), p. 278.

13 David Howell, *The Rural Poor in Eighteenth Century Wales* (Cardiff: University of Wales Press, 2000), p. 138.

14 Ibid., p. 139.

15 Ibid., p. 139.

16 See for examples Gwent Record Office, MS D43:5496, Letter from H.W. to Sir Charles Kemeys at Ruperra, undated, c. 1690; Cardiff Central Library, MS 4.30, Letter from Blanch Vann to Damaris Vann, 13 July 1691; Cardiff Central Library, MS 4.30(a), Letter from Tom Anwill to Robert Kanney, 25 May 1709.

17 Fox, *Oral and Literate Culture*, pp. 22–25.

18 NLW MS David Thomas Aberystwyth B14, Anon., Observations on the Parish of Caerwedros, Supplementary Information, p. 10.

19 Ibid., p. 11.

20 Fox, *Oral and Literate Culture*, p. 35.

21 Wellcome Library, MS 8241, Notes and Drafts for Unfinished Volume, 'The History and Lore of Cymric Medicine' by David Fraser-Harris, c. 1928.

22 Edwin Davies, *A General History of the County of Radnor* (Brecknock: Davies and Co., 1905), p. 321.

23 Ibid., p. 321.

24 D.L. Baker-Jones, 'Notes on the Social Life of Carmarthenshire during the Eighteenth Century', *Transactions of the Honourable Society of Cymmrodorion*, 2 (1963), p. 273.

25 John Chandler (ed.), *Travels Through Stuart Britain: The Adventures of John Taylor, the Water Poet* (Stroud: Sutton Publishing, 1999), p. 267.

26 Rhoda Murray, *The Making of Oxford: A Popular Account of the Growth of the City* (Oxford: B.H. Blackwell, 1912), p. 85.

27 Matthew Henry Lee (ed.), *The Diaries and Letters of Philip Henry, M.A. of Broad Oak, Flintshire A.D. 1631–1696* (London: Kegan Paul, Trench and Co., 1882), p. 157.

28 Ibid., p. 157.

29 Baker-Jones, 'Social Life of Carmarthenshire', p. 273.

30 Moelwyn E. Williams, 'The Economic and Social History of Glamorgan' in Glanmor Williams (ed.), *Glamorgan County History, Vol. IV: Early Modern Glamorgan* (Cardiff: Glamorgan County History Trust, 1974), p. 351; Carmarthenshire Record Office, Stackpole Correspondence, Bundle 2, John Campbell to Pryce Campbell, 28 October 1735.

31 Hugh Owen, 'The Diary of Bulkeley of Dronwy, Anglesey, 1630–1636', *Transactions of the Anglesey Antiquarian Society* (1937), p. 71.

32 Fox, *Oral and Literate Culture*, p. 112.

33 Ibid., p. 115.

34 T.R. Roberts, *The Proverbs of Wales: A Selection of Welsh Proverbs with English Translations* (London: Francis Griffiths, 1909), pp. 78, 84.

35 Ibid., pp. 15, 35.

36 Ibid., p. 64.

37 Wellcome Library, MS 8983, Notes and Drafts for Unfinished Volume 'The History and Lore of Cymric Medicine', by David Fraser-Harris, c. 1928, p. 10; Roberts, *Proverbs of Wales*, p. 79.

38 Geraint H. Jenkins, *Literature, Religion and Society in Wales, 1600–1730* (Cardiff: University of Wales Press, 1978), pp. 164–165. See entry for John Dod in the Oxford Dictionary of National Biography, available at www.oxforddnb.com/view/article/7729, accessed 26 June 2009.

39 Anon., *Old Mr Dod's Sayings* (London: Printed for A. Maxwell, 1680), p. 4.

40 Richard Suggett and Eryn White, 'Language, Literacy and Aspects of Identity in Early Modern Wales' in Fox and Woolf (eds), *The Spoken Word*, p. 74.

41 Ibid., p. 74.

42 Fox and Woolf, 'Introduction', p. 7.

43 Ibid., p. 21; Andrew Wear, *Knowledge and Practice in English Medicine, 1550–1680* (Cambridge: Cambridge University Press, 2000), p. 60.

44 Wear, *Knowledge and Practice*, p. 40.

45 Ibid., p. 29; R. Geraint Gruffydd, 'The First Printed Books, 1546–1604' in Philip Henry Jones and Eiluned Rees (eds), *A Nation and its Books: A History of the Book in Wales* (Aberystwyth: National Library of Wales, 1998), p. 56.

46 Elaine Leong and Sara Pennell, 'Recipe Collections and the Currency of Medical Knowledge in the Early Modern "Medical Marketplace"' in Mark S.R. Jenner and Patrick Wallis (eds), *Medicine and the Market in England and its Colonies c. 1450 – c. 1850* (Basingstoke: Palgrave Macmillan, 2007), pp. 138–139.

47 For example see Geraint H. Jenkins, *The Foundations of Modern Wales, 1642–1780* (Oxford: Oxford University Press, 2002 edition), pp. 87–88.

48 For examples see Wellcome Library, MSS 8236–8255, 8968–8989, Notes and Drafts for Unfinished Volume, 'The History and Lore of Cymric Medicine' by David Fraser-Harris, c. 1928; Geraint Jenkins, 'Popular Beliefs in Wales from Restoration to Methodism', *Bulletin of the Board of Celtic Studies*, 27:3 (1977), pp. 440–462; to a lesser extent also, Glyn Penrhyn Jones, 'Folk Medicine in Eighteenth Century Wales', *Folklife*, 7 (1969), pp. 60–74.

49 Fox and Woolf, 'Introduction', p. 21.

50 Ibid., p. 22; James Raven, 'New Reading Histories, Print Culture and the Identification of Change: The Case of Eighteenth-century England', *Social History*, 23:3 (1998), pp. 281–283.

51 Raven, 'New Reading Histories', p. 282.

52 Mary Fissell, 'The Marketplace of Print' in Jenner and Wallis (eds), *Medicine and the Market*, p. 112.

53 Ibid., p. 114.

54 Fox and Woolf, 'Introduction', p. 24.

55 Ibid., p. 24; Helen M. Dingwall, *A History of Scottish Medicine: Themes and Influences* (Edingburgh: Edinburgh University Press, 2003), pp. 56, 94.

56 Jenkins, *Literature, Religion and Society*, p. 35.

57 Ibid., p. 35.

58 Edward Lloyd, *Meddyginiaeth a Chyssur* (London: Printed for Roger Adams, 1722).

59 Thomas Richards, *Cyngor Difrifol i un ar ol bod yn glaf . . .* (London: J. Downing, 1730).

60 William Bevan, *Llyfr Meddyginiaeth, ir anafys ar chlwfus* (Chester: Printed by Roger Adams, 1733).

61 Suggett and White, 'Language, Literacy', pp. 63–64.

62 Wear, *Knowledge and Practice*, p. 83; John Gerard, *The herball or Generall historie of plantes. Gathered by Iohn Gerarde of London Master in Chirurgerie very much enlarged and amended by Thomas Iohnson citizen and apothecarye of London* (London: Printed by Adam Islip, Ioice Norton and Richard Whitakers, 1633).

63 For example, Robert Recorde, *The Judgement of Urines* (London: Printed and to be sold by Peter Parker, 1679); Robert Recorde, *The Urinal of Physick* (London: Printed by Reynold Wolfe, 1548).

64 Edward Edwards, *The Analysis of Chyrurgery . . .* (London: Printed by Thomas Harper, 1636); Edwards, *The Cure of All Sorts of Fevers* (London: T. Harper, 1638); Edwards, *The Whole Art of Chyrurgery* (London: Thomas Harper, 1639).

65 John Jones, *De Morbis Hibernorum . . .* (London: S. Keble, 1697); for the full list of Jones's publications, see John Cule, *Wales and Medicine: A Source List for Printed Books and Papers Showing the History of Medicine in Relation to Wales and Welshmen* (Aberystwyth: Privately Printed, 1980), p. 88.

66 Richard Suggett, 'Pedlars and Mercers as Distributors of Print in Early Modern Wales' in Peter Isaac and Barry McKay (eds), *The Mighty Engine: The Printing Press and its Impact* (Winchester: St Paul's Bibliographies, 2000), p. 23.

67 Raven, 'New Reading Histories', p. 276.

68 Nicholas Culpeper, *Herbal, neu Lysieu-Lyfr. Y Rhan Gyntaf . . . Wedi eu Casglu Allan o Waith N. Culpeper . . . Gan D.T. Jones* (Caernarfon: L.E. Jones, 1816); Cule, *Wales and Medicine*, p. 29.

69 Peter M. Dunn, 'Dr William Buchan (1729–1805) and his *Domestic Medicine*', *Archives of Disease in Childhood: Foetal and Neonatal Education and Practice*, 83 (2000), p. 71.

70 See biography of John Jones in Welsh Biography Online, available at http://wbo.llgc.org.uk/en/s-JONE-JOH-1578.html.

71 See Cardiff Central Library, MS 2.973, Thomas ap Ifan, Meddyginiaeth, 17th century.

72 Timothy Lewis (ed.), *A Welsh Leech Book or Llyfr o Feddiginiaeth* (Liverpool: D. Salesbury-Hughes, 1914), p. xii.

73 Ibid., p. xii.

74 British Library, BM Add. MS 15078, John ap Ifan, Welsh translation of Humfrey Llwyd's English version of 'The Treasury of Health', unknown date.

75 British Library, BM Add. MS 15049, Anon., Quarto Volume of Medical Remedies in Welsh, 17th century, p. 54.

76 Alexander Read, *Most Excellent and Approved Medicines and Remedies for Most Diseases and Maladies Incident to Man's Body . . .* (London: Printed by J.C. for George Latham Junior, 1651).

77 Harold Love, *Scribal Publication in Seventeenth Century England* (Oxford: Oxford University Press, 1993), p. 38.

78 Jenkins, *Literature, Religion and Society*, p. 249.

79 Ibid., p. 250.

80 Cule, *Wales and Medicine*, p. 24.

81 Suggett, 'Pedlars and Mercers', p. 32.

82 Ibid., pp. 28–29.

83 Matthew Griffiths, 'Land, Life and Belief: Wales, 1415–1642' in Gareth Elwyn Jones and Dai Smith (eds), *The People of Wales* (Llandysul: Gomer Press, 2000), p. 66.

84 Alun Withey, 'Medicine and Mortality in Early Modern Monmouthshire: The Commonplace Book of John Gwin of Llangwm', *Welsh History Review*, 23:1 (June 2006), pp. 66–67.

85 Suggett, 'Pedlars and Mercers', p. 30.

86 Alun Withey, 'Medical Knowledge and Practice in Early Modern Wales' (Cardiff University: Unpublished MA Thesis, 2006), p. 65; Owen Morris, *The 'CHYMICK BOOKES' of Sir Owen Wynne of Gwydir: An Annotated Catalogue* (Cambridge: LP Publications, 1997), p. 3.

87 Pembrokeshire Record Office, MS HDX/382/1, *A Collection of Choice Approved and Experienced Remedies*, signed by Pryce Hughes; NLW, Dolforgan MS 529, Audited Accounts of Lord Powis, 1709; NLW, Powis Castle DeedsMS 12206, Address to Jury at Poole signed by Pryce Hughes, 1710.

88 NLW MS 4545A, Edition of *The English Physician Enlarged* by Nicholas Culpeper, owned and annotated by William Bona of Llanpumpsaint, c. 1730.

89 Ibid., pp. 398–410.

90 Gwent Record Office, MS D43:4216, Commonplace Book of John Gwin of Llangwm, 17th century, p. 123.

91 Ibid., p. 22.

92 West Glamorgan Archives, MS D/DZ/123/1, Notebook of John Morgan of Palleg, c. 1728–68, pp. 66–71.

93 Ibid.

94 Cardiff Central Library, MS 2.126, Medical Book attr. Sansom Jones of Bettws, c. 1600, p. 3.

95 NLW MS 788B, Barddoniaeth Humphrey Owen, undated, c. 1665, p. 94.

96 Johannes Wecker, *Eighteen Books of the Secrets of Art and Nature Being the Sum and Substance of Naturall Philosophy* (London: Printed for Simon Millar, 1660), p. 49.

97 NLW MS 788B, Barddoniaeth Humphrey Owen, undated, c. 1665, pp. 53, 94.

98 Pembrokeshire Record Office, MS HDX 88/1, Anon., Medical Remedies headed '1698 Receipts'.

99 Glanmor Williams, 'Language, Literacy and Nationality in Wales', *History*, 56:186 (1971), p. 8.

100 Jenkins, *Foundations*, p. 104.

101 Geraint H. Jenkins, '"The Sweating Astrologer": Thomas Jones the Almanacer' in R.R. Davies et al. (eds), *Welsh Society and Nationhood: Historical Essays Presented to Glanmor Williams* (Cardiff: University of Wales Press, 1984), p. 164.

102 Ibid., p. 175.

103 Thomas Jones, *Almanack am y Flwyddyn 1681* (London: 1680).

104 Thomas Jones, *Newyddion mawr oddiwrth y ser. Neu almanacc am y flwyddyn o oedran y byd, 5648. ac am y flwyddyn o oedran Crist 1699* (London: 1699), pp. 10–11.

105 Thomas Jones, *Y mwyaf o'r almanaccau am y flwyddyn (naid) o oedran y byd-5641. Christ-1692* (London: 1691), pp. 18–19; Jenkins, 'Popular Beliefs', p. 456.

106 Jenkins, 'Popular Beliefs', p. 456.

107 NLW, Peniarth MS 521A, Diaries and Notebooks of Griffith Wynn of Bodfaen, 1668, p. 6.

108 Flintshire Record Office, MS D/HE/432, Diary of Dr Thomas Griffiths of Mold, 1726.

109 NLW, Peniarth MS 521A, Diaries and Notebooks of Griffith Wynn of Bodfaen, 1668.

110 Ibid.

111 NLW MS 1613a, Misc. Flintshire Notebooks and Diaries, Various Dates.

112 For fuller discussions of the importance of almanacs in early modern society, see Bernard Capp, *English Almanacs 1500–1800: Astrology and the Popular Press* (New York: Cornell, 1979); Louise Curth, *English Almanacs, Astrology and Popular Medicine, 1500–1700* (Manchester: Manchester University Press, 2007).

113 See David Cressy, *Literacy and the Social Order: Reading and Writing in Tudor and Stuart England* (Cambridge: Cambridge University Press, 1980); Fox, *Oral and Literate Culture*; Fox and Woolf (eds), *The Spoken Word*; Isaac and McKay (eds), *The Mighty Engine*.

114 Owen, 'Diary of Bulkeley', p. 32.

115 Fox, *Oral and Literate Culture*, pp. 36–37; Cressy, *Literacy*, pp. 14–15.

116 Fox, *Oral and Literate Culture*, p. 37.

117 Philip Jenkins, *A History of Modern Wales 1536–1990* (London and New York: Longman, 1992), p. 61.

118 Gwent Record Office, MS D43:4216, Commonplace Book of John Gwin of Llangwm, 17th century, p. 35.

119 Suggett and White, 'Language, Literacy', p. 73.

120 Ibid., p. 73.

121 Morfydd E. Owen, 'The Medical Books of Medieval Wales and the Physicians of Myddfai', *Carmarthenshire Antiquary*, 31 (1995), p. 37.

122 Mary J. Dobson, *Contours of Death and Disease in Early Modern England* (Cambridge: Cambridge University Press, 2002 edition), pp. 237–239.

123 Wear, *Knowledge and Practice*, p. 107.

124 Lucinda McCray Beier, *Sufferers and Healers: The Experience of Illness in Seventeenth Century England* (London and New York: Routledge and Kegan Paul, 1987), p. 133.

125 See for example Lee (ed.), *Diaries of Philip Henry*; Pembrokeshire Record Office, MS HDX/88/1, Anon., Medical Remedies headed '1698 Receipts'; Glamorgan Record Office, MS D/D/Xla, Anon., Medical Remedy Collection, 17th century; Cardiff Central Library, MS 2.126, Medical Book attr. Sansom Jones of Bettws, c. 1600; Cardiff Central Library, MS 2.998, Medical Remedy Collection of 'Mrs Spyors, 1725; Flintshire Record Office, MS Erddig D/E/1203, Medical Remedy Collection attr. Wynn family, c. late 17th century; West Glamorgan Archives, MS D/DZ/123/1, Notebook of John Morgan of Palleg c. 1728–68; John H. Davies, *The Letters of Lewis, Richard, William and John Morris of Anglesey (Morrisiaid Mon) 1728–1765*, 2 Volumes (Aberystwyth: Privately Published, 1907); Gwent Record Office, MS D43:4216, Commonplace Book of John Gwin of Llangwm, 17th century.

126 Ida B. Jones, 'Hafod 16: A Mediaeval Welsh Medical Treatise', *Études Celtiques*, 8 (1958–59), pp. 367–368.

127 Although I have not referenced individual words here, the derivations are taken from Gareth A. Bevan and Patrick J. Donovan (eds, *Geiriadur Prifysgol Cymru: A Dictionary of the Welsh Language*, 4 Volumes (Cardiff: Gwasg Prifysgol Cymru, 1950–2002).

128 Keith Thomas, *Religion and the Decline of Magic* (London: Penguin, 1991 edition), p. 229.

129 Ibid., p. 228.

130 T.H. Parry-Williams, *The English Element in Welsh: A Study of English Loan-Words in Welsh* (London: Honourable Society of Cymmrodorion, 1923), p. 5.

131 Ibid., pp. 67, 77, 141, 177, 131.

132 Ibid., p. 129.

133 Cardiff Central Library, MS 2.973, Thomas ap Ifan, Meddyginiaeth inc. extracts from Thomas Wiliems, 17th century, pp. 192, 201; Davies, *Morris Letters*, Volume 2, p. 286.

134 'Carthiad' (purgation), 'darfodedigaeth' (consumption).

135 Cardiff Central Library, MS. 2.973, Thomas ap Ifan, Meddyginiaeth, 17th century, p. 3.

136 Ibid., p. 2.

137 Taken from http://wbo.llgc.org.uk/en/s-EVAN-THO-1596.html?query=thomas +evans&field=name, accessed 21 January 2008.

138 Gwent Record Office, MS D43.4216, Commonplace Book of John Gwin of Llangwm, 17th century, p. 43.

139 West Glamorgan Archives, MS D/DZ/123/1, Notebook of John Morgan of Palleg c. 1728–68, p. 54.

140 Ibid., p. 38.

141 Davies, *Morris Letters*, Volume 1, p. 46.

142 Glanmor Williams, 'The Renaissance and Reformation' in Philip Henry Jones and Eiluned Rees (eds), *A Nation and its Books: A History of the Book in Wales* (Aberystwyth: National Library of Wales, 1998), pp. 45–46.

143 Peter Lord, *Words with Pictures: Welsh Images and Images of Wales in the Popular Press, 1640–1860* (Aberystwyth: Planet, 1995), p. 34. See also Mark Stoyle, 'Caricaturing Cymru: Images of the Welsh in the London Press 1642–46' in Diana Dunn (ed.), *War and Society in Medieval and Early Modern Britain* (Liverpool: Liverpool University Press, 2000), pp. 162–179; Lloyd Bowen, 'Representations of Wales and the Welsh during the Civil Wars and Interregnum', *Historical Research*, 77:197 (2004), pp. 358–376.

144 Jenkins, *Foundations*, p. 222.

4

An economy of knowledge: social networks and the spread of medical information

Through what channels did the people of early modern Wales obtain and pass on their medical knowledge? How far was Wales truly 'cut off' both internally and from the wider world? Medical knowledge was ubiquitous within early modern society, but this information did not exist in isolation. It was continually recycled, reinforced and reinvented through a multiplicity of informational pathways. In the previous chapter, the growing importance of medical books was argued to be an increasing source of orthodox medical knowledge, even amongst those who could not read the information for themselves. In order to fully understand the range and spread of such information, however, the ways in which medical information travelled and was received must be more fully elucidated. As we shall see, information passed back and forth freely through a variety of channels, with concerns for health being at the forefront of social relations. Health was also an issue which cut across normal social boundaries. A medico-social network could involve family, friends, employers and employees, but also even bring together people of such disparate social classes as would normally preclude communications between them. These social networks are vital to our understanding of medical knowledge in Wales, since they explain how information was able to move both up and down the social scale, and also around the geographically intractable terrain of Wales, with apparent ease. Such networks crossed social and geographical boundaries and question previous depictions of Wales as being insular and remote. This chapter explores these networks and highlights the variety of means by which medical knowledge could spread.

Crossing the boundaries: medical knowledge and authority

Fundamentally, people shared their medical knowledge freely and this sharing transcended boundaries of class, literacy, geography and even personal acquaintance. Although it is difficult to track the pathways of transmission, it is important to remember that much early modern medical culture was already in the public domain in the form of a cognitive 'knowledge bank' from which people could draw through social interaction.[1] As they travelled from person to person, certain remedies were augmented, added to and altered. Even amongst the literate, medical remedies probably travelled verbally first and foremost, their committal to paper being a secondary result of this initial transaction of knowledge. The compiling of medical information was obviously a logical and necessary means of accumulating sufficient medical acumen to tackle a range of conditions within the home. On the other hand, the ownership of medical knowledge was a powerful tool. A single volume of medical remedies could include information drawn from a wide range of sources, both within a community and from outside. It could include remedies from books which many in a rural parish could not read for themselves. The owner of the collection thereby effectively also owned the information within it, making them automatically a potential source of medical authority. In some ways, even, the book itself might be seen as a proxy healer, further bestowing its owner with a strong degree of social capital.

Recent analyses of a broad sample of English sources have shown how domestic remedy collections can reveal much about both medical relationships and the availability of medical knowledge in the early modern period. Jennifer K. Stine explored the range of ways in which remedy collections foreground women's roles as familial healers, while Mary Fissell has noted the ways in which remedy collections, and especially published examples, deal with popular concepts of the female body.[2] Elaine Leong and Sara Pennell have argued that medical remedies were valuable commodities for those who possessed them, and could be gifted or exchanged as transactions of knowledge.[3] Moreover, by looking at issues such as the attributions of remedies, they have shown how it is possible to gain access to the social networks through which people acquired medical remedies, and what implications this might have for social relations.[4]

Regardless of social status, the most important of all medico-social networks was the immediate circle of family and friends. Indeed, the family was a ready-made medical network. Especially in lower class households, family medicine made sense; it was local, readily available and cheap. It also had a range of beneficial associations, linked with a sense of place and the importance of local medicines, as well as the benefit of proven efficacy with blood relatives. Each household was effectively a storehouse of medical knowledge where inherited and trusted family remedies interfaced with information gleaned from a wide variety of sources, including family and kin, friends, servants, employers and practitioners. However, this kitchen physick was not necessarily the antipode of orthodox medicine. Even at the lowest levels of society, domestic medical knowledge could include anything from magical or folkloric medicines to the remedies and techniques employed by orthodox, learned physicians. As Mary Fissell has admirably demonstrated in her study of vernacular medicine in eighteenth-century Bristol, domestic remedies were a crossing point of popular and orthodox sources, with little separation between the two categories.[5] Equally, though, domestic medicine did not exist in isolation, and the knowledge inherent within each household was also an accumulation of community knowledge.

In terms of our understanding of socio-medical networks in early modern Wales, a useful conceptual model is that of the 'illness behaviour model' developed by social anthropologists to understand care seeking. Here, an individual sufferer draws upon a 'lay referral network' (family, friends, neighbours, kin) and makes value judgements based on their advice.[6] This model assumes (correctly, based on much of the evidence) that people were also as willing to supply information such as medical remedies as they were to seek it, making it a useful form of gift exchange. Early modern people were accustomed to the consultation of friends and neighbours as valid points of reference on a range of matters.[7] Remedies, therefore, which had been tested or proved by others were always more preferable, especially those of family, friends or kin who were connected by blood. Since, as Leong and Pennell have shown, the trustworthiness of a remedy was key to its value, such family ties were adjudged important in the selection process.[8]

It is clear from the large number of familial attributions given in Welsh medical sources that people trusted the remedies of their kin. When the children of John Gwin of Llangwm fell ill of smallpox in 1655, it was to a cure provided by his wife's cousin that Gwin turned.[9] Gwin's commonplace book also records cures derived from a variety of other local sources, including friends and employees, as well as physicians and medical texts, all of which became part of Gwin's personal store of medical references.[10] The number of attributions to friends and local acquaintances in the notebook of John Morgan of Palleg hints at the range of local sources from which medical authority could be derived, and this is mirrored elsewhere.[11] One seventeenth-century remedy in the papers of the Seys family of Ogmore, highlights the extent to which the medicine of the immediate domestic network was seen as particularly effective. Noting 'My aunts [remedy] for and forth continued swelling above a mouth', which had 'brought her present ease', the anonymous writer adds that one 'Mstrs Browne used noe other remedy but this', while a 'Mrs Lug' also found that the remedy brought her relief when other medicines failed.[12] In this instance, a remedy attributed to the writer's aunt, but in all likelihood deriving from information gathered from other sources, moved around a social network, gaining efficacy as the number of its advocates increased.[13] The importance of familial medicine was certainly not limited to oral exchange, and letter writing was an important means through which families could seek the medical advice of relations. In family correspondence, health was a regular topic of conversation, and a letter mentioning illness might well yield a favoured remedy.[14] Robert Gethin of Kernioge, Denbighshire wrote to his nephew, the apothecary John Bell at Wrexham in March 1662, complaining of sore or diseased kidneys and inflamed eyes. Bell replied with a list of remedies and regimens, advising his uncle to take a diet drink – effectively a tonic – for a week and purge regularly to cleanse his body.[15] Daniel Thelwall, part of the large Thelwall family of Ruthin, north Wales, also wrote to his friend Evan Edwards, describing his afflictions and treatments at the hands of medical practitioners while some even sent others to seek out cures on their behalf.[16] Records of Welsh elites also show that seeking medical remedies from family members was by no means limited to the middle or lower orders. The Welsh patriarch (and serial hypochondriac) Sir John Wynn of Gwydir often sought remedies from his family. In 1619, he wrote to his uncle seeking a remedy for a bout of the colic, which duly followed.[17]

People moved within a number of social networks at any given time and this increased their potential exposure to a range of information, often outside their own limited social sphere. Depending upon location and indeed social status, some were becoming increasingly mobile during the early modern period, and were also increasingly willing to travel outside Wales for their medical services. In the 1660s, John Gwin regularly travelled to Bristol from his Monmouthshire home to buy medicaments from an apothecary there, as well as purchasing medical books.[18] During the eighteenth century, travel to London became more and more popular with the well-heeled, and men like the Welsh doctor Thomas Griffiths of Mold travelled there on many occasions, conducting business as well as picking up useful medical books.[19] Again, it is not hard to imagine that such knowledge was put to use on Griffiths' own patients when he returned.

Consultations with practitioners provided another strong source of medical remedies and such remedies are much in evidence in Welsh collections. Many remedy books contain receipts which are attributed to practitioners. Attribution of remedies to doctors was a common practice, especially in printed remedy collections, making it sometimes difficult to assume that the compiler had personally met the doctor in person. Nevertheless, in many cases, there is direct evidence to show that the remedy was given in person. John Morgan of Palleg is one who was explicit in his record of a remedy to purify the blood which, he noted, was 'given by Jones, Doctor of Cardigan for William my son'.[20] Given the probable financial element of these consultations, people were not proprietorial with their medical knowledge. In Morgan's book are recorded the 'directions given by David Rees Doctor of Cayo in Carmarthenshire given to Thomas Phillips wife may 10, 1762' which were to be used for shortness of breath.[21] Morgan recorded not only the derivation of the remedy but also the date of the consultation, as if this in some way legitimised the reference. He also clearly felt that the remedy was useful and seemingly viewed as positive the duality of provenance from both a friend and a medical practitioner. This is mirrored in other sources. The 1705 remedy collection of Sydney Vaughan contains two receipts, 'Dr Pughs directions to Mrs Jones against the stone' and 'Dr Pughes directions to Humphrey Jones wn sick of ye intermittent fever'.[22] Linking the cure to the doctor implies that he had some reputation as a healer and tacitly that the remedy had been adjudged successful.

Such examples raise the further issue of trust in terms of medical knowledge. The inclusion of the derivation of remedies was one means of validation, linking them to familiar, and presumably trusted, acquaintances. Thus, 'For a man that cannot make water alle proved per Mrs J.L.', 'Ye spirit of Anneyseedsoyl of amber and oyl of mace per Mrs M.B.' and 'Ye milk matter by Mr Smith, Apothecary in Sallop' all held intrinsic value for one compiler through their personal associations.[23] In the same vein, Welsh elites also appeared to place a great deal of trust in the medical opinions of their fellow gentry.[24] Since such figures often travelled widely and could afford to consult the best physicians, this was more a logical than an emotional approach. In most cases, the relationship between donor and recipient was a known one and, as Leong and Pennell note, therefore a 'safe' one.[25] But, for medical remedies to be shared it was not always necessary for the donor and recipient to be personally acquainted, since a third party could act in proxy. When told by her maid Ann Mason of the illness of a fellow lady in 1697, Valentina Malyn wrote to 'make bold to recommend a plaister of mine which cured me', and despatched her maid to find ingredient components for the plaster.[26] This willingness to help others fits in with accepted female healing roles, although it also demonstrates something of the ways in which social networks could overlap. Here, a remedy crossed boundaries of association and also involved a member of a lower social class in the process, tacitly providing a link between upper and lower class medical networks. Having access to the remedy herself, the maid had the potential to add it to her own store of medical knowledge, and thus further disseminate it within her own network. Malyn ended her letter, 'pray think not the worse of my plaister because it come from a strainger', suggesting that the remedy might otherwise be seen as risky.[27]

Remedies from known and trusted sources were high value – they came with the endorsement of accepted members of the sufferer's lay referral network. Outside this immediate network, the implication is of risk or even rejection unless this could be mitigated by the involvement of a third party, in this case the maid who provided the link. Where people did not personally know the donor of a remedy, they seemed especially careful to note the paths through which it had moved. The collector of a seventeenth-century recipe for the 'weapon salve' noted that 'this receite I had from Sir John Trevor and hee from Mr Stiles'.[28] Leong and Pennell also note one remedy surviving in an English collection but involving Welsh nobles, which was annotated as being 'given me by Watkin Williams Esqr . . . who had it from Lord Nowel Somerset. Mr Williams assured me he had tryed it with great success'.[29] In this instance, although Somerset was clearly not acquainted with the compiler, the risks involved were negated by the personal recommendation of Watkin Williams. This brought the remedy within the personal lay referral network of the compiler and thus validated it.[30] But in some cases, the process of actually *needing* to ask for a remedy could also engender potentially awkward social situations.

In the autumn of 1628, Sir Peter Mytton of Llanerch Park near St Asaph, a powerful local figure, was evidently suffering from infected or damaged eyes. Eye complaints were one of the most common forms of seventeenth-century dis- ability due to a combination of poor hygiene, lack of ophthalmic knowledge and inadequate treatment and, whilst not fatal, caused much discomfort and concern. So, when reports reached Mytton of an old man living in nearby Conwy, who had 'by the meanes of ye powder of eyebright . . . recovered his long lost sight', he was keen to try and acquire the remedy for himself.[31] But, such a request would not fit comfortably with the usual patterns of deference. Early modern society was founded upon concepts of structure and status, and people were encouraged to know their place. Elites were encouraged to be hospitable and charitable to the lower orders and also participated in popular events such as fairs, festivals and wakes. This was, however, effectively one-way traffic. Elites bestowed charity and hospitality *upon* their local parishioners and poor; they saw their participation as part of their role and not necessarily as a personal choice. Mytton's ailment put him in a position of vulnerability. The 'old man' of Conwy possessed a poten- tially powerful piece of knowledge which Mytton needed, but the physical act of asking for the cure, at least in person, could have shifted the balance of power since it involved his tacit admission that the man's knowledge, a man of lower social status, was in some way superior. It could be argued that this situation was in reality no different than Mytton seeking the services of a workman or crafts- man. Yet it *was* different since there is no evidence that financial recompense was sought or offered. Equally, since the man was not in effect offering medical services, this was not therefore an equal or value-free relationship of exchange. Mytton ultimately took steps to bypass this potentially embarrassing situation. He despatched his servant to Conwy, who found the man and responded with evident satisfaction that he was enclosing the remedy which the man had duly (and freely) provided with hopes that it would render the same effect on Mytton that it had upon him. Here, again, the use of a known third party offset the lack of a personal connection. It is obviously unlikely that a request would have been met with a refusal in any case, but this solution spared Mytton the act of having to ask for the remedy himself and risk a negotiation or loss of face.

Such examples also highlight the fact that social status was not necessarily a barrier to the sharing of medical knowledge. A willingess to accept and involve social subordinates in decisions about personal health and medicine says much about the ways that potentially useful information could transcend, and even subvert, usual social roles. But this type of sharing was also two-way, since other sources show that the upper and middle orders were likewise prepared to share otherwise esoteric information with servants or employees. As the example of John Gwin, noted above, demonstrates, Gwin was perfectly happy to share remedies with family, friends and employees, facilitating both the introduction of potentially exclusive medical knowledge into his rural home village, and, most likely, its further dissemination.[32] Here again, his employees effectively gained access to the medical network of a prosperous yeoman farmer.

Crossing the boundaries 2: literate sources in Welsh remedy collections

Having explored the question of oral dissemination of remedies, we turn for a final time to the written word, and the ways in which remedy collections can also demonstrate the strong crossover between oral and literate forms of knowledge spread. Many collections contain remedies which have clearly been taken directly from printed works that the compiler either owned or had access to. But deviations from the printed form of these works point to various stages and removes between the printed original and manuscript text. Such examples strongly demonstrate the ways in which medical remedies could shift back and forth from print to orality, and back again to manuscript. This is crucial to our understanding of how English-language medical knowledge could enter and spread within Wales, since it reconciles the question of how a largely illiterate and monoglot Welsh population could gain access to literate, English medical texts.

In several cases, remedies in Welsh collections can be reliably traced to the published texts from which they derived. One anonymous seventeenth-century remedy collection in English and Welsh contains remedies 'to purge the bladder' which are similar in both form and ingredients to those for the same condition in the 1596 publication, *Practitioner in Physick* by A.T.[33] Another collection attributed to Thomas Wynn (possibly Thomas Wynn of Bodfaen, d. 1673) contains several receipts taken directly from the 1659 edition of *The Queen's Closet Opened* by W.M. (perhaps William Mathew), including 'a medisone for the dropsy' attributed to 'Lady Hobby' and 'Sir Edward Fertil's salve' although the original form is 'Sir Edward Tertile'.[34] 'Oil of swallows' – a remedy for shrunken sinews or 'bones out of joint' occurs in several Welsh remedy collections, although they are all

English-language examples.[35] The form in which the remedy appears is essentially the same as that from Gervase Markham's seminal work of 1615, *The English Housewife*, a popular work that was seemingly beginning to make an impact in Wales by mid-century.[36] But in a few cases, differences in the form of a remedy suggest that, although it had clearly originated in a printed volume, it had been filtered through another, possibly verbal, source. One example is a particular preventative medicine for the plague. The remedy for 'Dr Batten's Preservation against the plague' appears in two eighteenth-century Welsh sources, one the book of Catherine Nanney (d. 1733), wife of Colonel Hugh Nanney of Merionethshire, and the other a later eighteenth-century collection from Cardiganshire.[37] In both cases, the remedy appears almost identically in the following form:

> Take wood sorrel pick'd from the stocks and pound them very well in a stone mortar, then add to every pound of beaten sorrel, a pound of sugar finely beaten, and 2oz of mithridate; beat them very well together and put them in pots for your use. Take every morning before and after the infection for some time together, of this consume [as] much as the quantity of a small nut.[38]

For the sake of accuracy, the Nanney receipt book differs in the first line 'Take wood sorrel, pick it from ye stalk', and also the last, where the quantity is given as a 'walnutt'.[39] A search for remedies attributed to the name 'Batten' reveals none in any of the most popular remedy collections of the time.[40] In the *Queen's Closet Opened*, however, is an almost identical remedy for 'Dr Butler's Preservation against the Plague'. But the variation in the name of the doctor also makes it not implausible that a process of verbal dissemination at some stage altered the name due to a mishearing or mis-transcription. This theory is seemingly corroborated by the variations in 'stocks' and 'stalks' in the Nanney receipt book. These altered forms survive in two sources of both some physical and temporal distance. It may be possible that the remedy became entrenched verbally in its altered form and took time to embed more widely in manuscript. Other sources provide similar examples of remedies which are slightly different in form to the original printed texts. In the 'Llyfr Byr Llangadwaladr' remedy collection is the following remedy for 'ye liver that is corrupt &wasted'. 'Take a quantity of liverwort & boyle it in strong wort with a quantity of Rubarb [and] use ye medicine'.[41] This version appears to be précised from a remedy under the same heading in Thomas Moulton's sixteenth-century work, *The Mirror or Glasse of Health* although, with the presence of two other remedies from this book, the writer may have seen the original.[42] Nevertheless, the evidence here also points to the compiler having been given the remedy by another person, with the variations further implying that this was done verbally. In such instances, the compiler was in a position to write the remedy down for themselves, thus committing it back to paper. But more importantly, it also shows that the remedy could pass just as easily between those who could not write. In this way, a remedy derived from a printed work could become part of oral medical currency.

Even these limited examples tell us much: they demonstrate the means through which remedies could move from oral culture to print and back, but also from print and oral to manuscript. In this way, there was a constant dialogue between various forms of communication and, by way of conclusion to this chapter, this is key to our understanding of the availability of medical information in Wales and in English and Welsh. Illiterate Welsh-speaking people had potential access to English-language print, providing a direct link between Wales and English, and indeed broader, medical cultures. Medical information in Wales, as elsewhere, fell within the wider context of knowledge exchange through both oral and literate means since people derived their medical remedies from family and friends, neighbours, wider kin and medical practitioners. Equally, however, the growing impact of medical texts led to something of a unique paradox in Welsh medical culture, namely that it took a lively indigenous Welsh-language oral culture to disseminate English-language medical print culture. We can also now make a direct link between English medical texts and Welsh manuscripts. It is likely that English-language remedies entered Wales and were disseminated beyond literate and into oral culture, afterwards shifting back and forth between oral and literate. This shows how medical knowledge was able to bypass issues of literacy, and explains how even illiterate inhabitants of deeply rural areas had the propensity to have access to a wide range of medical literature. Despite seemingly intractable linguistic, literary and geographical barriers, therefore, Welsh people were inextricably connected to wider early modern popular and elite cultures. So far in this book, however, discussion has concentrated broadly upon disease and medical knowledge, and we have not yet interrogated anything of the actual experience of 'being' sick, nor engaged with the Welsh disease sufferer, their sickness behaviour or wider issues of care. Having discussed the 'economy of knowledge', then, we now need to address the question of how far Wales participated in a tangible, economic medical culture, through the individual sufferer themselves, availability and execution of care, and the material culture of medical goods in early modern Wales. It is to such issues that the third, and final, section of this book will now turn.

Notes

1 Elaine Leong and Sara Pennell, 'Recipe Collections and the Currency of Medical Knowledge in the Early Modern "Medical Marketplace"' in Mark S.R. Jenner and Patrick Wallis (eds), *Medicine and the Market in England and its Colonies, c. 1450 – c. 1850* (Basingstoke: Palgrave Macmillan, 2007), p. 134.

2 Jennifer K. Stine, 'Opening the Closets: The Discovery of Household Medicine in Early Modern England' (Stanford University: Unpublished PhD Thesis, May 1996); Mary E. Fissell, *Vernacular Bodies: The Politics of Reproduction in Early Modern England* (Oxford: Oxford University Press, 2004), pp. 189–191.

3 Leong and Pennell, 'Recipe Collections', pp. 133–134.

4 Ibid., pp. 138–141.

5 Mary E. Fissell, *Patients, Power and the Poor in Eighteenth-Century Bristol* (Cambridge: Cambridge University Press, 2002 edition), esp. ch. 2.

6 Byron J. Good, *Medicine, Rationality and Experience: An Anthropological Perspective* (Cambridge: Cambridge University Press, 2007 edition), p. 42.

7 Keith Wrightson, *English Society 1580–1680* (London and New York: Routledge, 2003 edition), p. 62.

8 Leong and Pennell, 'Recipe Collections', p. 134.

9 Alun Withey, 'Medicine and Mortality in Early Modern Monmouthshire: The Commonplace Book of John Gwin of Llangwm', *Welsh History Review*, 23:1 (June 2006), p. 57.

10 Ibid., pp. 61–63.

11 West Glamorgan Archives, MS D/DZ/123/1, Notebook of John Morgan of Palleg, c. 1728–68, pp. 21, 38, 57, 58.

12 Glamorgan Record Office, MS D/DF V/206, Medical Remedy attr. Seys Family, undated, c. late 17th century.

13 This is a process also noted in English sources. See Andrew Wear, *Knowledge and Practice in English Medicine, 1550–1680* (Cambridge: Cambridge University Press, 2000), p. 51.

14 Some parts of this analysis are based on Alun Withey, 'Medical Knowledge and Practice in Early Modern Wales' (Cardiff University: Unpublished MA Thesis, 2006), pp. 64, 66–67; see for example, National Library of Wales (hereafter NLW), Clenennau 2 (A) MS 521, Letter from William Griffith of Trefarthen to his daughter-in-law, '15th of 8'ber, 1640'; Gomer Morgan Roberts (ed.), *Selected Trevecka Letters (1747–1794)* (Caernarvon: The Calvinist Methodist Bookroom, 1962), p. 13.

15 NLW, Crosse of Shaw Hill MS 1037, John Bell to Robert Gethin, 2 March 1662.

16 B.E. Howells (ed.), *A Calendar of Letters Relating to North Wales 1533–circa 1700* (Cardiff: University of Wales Press, 1967), p. 235; Flintshire Record Office, Gwysaney MS D/GW/2115, Letter from 'J. Glynne', regarding powder to cure blindness, 18 October 1628.

17 J. Gwynfor Jones, *The Wynn Family of Gwydir: Origins, Growth and Development c. 1490–1674* (Aberystwyth: Centre for Educational Studies, 1995), p. 129.

18 Withey, 'Medicine and Mortality, p. 66.

19 Flintshire Record Office, MS D/HE/432, Diary of Dr Thomas Griffiths of Mold, 1726, pp. 72, 110.

20 West Glamorgan Archives, MS D/DZ/123/1, Notebook of John Morgan of Palleg, c. 1728–68, p. 8.

21 Ibid., p. 58.

22 NLW, Peniarth MS 348 (A), Remedy Collection attr. Sydney Vaughan, 1705, p. 135.

23 NLW MS 182-D, Remedy Collection and Miscellanea of 'Madam Lloyd' of Penpedust, undated, 18th century, pp. 68–71.

24 See for examples W.J. Smith, *Herbert Correspondence* (Cardiff: University of Wales Press, 1968), p. 130; John Ballinger (ed.), *Calendar of Wynn (of Gwydir) Papers 1515–1690* (Cardiff: National Library of Wales, 1924–26), p. 347; NLW MS 5309B, Medical Remedies in hand of Henry, fifth Baron Herbert, undated, c. late 17th century, p. 29; Flintshire Record Office, Gwysaney MS D/GW/2115, Letter from 'J. Glynne', regarding powder to cure blindness, 18 October 1628.

25 Leong and Pennell, 'Recipe Collections', p. 139.

26 Flintshire Record Office, MS Erddig D/E/1147, Letters of Valentina Malyn and Ann Mason, 13 April 1697.

27 Ibid.

28 Cardiff Central Library, MS 5.50, Flintshire Miscellany, c. 1650, p. 70.

29 Quoted in Leong and Pennell, 'Recipe Collections', p. 140.

30 Ibid., pp. 139–140.

31 Flintshire Record Office, Gwysaney MS D/GW/2115, Letter to Sir Peter Mytton from 'J. Glynne' regarding eyebright powder, 1628.

32 Withey, 'Medicine and Mortality', p. 62.

33 Cardiff Central Library, MS 2.622, Anon., Medical Recipes, c. 1700, p. 20; A.T., *Practitioner in Physicke: A Rich Storehouse and Treasury for the Diseased* . . . (London: Printed for Thomas Purfoot and Ralph Blower, 1596), pp. 102, 104.

34 Flintshire Record Office, MS Erddig D/E/1203, Medical Remedy Collection attr. Wynn family, c. late 17th century, pp. 29, 35; W.M., *The Queen's Closet Opened: Prestigious Medicines* (London: Printed for Nathaniel Brooke, 1659), pp. 11, 40.

35 See for examples Glamorgan Record Office, MS D/D/Xla, Anon., Medical Remedy Collection, 17th century; NLW MS 5309B, Remedies in the hand of Henry, fifth Baron Herbert, 17th century, p. 15.

36 Michael R. Best (ed.), *The English Housewife by Gervase Markham* (Quebec: McGill-Queen's University Press, 2003 edition), p. 249.

37 NLW, Peniarth MS 517D, Medical Remedy Collection owned by Catherine Nanney of Merioneth, c. 1730, p. 97; Cardiff Central Library, MS 2.655, Anon., Medical Remedy Collection, 1781, p. 15.

38 Cardiff Central Library, MS 2.655, Anon., Medical Remedy Collection, 1781, p. 15.

39 NLW, Peniarth MS 517D, Medical Remedy Collection owned by Catherine Nanney of Merioneth, c. 1730, p. 97.

40 For example, Best (ed.), *The English Housewife*; Nicholas Culpeper, *The Complete Herbal and English Physitian Enlarged* (London: Wordsworth, 1995 edition).

41 British Library, BM Add. MS 14900, Anon., 'Llyfr Byr Llangadwaladr', Miscellaneous sermons and remedies, 18th century, p. 85.

42 Thomas Moulton, *The Mirror or Glasse of Health, Necessary and Needefull for Every Person to Looke in* . . . (London: Printed by Hugh Jackson, 1580), p. liii.

Part III

Domestic sickness and care in the Welsh home

5

Care and the Welsh medical home

The role of the early modern home as both a storehouse of medical knowledge and physical space of healing has long been stressed. Medical self-help books reinforced lay and domestic medical practice to a certain extent, and it was implicitly assumed that people had at least a basic level of ability in terms of being able to prepare remedies. Far less clear however is the extent to which Welsh, and indeed early modern houses in general, had the necessary equipment to be able to manufacture medicines, even on a small scale. Much historiographical work concentrates on medical knowledge but sidesteps questions of the actual ability of householders to manufacture their own medicines. Roy Porter argued that 'most people in early modern England medicated themselves', while Mary Lindemann points out that medical practice for the whole of society 'almost always began at home', but exactly how this production was achieved, and what it involved, is often tacitly assumed rather than explicitly stated.[1] For others such as Andrew Wear, the 'technical and material conditions of life enabled housewives to act as distillers, brewers, cloth-makers, physicians and apothecaries' and he highlights the strong link between medicine and cookery.[2]

However, little work has yet been undertaken either to try to quantify amounts of medical equipment in the home, or to address important questions such as the storage of medicines. Equally neglected has been the question of the range of materia medica available from local shops, especially in rural areas, and not only in Wales. How far did the people of early modern Wales have access to the ingredients necessary to make compound medicines? This chapter will argue firstly that the majority of people, at all levels of society, had the ability to prepare at least some basic remedies within their homes. Furthermore, people of both rural and urban areas also had access to a range of medical goods, often within relatively short distances from their homes, and this included a growing number of exotic, foreign ingredients, as well as a variety of medical equipment. However, there appears to be little evidence to support arguments for a household store of medicines, and equally scant are traces of specific medical equipment in probate inventories. Whilst not conclusive, this points more to a pragmatic approach to medicines, buying or making them when necessary, rather than keeping a domestic medical 'chest'. This economic element is important since it highlights again the extent to which Wales was part of a wider, indeed global, medical economy.

The sample data for much of the following discussion is taken from a database of privately transcribed probate inventories from 82 parishes in the old county of Glamorgan, between 1600 and 1750. This area mainly comprises Cardiff and the Vale of Glamorgan, and also some parishes west of Cardiff, as far as Swansea. The documents form somewhere between 40% and 50% of the total number of such sources for the selected parishes of Glamorgan held in the National Library of Wales and consist of 1,372 domestic inventories plus 28 shops of various kinds. The percentage proportion of transcribed inventories varied widely between parishes. The somewhat arbitrary sampling renders it unsuitable for the kind of statistical rigour preferred by quantitative historians, but as some have argued that probate inventories, by their nature, are selective and unreliable for averaging, this should not devalue it.[3]

In general terms, Glamorgan makes a useful region to explore, not least because it has one of the largest surviving bodies of probate inventories. Within the county were several distinct regions, and Glamorgan was essentially divided in half horizontally by its own geography. In the northern half of the county was the upland *Blaenau* region which was generally relatively sparsely populated with hearth tax records yielding a figure of between zero and twenty households per 1,000 acres.[4] The settlement pattern here was one of isolated farmsteads and small hamlets, with few, if any, nucleated villages.[5] Conversely, although thinly populated, these parishes were also generally quite large, leaving a substantial body of records. This discussion, however, will concentrate mainly upon the lowland areas known collectively as *Y Fro*, which included large urban areas, such as Cardiff, but also a large number of outlying rural parishes in the Vale of Glamorgan. This area was far more populous with some parishes, such as Cardiff and Cowbridge, containing over 50 households per 1,000 acres, with the majority of the rest containing between 30 and 50 households per 1,000 acres.[6] *Y Fro* contained some upland parishes, but most were lower lying and a large number were located along the coast. Economically, this was also a county of contrasts. Overall, Glamorgan was not a wealthy county, but rather contained pockets of wealth around areas of trade and also the estates of the gentry. In terms of the general population, the majority (62%) of people who died between 1693 and 1760 were worth £40 or less, with around 17% worth less than £10.[7] The area was also rich in coastal trade, however, containing the large ports of Cardiff and Swansea, but also smaller trading ports such as Penarth and Barry. Such factors could greatly affect the availability of medicines and medical equipment and this study therefore allows us to explore medicine in a wide range of Welsh environments. The proximity of the area to so many potential trading routes and to the larger English town of Bristol in particular, may skew the results to some extent, but also invites further studies to draw comparisons. What, then, can these sources reveal about the medical habits of the 'ordinary' people of Glamorgan?

Domestic medical production in early modern Wales

Many seventeenth- and eighteenth-century self-help books extolled the virtues of a well-equipped kitchen. For the seventeenth-century medical writer Thomas Brugis, top of the list of desirable items for those people wishing 'to compound medicine themselves' were 'a great mortar of marble and another of brasse'. A long list of other items were included, from 'copper pannes to make decoctions' and 'glasses for cordiall powders' to a range of medical implements.[8] Gervase Markham entreated his idealised English housewife to 'furnish herself of very good stills, for the distillation of all kinds of waters . . . for the health of her household', and the emphasis all round lay firmly with a well-equipped kitchen, able to minister autonomously to sick family members.[9] To what extent, however, was this idealised domestic medical environment actually realised in early modern Glamorgan, and especially in 'ordinary' households? A brief survey of the documents shows some trends of the ownership of basic medical and culinary items.[10]

Taking the sample data as a whole, it is clear that the vast majority (91%) of inventories displayed at least one item of kitchen equipment and this figure remains fairly constant across the whole time period. In all probability, the true figure is much higher, given that at least half of the 124 inventories showing no kitchen equipment listed had an inventory value of more than £10, and many substantially more. In such cases they were probably present but simply not listed. Clearly, this statistic is not altogether surprising, since even the poorest households needed to be able to prepare at least basic meals, and the most commonly listed items were pans and crocks either of earthenware or brass. Nevertheless, it does demonstrate that, even in the poorest households, people had the ability to prepare some basic medical preparations. Boiling, for example, was an essential aspect of early modern medical remedies, occurring in around 20–30% of remedies sampled in a recent survey by Elaine Leong.[11] Generally, the larger the household, the better equipped was its kitchen. For the poor, with an inventory of only a few pounds or less, such as Rees Jones of Cardiff in 1680, or Gwenllian John of Llandaff, 1684, their entire possessions might include just one or two crocks or cauldrons.[12] At the other end of the scale, larger houses of more prosperous gentlemen or yeomen such as Edward Nicholl, a gentleman of Eglwys Brewis in 1690, included long lists of equipment spread throughout the house.[13] As well as basic pots, crocks and pans, some inventories also include more specialised equipment. Twelve Glamorgan inventories include utensils called chafing dishes, which were a type of small, portable coal grate for warming food, but also sometimes used in remedies.[14] In the 1628 commonplace book of Philip Howell of Brecon, a chafing dish was required to make a preparation 'to cure tooth atch and drawe woremes out of hollow teeth'.[15]

What of items more associated with medical usage? From a total of 1,248 inventories, a mere 141 testators (11%) had listed a pestle and mortar.[16] This was a basic culinary utensil, put to a wide range of uses from grinding herbs and crushing seedsto medical uses such as preparing pastes and electuaries. Obviously, the presence of a pestle and mortar does not automatically denote medical usage, and it would be wrong to identify a household as being medically productive simply because it contained one. What can be stated more definitely, however, is that the owner had, at the very least, the ability to produce a wider range of medical preparations within their own homes than did a neighbour with a simple pan or cauldron. In general the majority of examples of pestle and mortars tended to occur in households which, regardless of inventory value, contained larger numbers of kitchen equipment. A brewing still was another multi-purpose item which had utility in making medicines. Home-brewing was an important part of the domestic routine, and especially in larger houses. Cider-making was becoming increasingly popular during the seventeenth century and in some areas, such as Monmouthshire, cellars of larger houses were often adapted to the requirements of brewing.[17] It was also a useful way of supplementing income in poorer households. In medical terms, however, a still would have been a vital piece of equipment for distilling chemical oils as well as medical waters from simples such as lavender or hawthorn.[18] In fact, a recent survey of early modern remedies puts the number of remedies requiring the use of a still at around 10%.[19]

In terms of a still or 'limbeck', the early modern term, only 41 Glamorgan inventories sampled (some 3%), listed this item. There is plenty of circumstantial evidence from other parts of Wales to show that stills were put to medical usage in Wales, and especially as part of a growing interest in science and chemistry, part of the intellectual pursuits of wealthier gentlemen. In Flintshire in the 1690s, the prominent MP John Meller of Erddig Hall, Wrexham, kept detailed notes of his 'physical observations' which included experiments with chemical oils for medical uses. In one remedy for gripe water, Meller even specified that the still should be made of pewter.[20] The 1610 will of Hugh Powell, rector of Llangynidr in Breconshire, included an entry for 'my stillatory and all my water glasses', suggesting more than a passing interest in iatrochemistry, as well as simple brewing.[21] On the whole, however, numbers of specifically medical equipment are low, although we must be cautious since there are few other surveys with which to compare. Also, bare figures can be skewed by terms such as 'household stuff' or 'brass and pewter' which appear regularly in inventories, making it difficult to know whether individual items are present but simply not listed individually.

To provide a comparison with other areas of Wales, a further smaller sample of 430 inventories was taken from the northern Welsh county of Montgomeryshire. Montgomeryshire, although bigger in size than Glamorgan, was poorer and less populous. Unlike lowland Glamorgan with its urban market towns and proximity to the large English centre of Bristol, Montgomeryshire was largely upland and rural, and contained only one substantial market town. The results of this sample were even more striking. Whereas in Glamorgan 11% of testators listed a pestle and mortar, in Montgomeryshire the figure was only 2%. The difference between the two counties was even more marked for stills; compared to Glamorgan's 3%, only 0.2% of Montgomeryshire inventories listed the item. This must be qualified slightly by the higher numbers of Montgomeryshire inventories which included 'household stuff' as a blanket term but, even so, the comparatively low ownership of specialist items in rural areas seems clear. Overall, the results of these surveys might raise questions about the ability of the 'average' rural household to manufacture its own medicines.

So far then, the majority of sample inventories demonstrated the potential to make medical remedies in some form while, to a much smaller degree, some households also owned more specialised equipment. Did people in early modern Wales, though, keep stores of ointments, curative waters or preparations? Part of the problem in establishing the presence of medicines is that they would, in all probability, fall outside the normal parameters for the types of material to be recorded in an inventory. There was a fairly rigid set of guidelines for inventory compilers as to what could, or could not, be included in probate inventories. Perishable goods, such as many fresh foodstuffs, were mainly left out since they were transient and unlikely to retain value long enough to be a tangible asset.[22] Such phrases as 'other small things yt is not name[d] about ye house' appear frequently in inventories, leaving their identity frustratingly unknowable.[23] The recording of any items depended firstly on its intrinsic value, secondly on the diligence of the recorder and thirdly on its permanence or transience. Some medical remedies, once made, were designed to be kept and be useable for years. The famed 'weapon salve' remedy, included in one Flintshire miscellany, was believed to improve by being kept for two to three years.[24] In another case, a 'leaden salve for many diseases', appearing in a 1698 Haverfordwest remedy collection, claimed to 'last twenty yeares' once it had been prepared.[25] Likewise, preparations including expensive ingredients, such as pastes, plasters and chemical oils, were unlikely to be too readily disposed of. Others, however, and indeed probably the majority of remedies, were made on demand with readily available and perishable ingredients, such as butter, eggs and cream, and would therefore leave no trace in the historical record.[26] Does this mean, however, that domestic medicine is untraceable?

Of actual medicines or preparations, there is very little direct evidence within the sample inventories. The one exception is 'theriac', also known in early modern British pharmacopoeias as 'Venice Treacle'. Theriac was a compound medicine of ancient origins, composed of over eighty ingredients, and popular during the seventeenth century.[27] According to a remedy within the book of John Morgan of Palleg, amongst its other uses, treacle was 'good for the wind cholick'.[28] John New, a Cardiff tailor who died in 1740, kept a number of goods in 'Mr Richards storehouse', including butter, salt and half a hundredweight of treacle, valued at three shillings and sixpence.[29] In 1756, Llantwit shoemaker Isaac Griffeys' inventory contained 'treagle a casg [sic]' valued at ten shillings and sixpence, as well as tobacco worth nine shillings and sixpence.[30]

Other than this, however, no households from the sample provided any equivalent of a medical 'store cupboard', or anything to imply that medicines, if they were present, were regarded as anything other than part of normal domestic or culinary activity. They were not, in this sense, sufficiently extraordinary to record. But, to borrow the astronomical maxim, absence of evidence is not evidence of absence. If we cannot necessarily find explicit evidence of medicines within the home, it might be possible to infer their presence through other means. Firstly, inventories sometimes mention items which could potentially be regarded as medical, of which one example is tobacco, and there are many instances in the Glamorgan sample. The 1683 inventory of John Morgan of Cardiff, a weaver, contained 'two roules of tabaco', while William Thomas of Llanblethian had twelve rolls of tobacco in his chamber when he died in 1666.[31] In 1713, Philip Herbert of Cogan even owned a large box of tobacco valued at £1.[32] Tobacco was originally thought to have medicinal properties; the smoking of it was reported to have more value for medicinal purposes than for pleasure.[33] It was also used in particular medical preparations, such as for toothache, and appears in a doctor's remedy for diseased teeth addressed to Elizabeth Bridges of Woodchester, later part of the Seys family of Ogmore in South Glamorgan.[34] Richard Evans, a surgeon from Llanmerchedd in Anglesey, was sufficiently impressed by the medicinal (and social) pleasures of snuff tobacco, that he wrote or copied a poem entitled 'six reasons for taking a pinch of snuff' into his commonplace book, including such memorable verses as: 'When strong perfumes and noisome scents the suffering nose invade, Snuff, best of Indian weedspresents its salutary aid'.[35]

Honey, too, was a common medicinal ingredient, useful for a range of purposes from burns to colds. Several inventories such as those of Thomas William of Llanwonno in 1714 and Henry Thomas of Whitchurch in 1708, contain quantities of honey, the former himself keeping bees valued with the honey and wax at ten shillings.[36]In each case here – treacle, tobacco, apiary products – the value and quantity of the items appears relatively large. These were clearly expensive commodities, worth keeping, further highlighted by the fact that items such as tobacco and honey received individual listings.

Aside from individual ingredients, there are other items which may also point to the production or storage of medicines within the home. A large number of inventories included glass bottles or jars. The number of these varied, from one or two, to the thirty-two glass bottles listed in the £276 inventory of Joseph Meredith of Roath, Cardiff.[37] The problem lies in not knowing the contents of the bottles. In some inventories, they are specifically recorded as being empty, but ten bottles 'of all sorts' might just as easily indicate a range of contents as the types of bottles, and, if so, there is no reason why this might not include medical waters, or healing drinks.[38] In other cases there are fleeting references to medical activities. The 1675 inventory of Henry Meredith, a 'gentleman' of Cardiff, contains a 'Nurceing chair' listed amongst goods in the kitchen. Such items were low chairs, specially constructed to facilitate the feeding of infants. They were a specialist piece of equipment and, as such, one which might be expected to be found only, as in this case, within larger valued inventories.[39]

A great many inventories also list books. In nearly all cases, book titles are unfortunately not provided, with inventories simply making reference to collections of books, from the extensive 'study of bookes' of David Price MA, prebend of Llandaff Cathedral, to the 'few old books' belonging to Lewis Rees of Lisvane.[40] One seemingly promising example of a 'booke of doctor Fishers' belonging to Thomas Lewis of Cardiff in 1690 is most likely the work of Doctor John Fisher, author and erstwhile Bishop of Rochester, since no printed medical works can be located with this author. There is, in fact, only one identifiable medical work amongst the probate inventories, an edition of the 'Compleat Housewife' by Gervase Markham, in the inventory of the wealthy landowner John Nicholl of Saint Athan.[41] Even this one example, however, does highlight the potential importance of medicine and medical books, especially as a part of an interest in medicine amongst the literate and wealthy.

Indeed, within some higher status households, there are other very strong indications of an interest in medicine. Most commonly, inventory makers were men of a fairly wealthy status, which again points to the note made earlier, of a growing interest in medicine as an intellectual pursuit. One example lies in the 1752 inventory of John Thomas (alias Deere) of Wenvoe.[42] Deere was obviously a wealthy man, living in a house of sixteen rooms, and his inventory hints at more than a passing interest in science and medicine. He seems to have had a strong interest in meteorology and astronomy, owning a large number of books, a weather glass and even a telescope. Deere also owned a pestle and mortar and still, but amongst his other possessions were scales and weights, a pepper box and a nutmeg grater – both spices had medicinal uses. Further, in a small room adjoining the main hall could be found thirteen dozen bottles and a chest containing six small casks. Although the contents are unknown, medical preparations are certainly a possibility. Another example is more suggestive. The 1691 inventory of William Price of Saint Donat's, in the Vale of Glamorgan, contains a large number of goods including many kitchen utensils, such as a still, bottles and casks, and also a number of books valued at around ten shillings.[43] Intriguingly, however, his inventory also includes an entry for 'tenne Alchymy spoons'.[44] Such items were usually so-called because of their construction from a chemico-metal alloy; but, they might also denote measuring spoons for use in alchemical preparations. They are in fact listed here amongst the kitchen goods, but the explicit reference to alchemy is nonetheless noteworthy. Given the large value of the inventory, over £129, Price was a man of substantial wealth with an apparent interest in the 'New Science'. Clearly, such references are few and far between, and also not representative of the majority of people, but the number of other incidences from across Wales does suggest that the Welsh middle and upper orders were no less interested in such matters than were their English counterparts.

The market for medicines in early modern Wales

Although most people to a greater or lesser extent, then, clearly had the wherewithal to prepare at least basic medical remedies domestically, they did not necessarily keep large stores of medicines within their homes. It is entirely possible that medicines were simply too small or too impermanent to merit listing in probate inventories, but the almost total lack of evidence for explicit medical preparations is nonetheless noteworthy. What did people do when they fell ill? There are three plausible explanations, none of which is mutually exclusive. The first is that people simply 'picked their own' ingredients as and when needed. 'Simples', i.e. remedies made from single, unadulterated herbs, are well represented in Welsh remedy collections, and these would have been readily available locally, even within domestic gardens. They were free and quite likely the only method of recourse for those who could not afford commercial medicines or practitioners, but equally left little trace in the historical record. Secondly, people might pay for the services of the local medical practitioner, however defined. This had the benefit of yielding ready-prepared compound or patent medicines, thus negating the need to concoct the remedies at home, and also therefore bypassing the need for specialised equipment.[52] There is no doubt that this was an important aspect of day-to-day medical life, and one which will be addressed later. But the third (and for Wales almost entirely ignored) option is the purchase of medicines from a range of local shops and providers. A wide variety of medical goods were available in Welsh shops and these included ingredients far more complex than rural 'simples'. In fact, the evidence points to a strong demand for medicines at a local level in Wales, and also one which thrived both within, and away from, urban centres. Probate inventories for shop owners often provided detailed lists and individual valuations of their shop goods. This is useful, since it affords a glimpse into the range of goods and also a rough guide as to their price, although the valuation might not necessarily reflect the retail value accurately. Beginning with general and village shops in Glamorgan, it is clear that a wide range of both medical goods and ingredients were available.

Examples of rural village shops are relatively rare and, indeed, within the sample are only seven inventories relating to such premises.[45] Nevertheless, much can be learned even from this small sample. The 1696 inventory of Jane Lewis of Llanblethian provides a great deal of information about the types of goods available in a rural Glamorgan village. Lewis sold a wide range of consumer goods, from clothing material to millinery, soap and candles and foodstuffs, including many potential medical ingredients. Amongst her goods was a range of exotic spices, such as 'Jamaica pepper', at one shilling and twopence a pound, turmeric and 'beaten ginger'.[46] But 'half a hundred of treacle' in the shop, valued at eight shillings, highlights the sale and availability of compound medicines even in a village shop.[47] As with domestic inventories, the shop goods of Jane Lewis hint at a large demand for tobacco, her inventory containing eighteen pounds-worth, either cut, rolled or pressed.[48] Tobacco, sugar and currants were all to be found in the shop of James Leckey of Llantwit Major in 1708, while soap and spices adorned the shelves of David Lewis of Saint Athan in 1642.[49] Even soap could have medical uses, being used in one Welsh medical reference to make pills to dissolve a stone.[50] Trade in spices from the Mediterranean and the New World had increased markedly during the sixteenth and seventeenth centuries, with such commodities starting as expensive and exclusive ingredients of the wealthy but, by the early modern period, also appearing more regularly in humbler households.[51] Port books for this period confirm that Welsh ports were part of this global trade network, and traded along a variety of coastal and international routes, importing a vast range of goods.[52] In one intriguing instance at the turn of the seventeenth century, the *Cuthbert of Chester* arrived at Beaumaris in Caernarvonshire with a cargo including a chest of 'surgery wares', perhaps specialist goods needing to be imported from elsewhere.[53] But the consistent appearance of exotic foreign medicines chimes with contemporary debates about the nature and efficacy of foreign medicines upon British (and by extension Welsh) bodies. As Andrew Wear has shown, foreign herbs and spices became more popular as they gained a reputation for strength or effect. This gradually supplanted older arguments that local was necessarily best and bestowed an extra value upon these foreign substances.[54] It is indeed noteworthy to find so much evidence for these ingredients in rural Welsh shops, and acts as a reminder that even rural Wales was part of the increasing globalisation in trade, including medicines.

Turning to the shop inventory of one John Thomas of Llandaff, direct evidence of the presence of medicines for sale can be seen.[55] One entry recorded 'halfe a bottle of syrup of Buckthorn', a strong purgative syrup, and one which was often used in pharmacopoeia and medical self-help publications, and until well into the twentieth century.[56] Syrup of buckthorn was actually a compound medicine, having other ingredients such as cinnamon and nutmeg added to disguise its sour taste. This was valued, along with five sticks of wax, at one shilling and sixpence, and since half of it was already gone, we might surmise that there was at least some local demand for it. Although no still is listed, it is possible that Thomas did own one and distilled his own medicines, since his inventory contains a reference to 'other distill'd liquors' alongside a quantity of brandy and 'a small quantity of oyle'.[57] Another reference within the inventory points at one of the possible sources of shop goods. In an entry for 'fresh goods', the compiler noted that they were 'bought att St. Pauls faire in Bristoll'.[58] Bristol was one of the main urban and trading centres for south Wales and was effectively a regional capital for the area.[59] Given that there were certainly regular fairs and markets in Cardiff and Cowbridge at the time, Thomas still clearly preferred to make the longer journey to Bristol.

Other shop inventories display a similar availability of compound medicines. One Elizabeth Lambert sold quantities of 'Annyseed water' in her Cardiff shop in 1685 which, in joint valuation with brandy, was valued at no less than ten pounds.[60] Anstance Wells of Cardiff also sold 'plague Water' in her shop in 1705, valued at three pounds. The collective memory of plague was obviously still fresh in Glamorgan minds many decades after the last outbreak.[61] The inventory of shop owner and salter Rowland Davies, also contains a 'blood dish' listed in his 'dwelling house' rather than the shop.[62] Given that bloodletting was not normally an activity carried out upon oneself, it seems fair to assume that he performed bloodletting for his customers. Evidence from other parts of Wales also shows that medical services were performed by non-medical providers, such as shopkeepers, traders and artisans. Walter Hart, a blacksmith from St Andrews, near Cardiff, sold 'Annyseed Water' amongst his items of ironmongery and metalware.[63] In fact, Hart had a gallon of the water, valued at over one pound.[64] Richard Lewis of Llandaff was a pedlar whose inventory included

'anniseed water', while Florence and William Hiley sold a great deal of medical goods, including 'a glass of pomatum', snuff, tobacco and spices from their
Cardiff mercer's shop.[65]

Urban areas, as might be expected, were generally better served by shops with
a greater variety of medical goods and ingredients, and even medical services.
The inventory of Henry Hammond of Cardiff contains over forty separate types
of goods, amongst which were tobacco, spices such as cinnamon, aniseed and
ginger, and raisins, and, again, evidence of compound medicines in the form
of Venice treacle.[66] Hammond owned a pestle and mortar and a still, but also
appears to have had a pestle and mortar for sale in his shop, valued at one shilling.[67] In fact, out of fifteen general shops in Cardiff between 1685 and 1740, thirteen sold items which were either specifically medical, or capable of medical use,
and very often of a similar type to those noted above.[68] Cardiff was not unique,
and similar evidence can be found in other parts of Wales. The 1692 inventory of
James Harries, owner of a general shop in Usk in neighbouring Monmouthshire,
contained an extensive list of various goods but, most notably, a box of 'Druggs
and spice in ye boxes' valued at eight shillings and 'Apothecaries Druggs' at one
pound, thirteen shillings and seven pence.[69] Local shops were clearly important
purveyors of medical goods. That the drugs were specifically identified as being
'in ye boxes' however may also be significant. This implies ready-prepared, or
even commercially produced, patent medicines, for which there is otherwise little
evidence in Wales.

Apothecary shops

So far, the discussion has centred on local, general shops, but the sale of goods
from specific medical outlets, apothecary shops, must also be considered. The
number of apothecaries in Wales is extremely difficult to gauge with exact-
ness. According to Mary Lindemann, apothecary shops could be found in 'all
cities, most towns and some villages' across Europe, and in terms of Glamorgan,
there are 5 surviving apothecary's inventories, in Cardiff, Coety, Neath, Pyle and
Swansea, covering a date range of between 1684 and 1746.[70] But, if we widen the
search across Wales, the number of surviving wills and inventories for those
described as apothecaries totals over 70. To this we can add a further 48 incidental references to apothecaries in the National Library of Wales catalogue, referring to those named apothecaries and their presumed place of business, giving
a total of at least 124 identifiable apothecaries across Wales between 1600 and
1762.[71] Given that many of the documents are probates, then it seems fair to
assume that the individuals concerned traded for years or decades before their
deaths, giving a fairly even coverage across the time sample. Moreover, this figure

must be assumed as a bare minimum, since a large number of ad hoc apothecaries probably existed in small towns and villages without ever leaving documentary proof of their existence.

Apothecary shops were widespread across many areas of Wales. At a county level, apothecary shops can be located in each of the thirteen counties of Wales, while towns just across the border, such as Chester and Oswestry, were also noted. Denbighshire, Monmouthshire and Glamorgan yielded the most apothecary references, with 21, 21 and 18 respectively, while Radnorshire and Anglesey contained just one and three examples. Individually, as might be expected, the vast majority of apothecary shops were located in or near towns. In Denbighshire, all examples were located within the three largest towns of Wrexham, Ruthin and Denbigh. In Glamorgan, Cardiff and Swansea held the most apothecary shops, while Welshpool in Montgomeryshire, Chepstow in Monmouthshire, Oswestry in Shropshire, and the county towns of Brecon and Carmarthen proved similar in terms of urban basing. In several instances though, apothecary shops were also located in rural parishes, giving such people direct access to their services. The shop of John Davies, died 1723, was located in Maesmynys, Breconshire, around three miles from the nearest town of Builth.[72] The shop of Henry Williams of Clynnog was nine miles from Caernarvon, while Thomas Kelly's Llandeilo Fawr premises were a full fifteen miles from the nearest town of Carmarthen.[73] What services, then, did such operators offer to their local communities?

It is clear that Welsh apothecaries sold a range of medicaments, and these goods are often listed separately, offering a unique insight into medicines for sale. The inventory of John Reynolds, apothecary of Llanbeblig near Caernarvon, for example, contained 'drugs, plaisters, cordial waters [and] syrrops', together valued at five pounds.[74] 'Old drugs, syrups, emplaisters and electuaries' formed the basis of the shop wares of John Davies of Maesymynys, Breconshire in 1723, while many others, such as Benjamin Price of Neath, listed more generic terms such as 'apothecary druggs and other shop goods'.[75] In some cases, even specific preparations are included, the 1681 inventory of James Preston of Wrexham containing a reference to 'Egyptiacum', also known as the 'Egyptian ointment', which was noted in early modern pharmacopoeia as a salve or ointment to soothe rotten or corroded flesh.[76] There are also several examples of chemical medicines for sale in apothecary shops around Wales, demonstrating not only that Paracelsian and Helmontian preparations were available in Wales, but also that they were sufficiently in demand to appear in local apothecary's shops over a fairly long period. Here, the inventory compilers clearly drew a distinction between chemical medicines and 'ordinary' preparations. The earliest example of such medicines appears in the 1665 inventory of John Bell of Wrexham. Bell's shop in fact contained several listings including 'Chymicall oyles' and 'a rounde box with some chemical

medicines'.[77] Similar sorts of 'Chemical Preparations' were noted in the inventories of John Farmer of Carmarthen in 1679 and Richard Philpots of Swansea in
1684, while the 1723 inventory of John Davies of Maesymynys, already mentioned,
contains an entry for 'chymicall preparations of all sorts' valued at five shillings.[78]

Turning to the question of social status it seems that, on the whole, Welsh
apothecaries could earn a good living from their trade. The total value range
shown in apothecary inventories was between £4 and £731, with a peak range of
between £10 and £20. Twenty-two out of 39 inventories were valued at under
£100, indicating a modest, if not wealthy, social group. Where individual valuations are given for shop goods, we can make some assessment of the value of
medicines in terms of the total wealth of the apothecary. The largest number
of valuations of shop goods fell between £1 and £10, all falling broadly within a
range of £1 and £80. Only one apothecary inventory exceeded £100, that of Elisha
Beadles, a Quaker apothecary from Pontypool who died in 1734, and whose total
inventory value was £691.[79] Somewhat frustratingly, Beadles' inventory merely
values 'shop goods' without giving individual listings of what his obviously large
premises offered to people in his locality. As a percentage of individual wealth,
in the majority of cases (14 out of the 30 inventories that included separate shop
valuations), the shop valuation accounted for between 1% and 25% of the total
inventory value, with a further 8 examples falling between 26% and 50% of the
total. In only 8 cases did the shop valuation exceed 50% and these varied from
the relatively poor, such as William Williams of Llandingat, Carmarthenshire,
whose 'shell and counter of an apothecary's shop' was valued at five pounds,
while his total wealth amounted to seven pounds, to the extremely prosperous
Elisha Beadles.[80] In general, it seems that most personal wealth was not tied in
to shop goods, and also hints at the potential profitability of these businesses.

The inventories of many Welsh apothecaries indicate that they possessed
medical books. The shop goods of William Williams of Builth Wells included
'physick books' while the inventory of David Jones of Oswestry set out a parcel
of 'about 100 bookes'.[81] In one unique case, however, listings of individual books
are provided, and these say much about the importance of English medical texts
for Welsh apothecaries. The recorder of the possessions of Henry Williams of
Clynnog, Caernarvonshire, was indeed diligent in his task. Alongside lists of
household items, a substantial list of books is also included, even subdivided into
categories of religion and finally 'physicke books'.[82] This portion of the inventory is transcribed in Figure 4.

The ownership of these ten books reveals much. Several were didactic volumes of medical practice, providing advice by well-known London professionals
on a range of conditions. These were books to which a lay practitioner might
logically be expected to refer in the course of his work. Amongst these were a

	Li	s	d
Item The new herbal or the Treasury of Plants by Doctor Rembert Dodoens Phisicium to the Emperor translated into ffrench then into English[83]			
It: The Method of Physick by phillip burrough[84]			
It: Two Treaties, one of the Venerall pox, the second of the Gout by Daniell Senertus, Med: Doct[85]			
It: Rivery Praxis Medica[86]			
It: The Art of Distillation by John French M:D:[87]			
It: Doctor Willis his London Practice[88]			
It: A perfect discovery of the French Pox[89]			
It: A discourse of the Whole Art of Chirurgery[90]			
It: An Ould book to all young practizers in Chirurgery[91]			
It: The Optick Glasse of Humours[92]			
	00	10	00

4 Selected data from probate inventory of Henry Williams of Clynnog

general herbal compendium, Thomas Willis's *Practice of Physick*, which provided both advice and remedies, and Peter Lowe's discourse on surgery.[93] In some cases, these works were deliberately tailored towards the needsof lay practitioners whose pharmaceutical knowledge was not necessarily backed up by university training. One such example in Williams's possession was the *London Practice of Physick* which was deliberately published with some of the more theoretical elements removed.[94] Other works owned by him, such as Dodoens's *New Herbal*,were similarly engineered for easy data retrieval by the laity, especially apothecaries, containing indexes of Latin, Arabic and English plant names, the virtues of herbs and plants and their uses for particular ailments.[95] John French's instructional work on distillation can likewise easily be explained within the remit of an apothecary's trade.[96] But other titles point to a deeper interest in the mechanics of medicine. Thomas Walkington's *Optick Glasse of Humours* described the properties and effects of humours upon the body but was couched in esoteric, philosophical language and references.[97] This was manifestly not a straightforward work of instruction, but required an understanding of Greek philosophy, mythology and astrology.[98] Two titles specifically concerned the 'french pox', one of which was authored by Gideon Harvey, actually an outspoken critic of apothecaries and their deliberately exclusive relationship with physicians.[99] Whilst it may be unfair to accuse the inhabitants of Clynnog of excessive promiscuity, the fact that two volumes were obtained for this specific condition might still indicate a particular need for such remedies amongst Williams's clientele.

More widely, the presence of such volumes, and their number and scope, show more than a passing interest in the mechanics of medicine. Williams's books were not merely rustic pamphlets, but largely authored by eminent physicians and aimed at an English audience. That a Welsh rural apothecary, nine miles from his nearest town, both desired and obtained these works says much. Welsh medical retailers were clearly capable of providing a fully 'orthodox' medical service to their locality. Equally, the ownership of books could be conjectured as a conscious attempt at self-edification, an attempt to keep up with wider developments in medicine. The need to purchase such books perhaps also points to a local demand for the services of a 'regular' practitioner. Moreover, it provides a further example of the availability of medical literature in early modern Wales, and clearly by no means was this restricted to a handful of titles. This potential for literacy and education amongst Welsh medical providers, even in rural areas, does much to belie an image of rustic simplicity.

The inventory of Richard Philpots of Swansea

To fully understand the potential breadth of knowledge and praxis of Welsh apothecaries, it is worth exploring a single inventory in more detail. To this end, the best single example for analysis is that of one Richard Philpots, a Swansea apothecary, whose will was proved in 1684. Philpots's inventory is especially rare since it provides a detailed breakdown and individual valuations for all his shop goods. This offers us a unique glimpse into an early modern apothecary's shop, and tells us much about the types of medicines available to ordinary people in a fairly typical Welsh port town.

Philpots's shop was certainly equipped to minister to the needsof those who wished to mix or make their own remedies.[100] One marble mortar is listed at two shillings and sixpence, but '4 brasse morters, 2 pistles [and] one little brasse pan' in another entry are valued at three pounds and five shillings in total, suggesting a higher value and price.[101] Bottles could be used for storage of medical preparations, and Philpots's shop contained '11 dozen bottles' while '6doz of gallypotts' provided another means of storage.[102] This, and the number of domestic inventories containing bottles, does add weight to an argument for some houses having at least some quantities of stored medicines, even if they were not explicitly listed. Importantly too, jars and bottles could perform a useful function of display in shops, projecting an image of orderliness and medical authority, useful in attracting custom.[103] A quantity of serge cloth might have found usage in binding wounds, while 'emplaisters' were a ready-to-use alternative. The presence of several reams of paper within the context of a medical outlet provided at least one source for those wishing to record remedies for themselves.[104] A range of culinary and potential medical ingredients were also for sale. Amongst the examples in the inventory are 'Spanish white', probably a wine used for medicines as well as home consumption, capers and anchovies, various kinds of sugar and also 'common turpentine', all of which had culinary, as well as medical usage. Indeed, given the close relationship between medicine and cookery, it is likely that the apothecary served a dual purpose in terms of supplying ingredients.

The weight of evidence from this inventory, however, points more to a strong demand for ready-prepared medicines from those who could afford it, and such people were as likely to purchase medicines from a supplier as they were to make them at home. One entry, for example, lists 'conserves, unguents, syrops, electuarys and oyles' valued at one pound and ten shillings, and another, 'pills, species and powders' to ten shillings.[105] These were a wide range of medical preparations to cover a variety of ailments, their number and value further hinting at a ready demand. Neither were these remedies necessarily simple kitchen physick. An entry for 'Chimicall preparations and salts', valued at one pound and ten shillings, provides yet more evidence that the people of early modern Wales knew of, and embraced, new and alternative types of medicines.[106] It also demonstrates that alternative types of medicine, in this case the herbal remedies of the Galenists, and the chemical remedies of Paracelsian and Helmontian practitioners, could exist side by side under the general umbrella of local medical provision. Evidence also exists for direct trade in medical goods between south Wales and London by the early eighteenth century, providing a strong link with what was, in effect, the medical centre. The inventory of one Jenkin Thomas, who owned two apothecary shops in Bridgend and Llantrissant by 1714, makes provision for a cask of butter worth thirty shillings, to be sent 'without fail' to Roger Willey, 'apothecary of Fish Street near the Monument in London', presumably in satisfaction of a debt.[107] Another Welsh apothecary, Elias Preston of Wrexham, died 1694, owed money to 'Mr Steal of London for Pills', as well as to other creditors around England and Wales.[108]

Philpots himself may have been responsible for mixing and preparing many of the remedies for sale in his shop. In the contents of other rooms in his house, are listed a wealth of equipment for use in preparing medicines. In his inner kitchen were three stills, eighteen bottles and a pestle and mortar, alongside a range of pots, pans and kettles, all pointing towards the activities of an owner-supplier of medicines.[109] This is supported in other apothecary inventories, such as in the household goods of one Benjamin Price of Neath which include a still and brewing vessels alongside his shop wares, recorded as 'apothecary druggs and shopp goods'.[110] In a sense, this closes the circle between domestic and commercial remedies, since the medicines which Philpots prepared and sold from his shop were still inherently local and thus, at least according to the tenets of Galenic medicine, should have been beneficial to the humoral temperament of his customer base. They were presumably made from local ingredients, making them potentially as efficacious to local people as medicines they had made themselves.

Perhaps the most compelling entry in the inventory is 'drugs, simple and compounds', valued at the relatively large sum of ten pounds; such terms were loaded. 'Simples' were the baseline of early modern medical preparations. They were readily available to almost everybody, and the picking of herbs, and knowledge of their use, was proverbially one of the domestic tasks of women.[111] Yet, as in England and elsewhere, here is clear evidence that remedies based around simples were commercially available at a local level, meaning that they were not merely something connected with the back garden and, more importantly, showing that the people of early modern Wales had some recourse to commercial medicine. There is also, in fact, increasing evidence to demonstrate that English proprietary medicines were available in Wales. In 1674, the accounts of Anthony Daffy – creator of Daffy's Elixir – show that he sent more than thirty half-pint bottles of the elixir to Charles Taylor of the King's Arms public house in Monmouth, evidently for retail by Taylor.[112] Unfortunately, Daffy never appears to have received the four pounds payment for the consignment, meaning that Taylor's status as medical entrepreneur may have been short-lived. Proprietary medicines such as 'Nendick's Pill' could be purchased from a bookseller in Carmarthen, while apothecaries in market towns such as Monmouth, Ruthin and Hay, Breconshire, also sold London medicines under licence.[113]

Compound remedies were part of the domestic economy, and could be manufactured at home but, as Philpots's inventory shows, equally often they might be purchased ready-prepared. Moreover, the large value of these types of medicines in Philpots' stock also points to a healthy local demand for these 'off-the-shelf' drugs. Historians have long since identified the operations of the medical marketplace and the fact that medical production was interchangeable between home and supplier. The purchase of ready-prepared remedies was just one of a range of choices available to the early modern disease sufferer.[114] Historians have yet to acknowledge the mechanisms, or indeed even the presence, of any sort of medical market in early modern Wales, however. There has been a tendency to disregard individual regions within Wales, and the potential effects of geographic location upon the availability of medicines, as well as a more troubling failure to relate Wales to the wider early modern medical environment. Clearly this was a limited market for those who could afford it, and it must be stressed that those who could afford it were probably the minority. Equally, the apothecary inventories are, for the most part, in fairly substantial towns, making it difficult to generalise for rural areas. Even so, increased wealth perhaps brought a greater willingness to buy remedies, rather than go to the trouble of making them in-house. Given the reciprocity between town and countryside, it also means that even those from outlying rural areas had the potential to purchase the latest types of medical remedies, even if they did not have the equipment to make them for themselves.

Notes

1 Roy Porter, 'The Patient in England c. 1660 – c. 1800' in Andrew Wear (ed.), *Medicine in Society: Historical Essays* (Cambridge: Cambridge University Press, 1998 edition), p. 98; Mary Lindemann, *Medicine and Society in Early Modern Europe* (Cambridge: Cambridge University Press, 1999), p. 199.

2 Andrew Wear, *Knowledge and Practice in English Medicine, 1550–1680* (Cambridge: Cambridge University Press, 2000), p. 50.

3 Mark Overton et al. (eds), *Production and Consumption in English Households, 1600–1750* (London and New York: Routledge, 2004), p. 29.

4 Glanmor Williams (ed.), *Glamorgan County History, Vol. IV: Early Modern Glamorgan* (Cardiff: Glamorgan County History Trust, 1974), Appendix 3.

5 Ibid., p. 6.

6 Ibid., Appendix 3.

7 Moelwyn E.. Williams, 'The Economic and Social History of Glamorgan, 1660–1760' in Williams (ed.), *Glamorgan County History, Vol. IV*, p. 316.

8 Quoted in Wear, *Knowledge and Practice*, pp. 53–54.

9 Michael R. Best (ed.), *The English Housewife by Gervase Markham* (Quebec: McGill-Queen's University Press, 2003 edition), p. 125.

10 For a far more detailed quantitative analysis of the presence of medical and culinary items, see Alun Withey, 'Health, Medicine and the Family in Wales, c. 1600 – c. 1750 (Swansea University, PhD Thesis, 2009).

11 Elaine Leong, 'Making Medicines in the Early Modern Household', *Bulletin of the History of Medicine*, 82:1 (2008), p. 162.

12 National Library of Wales (hereafter NLW) MSS Rees Jones, LL/1680/18; Gwenllian John, LL/1684/66.

13 NLW MS Edward Nicholl, LL/1690/31.

14 NLW MSS William Jones, LL/171/77; Miles Rees LL/1715/92; John Thomas

Care and the Welsh medical home

LL/1639/66; James Robin, LL/1692/126; Edward John, LL/1745/80; John Wilkins, LL/1654/43; William Richard, LL/1696/171; Edward Jay, LL/1725/155; Richard Wade, LL/1645/33; Nicholas Kidnor, LL/1689/21; John Dembri, LL/1644/38; John Thomas, LL/1684/65.

15 Cardiff Central Library, MS 3.42, Commonplace Book of Philip Howell of Brecon, 1628–38, p. 76.

16 This figure of 1,248 represents the number of inventories displaying some kitchen equipment. See the discussion on frequency calculations in Overton et al. (eds), *Production and Consumption*, pp. 18–19.

17 Cyril Fox and Lord Raglan, *Monmouthshire Houses Part III: The Renaissance* (Cardiff: National Museum of Wales, 1954), p. 19.

18 For example see Nicholas Culpeper, *The English Physician Enlarged* (London: Wordsworth, 1995 edition), pp. 127, 147.

19 Leong, 'Making Medicines', p. 161.

20 Flintshire Record Office, MS Erddig D/E/2547, John Meller, 'My Own Physical Observations', 1697, p. 18.

21 Quoted in Christabel Powell, *Walter Powell's Gwent: An Architectural Biography of a 17th Century Diarist* (Risca: Starling Press, 1985), p. 42.

22 Overton et al. (eds), *Production and Consumption*, pp. 14–15; Tom Arkell, 'Interpreting Probate Inventories' in Tom Arkell et al. (eds), *When Death Do Us Part: Understanding and Interpreting the Probate Records of Early Modern England* (London: Leopard's Head Press, 2004 edition), p. 93.

23 NLW MS Philip Williams, LL/1691/102.

24 Cardiff Central Library, MS 5.50, Flintshire Miscellany, c. 1650, p. 70.

25 Pembrokeshire Record Office, MS HDX/88/1, Anon., Medical Remedies headed '1698 Receipts', p. 20.

26 Leong, 'Making Medicines', p. 158.

27 Wear, *Knowledge and Practice*, pp. 68, n.55, 92.

28 West Glamorgan Archives, MS D/DZ/1231, Notebook of John Morgan of Palleg, c. 1728–68, p. 54.

29 NLW MS John New, LL/1740/31.

30 NLW MS Isaac Griffeys, LL/1756/69.

31 NLW, MSS John Morgan, LL/1683/19; William Thomas, LL/1666/42.

32 NLW MS Philip Herbert, LL/1713/38.

33 Lindemann, *Medicine and Society*, p. 89.

34 Glamorgan Record Office, MS D/DF V/205, Anon., Letter to 'the Worthy Gentlewoman Mrs Elizabeth Bridges at Woodchester to this Present', undated.

35 NLW MS 15-C, Commonplace Book of Michael Hughes of Lligwy/Richard Evans of Llanmerchedd, c. 1730, p. 117.

36 NLW MSS Henry Thomas, LL/1708/242; Thomas William, LL/1714/-- (last part of reference missing); see also NLW MSS Jenkin Llewellyn, LL/1682/47; William Richard, LL/1687/69.

37 NLW MS Joseph Meredith, LL/1709/187.

38 NLW MS Robert Deere, LL/1680/122.
39 NLW MS Henry Meredith, LL/1675/11.
40 NLW MSS David Price, LL/1687/48; Lewis Rees, LL/1730/130.
41 NLW MS John Nicholl, LL/1774/91.
42 NLW MS John Deere, LL/1752/144.
43 NLW MS William Price, LL/1691/118.
44 Ibid.
45 Peter Bowen, *Shopkeepers and Tradesmen in Cardiff and the Vale, 1633–1857* (Cardiff: Peter Bowen, 2004), pp. 17, 32–47; NLW MSS David Lewis, LL/1642/44; Thomas Mawrice, LL/1673/21; Walter Hart, LL/1696/183; Jane Lewis, LL/1696/143; Margrett Richard, LL/1708/-- (reference missing); James Leckey, LL/1708/157; John Thomas, LL/1710/54.
46 NLW MS Jane Lewis, LL/1696/143.
47 Ibid. For a typical remedy using these ingredients, see NLW MS 182-D, Remedy Collection and Miscellanea of 'Madam Lloyd' of Penpedust, undated, 18th century, p. 70 – 'For a cold of long continuence with a Drye cough'.
48 Ibid.
49 NLW MSS David Lewis, LL/1642/44; James Leckey, LL/1708/157.
50 West Glamorgan Archives, MS D/DZ/1231, Notebook of John Morgan of Palleg, c. 1728–68, p. 54.
51 Wear, *Knowledge and Practice*, pp. 68–69.
52 See the listings for individual ports in E.A. Lewis (ed.), *Welsh Port Books 1550–1603* (London: Honourable Society of Cymmrodorion, 1927).
53 Ibid., p. 279.
54 Wear, *Knowledge and Practice*, pp. 77–78.
55 NLW MS John Thomas, LL/1710/54.
56 For example Robert Johnson, *Praxis Medicinae Reformata or The Practice of Physick Reformed* (London: Printed for Brabazon Aylmer, 1700), p. 124; John Pechey, *The Storehouse of Physical Practice* . . . (London: Printed for Henry Bonwicke, 1695), p. 30.
57 NLW MS John Thomas, LL/1710/54.
58 Ibid.
59 Philip Jenkins, *A History of Modern Wales 1536–1990* (London and New York: Longman, 1992), p. 4.
60 NLW MS Elizabeth Lambert, LL/1685/33.
61 NLW MS Anstance Wells, LL/1705/32.
62 NLW MS Rowland Davies, LL/1686/33.
63 NLW MS Walter Hart, LL/1696/183.
64 Ibid.
65 NLW MSS Richard Lewis, LL/1684/67; William Hiley, LL/1724/27; Florence Hiley LL/1724/26.
66 NLW MS Henry Hammond, LL/1700/26.
67 Ibid.
68 NLW MSS Elizabeth Lambert, LL/1685/33; Rowland Davies, LL/1686/33;

Evan William, LL/1694/29; Henry Hammond, LL/1700/26; Thomas Edwards, LL/1704/24; Anstance Wells, LL/1705/32; Wenllian Hedges, LL/1708/45; William Ford, LL/1717/20; Mary Lewis, LL/1720/41; William Hiley, LL/1724/27; Florence Hiley, LL/1724/26; Thomas Holiday, LL/1729/58; John Griffith, LL/1735/20; Florence Brewer, LL/1740/25; Margarett Shiers, LL/1740/32.

69 Inventory reproduced in Bowen, *Shopkeepers and Tradesmen*, pp. 240–249.

70 Lindemann, *Medicine and Society*, p. 215; NLW MSS Evan Pritchard, LL/1746/20; Jenkin Thomas, 1614/25; Benjamin Price, LL/1706/131; Charles Williams, LL/1709/182; Richard Phillpott, SD/1684/295.

71 This was done by controlled searches under the term 'apothecary' on the NLW online catalogue, with a specific date range of between 1600 and 1770. It must be pointed out that these particular documents have not been physically examined.

72 NLW MS John Davies, BR/1723/95.

73 NLW MSS Henry Williams, B/1690/49; Thomas Kelly, SD/1713/59.

74 NLW MS John Reynolds, B/1716/54.

75 NLW MSS John Davies, BR/1723/95; Benjamin Price, LL/1706/131.

76 NLW MS James Preston, SA/1681/216; for references to 'Egyptiacum' see, for example, Moses Charras, *The Royal Pharmacopea, Galenical and Chymicall* . . . (London: Printed for John Starkey, 1678), p. 234.

77 NLW MS John Bell, SA/1665/157.

78 NLW MSS John Farmer, SD/1679/223; Richard Philpots, SD/1684/295; John Davies, BR/1723/95.

79 NLW MS Elisha Beadles, LL/1734/123.

80 NLW, MSS William Williams, SD/1772/77; Elisha Beadles, LL/1734/123

81 NLW MSS William Williams, BR/1705/9; David Jones, SA/1730/185. See also NLW MSS Richard Morgan, LL/1682/32; John Lock, BR/1681/7; Elias Preston, LL/1694/210.

82 NLW MS Henry Williams, B/1690/49.

83 Rembert Dodoens, *A New Herbal or Historie of Plants* . . . (London: Printed by Edward Griffin, 1619).

84 Various editions of this book were produced in the sixteenth and seventeenth centuries. See for example Philip Burrough, *The Method of Physick, Containing the Causes, Signes and Cures of Inward Diseases in Man's Body, From Head to Foot* . . . (London: Printed by Abraham Miller, 1652).

85 Daniel Sennert, *Two Treatises, the First of the Venereal Pocks* . . . *the Second of the Gout* (London: Printed by John Streeter, 1673). An earlier edition, with a much longer title, had been published in 1660.

86 Lazare Rivière (1589–1655) whose edition of *Praxis Medica cum Theoria* was published in Latin in 1657.

87 John French, *The Art of Distillation or, A Treatise of the Choicest Sparigicall Preparations* (London: Printed by E. Cotes, 1653).

88 Thomas Willis, *The London Practice of Physick or, The Whole Practical parts of Physick contained in the works of Doctor Willis* (London: Printed for Thomas Basset, 1685).

89 Almost certainly Gideon Harvey, *Little Venus Unmask'd or, A Perfect discovery of the French Pox comprising the opinions of most ancient and modern physicians* (London: printed for William Thackeray, 1670).

90 Again, there are several editions of this title, by Peter Lowe. See for example Peter Lowe, *A Discourse of the Whole Art of Chyrurgery, Wherein is exactly set down the definitions, causes, accidents, prognostications and cures of all sorts of diseases* . . . (London: Printed by R. Hodgkinsonne, 1654).

91 Untraced. The EEBO (Early English Books Online) database contains no titles under these words.

92 Several editions appear of this work, the latest being Thomas Walkington, *The Optick Glasse of Humours or, The Touchstone of a Golden Temperature* . . . (London: Printed by G. Dawson, 1664).

93 Dodoens, *A New Herbal*; Willis, *London Practice*; Lowe, *Whole Art of Chyrurgery*.

94 Wear, *Knowledge and Practice*, p. 441.

95 Ibid., p. 83.

96 French, *The Art of Distillation.*

97 Walkington, *Optick Glasse.*

98 Ibid.

99 Harvey, *Little Venus Unmask'd*; Sennert, *Two Treatises*; Wear, *Knowledge and Practice*, p. 47, n.3.

100 NLW MS Richard Philpots, SD/1684/295.

101 Ibid.

102 Ibid.

103 Patrick Wallis, 'Consumption, Retailing and Medicine in Early Modern London', *Economic History Review*, 61:1 (February 2008), pp. 35–36; Jon Stobart, 'Sites of Consumption: The Display of Goods in Provincial Shops in Eighteenth-Century England', *Cultural and Social History*, 2 (2005), p. 171.

104 NLW MS Richard Philpots, SD/1684/295.

105 Ibid.

106 Ibid.

107 NLW MS Jenkin Thomas, LL/1714/25.

108 NLW MS Elias Preston, SA/1694/210.

109 NLW MS, Richard Philpots, SD/1684/295.

110 NLW MS Benjamin Price, LL/1706/131.

111 Wear, *Knowledge and Practice*, pp. 48–49.

112 David Boyd Haycock and Patrick Wallis (eds), 'Quackery and Commerce in Seventeenth-Century London: The Proprietary Medicine Business of Anthony Daffy', *Medical History Supplement No. 25*, 2005, p. 125.

113 British Library, MS C.112.f9, Collection of Medical Advertisements, 17th century, p. 54; British Library, MS 551.a.32, Collection of Medical Advertisements, 17th and 18th century, pp. 17, 222; T. Douglas Whittet, 'Welsh Apothecaries' and Barber-Surgeons' Tokens and their Issuers', *Archaeologia Cambrensis*, 138 (1990), pp. 104–105.

114 For example, Wear, *Knowledge and Practice*, p. 55.

6

Sickness experience and the 'sick role'

Much historical work over the past two decades has aimed at restoring a sense of balance to the patient/practitioner relationship, ensuring that the patient has been 'written back in' to history after a long period of relative neglect. This has been apparent in a spate of books and articles detailing the range of choices available to early modern patients, their networks of care, as well as important questions such as gender and the healing role within the domestic environment, and especially within urban areas.[1] The shift from domestic towards institutional public medicine during the later eighteenth century, has been explored, as well as its effects upon attitudes to sickness, giving some insight into early sickness experiences within hospitals.[2] Also, the sick person as an agent within the burgeoning Georgian medical marketplace, and their experiences at the hands of unscrupulous quack practitioners, has been charted by Roy Porter.[3] For all this recent work, however, little attention has yet been paid to the actual experience of 'being' sick, or to more general questions of familial therapeutic care within the home. Although a range of community healers has been readily identified, the actual processes of care, the conventions of sickness, the burden or disruption of caring for a sick person and community responses to the sick, have all yet to be fully addressed. We still know but little about the rural sickness experience, and the ways in which local tradition and belief could impinge upon personal views of illness: for early modern Wales, we know virtually nothing at all. How did Welsh people describe their symptoms? How was sickness experienced at different levels of Welsh society, and also how, if at all, did it change over time?

Illness, as Robert Ralley has noted, presented the early modern disease sufferer with a quandary.[4] What was it? What could it mean? How should it be dealt with? Illness therefore elicited a response – it meant something but equally required something to be done. It is perhaps stating the obvious, but people presumably knew when their bodies were not functioning 'normally' and had some concept of a different state of being, even if their diagnoses and concepts of causation were sometimes hazy. The ethnographer Byron J. Good has described illness as a 'syndrome of experience'.[5] Good sees this as a mix of words, experiences and feelings which 'run together in people' to create a view of illness.[6] Experiences of the body, health and illness are all inherently subjective. Only an individual knows how they 'feel' and, since it is impossible to divorce 'feeling' from the corporeal body, the experience of illness must begin with the body. Nevertheless, as social-constructionist historians argue, each society and culture constructs its own framework for conceptualising and experiencing illness and disease, and these are perpetuated through shared experiences.[7] Importantly, though, even within single cultures, many different systems can operate which overlap and contribute to a wider semantic network.[8] This can influence many issues from what constitutes a 'disease' to causation and also those who are able to treat it. In any given society, including that of the past, 'explanatory models' are employed by people to help them internalise their symptoms, including what symptoms are 'normal' for particular diseases and how to recognise them, how to act when ill and also when others are ill.[9] Illness and the body, therefore, begin with the individual but cannot be separated from the prevailing culture of which the person is a part, making sickness as much a social as an individual concern.

Sickness in the early modern period no doubt involved a great degree of convention and conformity, on the part of the sufferer and also their family, friends and neighbours. In many ways, the sufferer was, at least for the period of their symptoms, an important figure. Early modern patients were seldom passive, and exercised a great deal of choice in their own treatments. The sickness sufferer frequently became the subject of local attention and concern, and was able to invoke moral and religious obligations from local people, from visiting to physical care. Sickness, in this sense, could be empowering, but it could also prove limiting. The sufferer too had to demonstrate conformity and was expected to play their 'part'. From withdrawal from social duties to submitting to the care of others, the sufferer also had to yield to the opinion of others. The power relationships of early modern sickness, then, were in constant flux. Likewise, individual sickness experiences could be affected by a multiplicity of interlinking factors, such as social status, location, religion and gender. How people behaved during sickness depended greatly on the individual sufferer. It is clear that sickness involved fundamental alterations to the habits, routines and even the persona of the sufferer. It involved the undertaking of domestic and social conventions, but also necessitated the adoption of strategies of self-representation, which could be deployed, for example by the poor, to garner sympathy and more tangible support. Sociologists, historians and anthropologists have utilised the 'sick role' model to explain sickness experiences, and the personas and identities of sufferers will play a strong part of this chapter. Before moving on, it is useful to explore this 'sick role' and its deployment by medical historians, in more detail.

Sickness behaviour and the 'sick role'

The concept of the sick role was first put forward in the 1950s by the American sociologist Talcott Parsons, who held that sickness represented a deviation from 'normal' conditions, and that sickness behaviours were therefore ultimately reducible to expectations of social conformity. For Parsons, there were four important premises to the sick role. Firstly, a sick person is exempted, by their illness, from performing normal social duties; secondly, they manifestly *have* a condition, which is not their 'fault'; thirdly, they are expected to seek or submit to external help in order to recover; and fourthly, they should not remain in this role any longer than is necessary.[10] As John Burnham notes, although the model was roundly critiqued by sociologists, anthropologists and historians alike, its utility both in focusing on the individual, and also in placing them within prevailing social and cultural norms, was important and its influence can be seen in many of the works noted above.[11] Perhaps the main problem, however, lies in the fact that historians are still often too uncritical in their usage of the concept and terminology, and this has led to some problematic assumptions and omissions. Most commonly, the model has tended to be deployed fragmentally, with discussions of the 'sick role' strongly weighted towards the dynamic relationships between patient and practitioner. This potentially misses one of the primary stages of sickness, that of the somatic, physical experience of *being* a sufferer. Thus, elements such as coping strategies, and also the ways in which sufferers construct and deploy their conditions, can become lost or subsumed within wider discussions of the 'sick role'. In fact, if we address arguments against the original Parsonian model in more detail, it is possible to highlight some more general aspects of the sickness experience which have been largely ignored in early modern medical historiography.

Firstly, there are actually few works which explore sickness experience in any great detail, and those that do tend to be too reliant on the Parsonian model. Dorothy and Roy Porter's comprehensive study of the sufferer provides much evidence of the diverse range of individual approaches, dealing in detail with how illness was conceptualised, sufferer identities formed, and also with the effects of wider social factors.[12] Nevertheless, there are problems with their approach. Most troublesome is their apparent binary deployment of a sick role. In other words, a patient was either *in* the sick role or not. Lucinda McCray Beier was one of the first medical historians to explore the ways in which the 'sick role' could be adapted from anthropological and sociological frameworks and applied to the history of medicine. Beier's pioneering analysis of how the family of the seventeenth-century Puritan diarist Ralph Josselin expected themselves and others to behave when ill could almost be a direct summary of the Parsonian 'sick role'.[13] But Beier's approach, and that of the Porters, seems to suggest that one, universal, behaviour applied in all cases and, following logically on, that people responded to sickness in broadly similar ways. The question of exactly when somebody considered themselves to be sick is underdeveloped. This is important and points to the wider issue that many works appear to concentrate more upon responses *to* sickness, rather than the actual experience of *being* sick and how this was articulated and manipulated by sufferers.

Beier's study in fact highlights a second, important, issue in examining sickness behaviours – that of gender. Whilst the sicknesses of women are explored in both the above volumes, it is not done in context of the gender roles of women. One common criticism of the Parsonian sick role is that it is not gender-specific and even privileges men inasmuch as it was they who most easily fitted the model of physical withdrawal from the workplace. In the case of women, whose workplace was most often the home, the dynamics of sickness may well have been different, as their 'withdrawal' is less socially defined. Since women might still be capable of carrying out some or all of their domestic duties (at least with mild symptoms), we might question the actual extent to which they were exempted. As we shall in fact see, there was a marked distinction drawn in the case of female sickness between simply having an illness, and physically withdrawing to the bedchamber. Moreover, pressure on domestic life could also be increased when women fell ill, since men were forced into caring roles, for which they had few models or frames of reference. This, again, reminds us that we need to be more careful in inferring a unity of sickness coping behaviours that may not be justified. As this chapter will argue, there were, in reality, multiple 'sick roles', contingent on a number of different factors from age to sex, social status to religious belief and so on.

The individual agency of the sufferer in determining their own boundaries and responses to illness is another factor largely overlooked in the original Parsonian 'sick role' model. For Parsons, the boundaries of illness for the sufferer were, in effect, delimited and constrained by external social pressures to return to a state of normal productivity. And yet, if sickness itself was not desirable, it should not be overlooked that there were still potential social benefits to be gleaned from being in a state of sickness. One aspect of sickness behaviour which is most often neglected is that of self-representation. This is in fact a vital element since it highlights the considerable agency of the sufferer and their ability to deploy narratives of health and illness in a variety of self-serving contexts. The deployment and manipulation of sickness and symptoms could be a powerful weapon for the poor in seeking support. The Porters explored the social stigma of the shamming patient who cunningly and wilfully used the sick role to their advantage, but largely ignore the fact that those who were 'legitimately' sick could also use their sickness tactically.[14] How people represented themselves as sufferers to others, then, is also important since it foregrounds the increasing importance of literacy (and in particular the letter) in shaping representations of the sickness experience– what might be termed an 'epistolary sick role'. Here, sickness self-representation depended greatly upon context: who was sick, who were they addressing and what was the most appropriate mode of expression? Some recent work has begun to explore the epistolary rhetoric employed by sufferers, but only in context of letters between patients and doctors.[15] The ways in which sufferers represented themselves to others, such as family and friends, and the ways in which they constructed and narrativised their sickness, need to be further explored. Here, if anywhere, may be a more apt application of a sick 'role'.

Finally, there were many different stages of sickness, from mild and non-acute conditions to severe and disabling ones, but reactions to them were not uniform. If there was a fairly universal indicator of severity, it was withdrawal to the bedchamber, signifying literal withdrawal from daily life and duties. Here again, the 'sick role' model privileges the practitioner stage, while source evidence, as we shall see, places greater emphasis upon taking to one's bed. But even this could be subverted, and some people went to great lengths to avoid, and even deliberately flout, social conventions of sickness – effectively a 'sick role' in reverse. Neither, too, was the 'sick role' static, since it could vary greatly in degrees of severity but also in the personal tolerance thresholds of individuals. For Parsons, sickness seemed almost to be limited to a single event, with a definite beginning and end. But was this truly the lived experience for many people? What of conditions such as agues, which were of indeterminate length and could involve days of severe ague 'fits' followed by days of relative ease and recovery? Where did social expectations of the comportment of the sufferer lie on these 'good' days?

The following discussion will therefore focus upon self-representation, and the ways in which sufferers presented themselves to others. Key to this process was the growing importance of literacy which afforded new opportunities for sickness self-fashioning, and adds another dimension to our understanding of what it was like to *be* sick in the early modern period.

'Choosing' sickness

When and why did people cross the boundary between states of 'wellness' and 'illness'? Disease could manifest itself in any number of minor or chronic symptoms, but the establishment of a state of sickness within an individual was contingent on very rigid criteria. In her work detailing the relationship between patients and practitioners, Lucinda McCray Beier implied there were in essence two different types of sick roles.[16] The first was that of the 'patient', and might be considered as a minor sick role. Here, the sufferer displayed symptoms and would typically seek the opinions of others. This indicated to them the person was potentially sick, but did not entail a retreat from normal social duties.[17] The full sick role, however, usually confined the sufferer to their bed. It signalled a change in status in the sufferer from one actively involved in domestic and social responsibilities to one effectively confined to their homes and under the care of others. Beier's study of the Essex minister Ralph Josselin points to a definite distinction between sickness which entailed bed-rest, and less chronic ailments which entitled the sufferer to complain, but nevertheless carry on with normal duties.[18] The problem lies in the fact that this boundary between wellness and sickness, between a minor or full sick role, was mutable and entirely contingent upon the individual sufferer.

For some people, such as Robert Bulkeley of Dronwy, Anglesey, the boundaries of sickness were clearly based on practical considerations such as the duration of the sickness event and its impact upon his daily routines. Racked with toothache in May 1632, Bulkeley recorded his symptoms in a diary entry. 'I offered a peny at ye buriall of Rich[ard]: . . . his wife coing [sic] home I Sp[ent]: 6d at Sr John & 4d at d[avi]d ap Owen . . . east wind, tooth ach'.[19] Here, the symptom appeared almost as an addendum, and thus apparently not seen as chronic or severe. Over the coming days the toothache continued to vex him. The following day, he visited a barber and was trimmed, before noting that he 'paid a vagabond a penny' to cure his toothache while, on 20 May, he was again abroad, this time visiting an apothecary to purchase tobacco after the pedlar's cure had failed him.[20] Such instances reflect a minor, if no less troublesome, complaint, but one which did not prevent Bulkeley from continuing with his daily routine. On other occasions, however, there were more severe ailments. In April 1631, he noted that he was 'all day sicke of an ague'.[21] In the spring of 1634 he suffered a more prolonged bout of illness noting on 5 April that he 'fell sicke about 9 a clocke at night' and, the following day, he 'continued very sicke all day'.[22] Emphasis was clearly laid upon the 'all day' duration of the episodes, which certainly hints at a significant disruption to normal routines and confinement to his house, a possibility seemingly confirmed by the fact that no activities are noted for either day. For Bulkeley, there was also a clear distinction between 'falling' sick and 'laying' sick (i.e. requiring bed-rest). There can be little doubt of the severity of the condition of his wife Besse, 'who lay sicke these ten dayes', and was clearly confined to her bed.[23] This distinction can be clearly found in other sources.

Sickness experience and the 'sick role'

For the Flintshire Puritan Philip Henry, serious sickness was certainly demarked by withdrawal to the bedchamber. In November 1663, a fit of distemper meant that Henry 'kept ye house', while again in 1671, he contracted an ague which for several days made him 'a prisoner to house though not to bed'.[24] This grading was important because it clearly signalled that the situation was, although serious, probably not dangerous. Simply 'keeping the house' was not, for Henry and Bulkeley at least, necessarily the sole marker of illness: rather, it was the physical act of removing to the bedchamber which really drew the distinction. Likewise, if one was confined to house but not to bed, did this necessarily entail exemption from social duties, since some types of business might still have been able to be conducted from home? This last point bears further analysis, and especially since it raises the question of gender.

On the evening of 5 August 1682, Katherine Henry began to display the first symptoms of a tertian ague. This was to last almost continuously for the following three weeks and she was often confined to the bedroom, effectively signifying her withdrawal from normal familial duties. This withdrawal to the sickbed was a strong part of the sick ritual, and one especially familiar to women, for whom confinement to the house after childbirth was symbolically ended with the public ritual of 'churching'.[25] On 6 August Philip Henry noted that 'shee was Pretty wel and below stayres' and again, two days later, that 'shee was refresht, gott up and walkt about ye chamber'.[26] This was clearly seen as a positive sign and meant a reprieve, if only a temporary one. The regularity of Katherine's ague fits evidently allowed for a certain degree of planning for days between fits, but even this could be disrupted, as on 18 August, which 'should have been her better day but prov'd otherwise'.[27] On these 'better days', it seems that Katherine was keen to be 'below stayres' with the family, with some semblance of normal routine. Bed-rest was *the* defining element of full-blown sickness and the ultimate signal of a potentially serious situation. Some elements of alternative medicine in the early modern period, such as the astrological medicine of Nicholas Culpeper, in fact laid great emphasis upon 'decumbiture' – the need, for accurate diagnosis, to record exactly what time the patient fell ill and physically lay down.[28] But, in being 'below stayres', was Katherine tacitly back in her domestic productive role? It is clear that she crossed and re-crossed the notional boundary of sickness several times but, again, where were the boundaries of the 'sick role' here? I would argue that the importance of gender in determining sickness behaviours and experiences has been underestimated, and especially within the domestic realm. It is possible that the dynamics of female withdrawal into a 'sick role' were different, since women effectively remained within their sphere of work. This would certainly explain the notional emphasis on being 'downstairs' and thus active. From establishing the boundaries of sickness, the discussion now turns to the issue of coping with its effects.

To state the obvious, sickness for most people was certainly an unwelcome state and, for the very poorest in society, a severe sickness episode requiring bed-rest was undesirable, if not potentially catastrophic. The physical ability to be exempted from a usual social role relies on actually having a role to withdraw from. Large numbers of the lower orders of Welsh society, through poverty, simply did not have this option and many doubtless suffered the same fate as Owen Humphrey, a youth from Llanwrin in Montgomeryshire, who died on the road in the winter of 1739. Owen's post-mortem reported that he was 'of a sickly constitution and very poor' and 'was accustomed to walk about in the country to beg his bread and very subject to sleep out of doors'.[29] Through a combi-nation of 'his poverty, sickness and sleeping on the ground', recorders noted that he 'then and there perished and starved to death'.[30] For Owen, as doubt-less for many others, there was no opportunity for a 'sick role', and the onset of illness, combined with extreme poverty, could have desperate consequences. Livelihoods could be lost through sickness, as able men were forced to stop working when their health deteriorated. As Margaret Pelling's analysis of the censuses of Norwich has demonstrated, poor people in fact often elected not to disclose minor ailments, for fear of losing their positions, and even the seriously disabled or afflicted often continued to undertake paid employment to avoid becoming dependent on the charity or, worse, begging.[31] Unfortunately, there are few records from which we can draw inference about the actual experience of sickness in a poor household, but even occasional glimpses can be revealing. For people like Joan David, a widow of Saint Athan, who died in 1735 leaving an estate worth little more than six pounds, the possessions left in her will tell of an impoverished and miserable final few days. In a cold, hard winter in which several of her small group of livestock had already perished, she lay dying in 'old and ordinary' clothes on 'an old feather bed where there was but little feathers', with her few possessions of 'an old iron pott' and 'a small brass kettle broken and old'.[32] For Joan, and others like her, the 'sick role' probably consisted of little more than a painful wait for the *coup de grâce*.

But if the poor could not take up a 'sick role' through necessity, there were others who simply refused it. Some, for example, were clearly keen to maintain some semblance of normality even despite potentially serious conditions. For religious men, such as Philip Henry, a willingness to carry on with daily life regardless of physical suffering reflected his Puritan need for stoicism during the trials of sickness. In the majority of his sickness episodes, it seems that Henry did not retreat from his normal social duties and in fact appeared resolved to carry on with his responsibilities in spite of his illness. On more than one occa-sion he continued with his preaching duties whilst sick and only once explicitly recorded absence from his preaching through illness.[33] Sometimes, it is obvious that he persisted even in the face of quite severe symptoms. An entry in his diary in February 1680 records that he 'quakt of ye ague from 8. to 11. yet preached, neither eat nor drink inbetween'.[34] In September 1661, he visited Chester where he had 'cold and tooth-ake yet assisted in study, blessed bee God'.[35] Extracts from the diary of his daughter, Sarah Savage, provide further evidence. In one graphic entry in 1692, Savage notes that her (by now elderly) father, 'notwithstanding his illness . . . went on Sabbath June 12, limping to the pulpit'.[36] As mentioned, it is likely that Henry was keen to present a façade of stoicism in the face of illness, but other entries show the extent to which personal sickness could be turned towards didactic means. Henry recorded the case of Matthew Jenkyn, a local conformist minister who, suffering from 'a pining sickness . . . preacht to the very last, being carry'd in a chaiyr from his house to the pulpit'.[37] It is possible that Henry simply noted this example since he was impressed by the strength of the man's calling, and fortitude in the face of his suffering. His further comment that Jenkyn was 'burthensome to those with Wch hee had to doe' does, however, portray Jenkyn as a difficult, and perhaps strong-willed, man.[38] In involving others, Jenkyn was apparently keen to make a public show to his flock. Didactically, if even *he* could make it to church in this condition, then his parishioners surely had little excuse not to attend. But it was not only religious figures who might carry on regardless, perhaps even viewing the adoption of a sick role as inviting misfortune in the same vein as superstitions regarding the making of wills. In 1728, Thomas Edwards, a bailiff from Llanfechell on Anglesey, was 'indisposed . . . tho' getts up every day, yet can hardly crawl from his room to the house & back agen immediately upon the bed'.[39] Despite his obvious pain, Edwards clearly felt obligated to continue his duties and not withdraw from public life.

Such examples again raise the issue of the importance of gender and, in particular, the status of masculinity or manliness in terms of fending off sickness. Certainly in prescriptive literature, men were exhorted to give outward demonstrations of their spiritual piety and strength of character.[40] But could there be other reasons for such behaviour? In deliberately eschewing the opportunity to withdraw to the house or bedchamber, might there have been an element of the assertion of masculinity? As Alexandra Shepard points out, men's bodies were seen (at least by male writers) as exemplars of 'bodily perfection', with a resulting balanced constitution. This, she argues, played a strong part in the justification for the precedence of men in social and political life.[41] Even despite the wide range of variations from the 'perfect' or ideal male body, illness represented a departure from these masculine norms. Thus, masculine religious and social imperatives could have put pressure on men to avoid or downplay their own sicknesses as an outward means of demonstrating physical, moral or spiritual fortitude.

But the potential benefits in terms of the social power engendered by sickness were legion, and open to exploitation. There is certainly evidence, for example, that feigning sickness for a few days off work is not solely a modern phenomenon. Some employers became suspicious, especially when the sickness episodes of their hired hands were repeated. In 1724, Thomas Ffoulkes of Martyn, near Holywell in Flintshire, appeared to be keeping a very close eye upon his maid's sick days. On 6 January he noted that 'My mayd Marg't Jones fell sick this day and next day, did not gett out of bed'.[42] On the following Monday, 'she went unknown to me to her mother's & did not returne till Friday the 12th at noon. She went *rambling* [my emphasis] home severall other times'.[43] In October, Ffoulkes pointedly recorded more periods of sickness, seemingly indignant at the amount of time that Margaret was losing. Clearly we have only Ffoulkes's apparent suspicion to question the genuineness of the maid's condition, but this does raise questions of the power relations of sickness. On the one hand, Margaret may simply have been an early modern exponent of the sickie! On the other, however, it is also possible that sickness was one means through which servants could gain some measure of power over their masters and even use it as a means of challenging authority or gaining agency.[44] Clearly, in some ways, feigning sickness was self-defeating inasmuch as it could easily lead to loss of pay. Even more patient masters like William Davies of Clytha had a limit to their indulgence. When his servant William Prosser was ill in 1718, Davies noted that he 'gave [Prosser] one shilling when you were sick'.[45] When Prosser again fell sick in April 1719, Davies recorded that he lost seven days' work, but appears not to have paid him this time. Likewise, time to visit sick relatives, such as the one day lost when Prosser 'went to see [his] Sister when shee was sick', was similarly unpaid.[46] The health of servants was clearly important and, as we shall see in the next chapter, Welsh employers seemed generally willing to give the benefit of the doubt and even to provide some care. The extent to which their sickness was ministered to, however, almost certainly depended greatly on the individual household.

Self-representation and the 'epistolary sick role'

Once sickness had been established, the sufferer could undertake a variety of different behaviours and coping strategies. Withdrawal to the bedchamber, and from familial roles or duties, was one means through which this could be achieved. But the physical behaviour of the sufferer, their thoughts and actions, but especially their speech, were also subject to scrutiny. As Ralph Houlbrooke has convincingly shown, the comportment and speech of the sick could be incredibly important to family and friends.[47] Speech was a self-conscious representation of sickness, a verbal manifestation of inward suffering certainly, but importantly also one delivered with others in mind. It might begin, as with the response of Thomas Ffoulkes noted above, with a simple acknowledgement that the sufferer considered themselves to be in a 'state' of sickness. It might, though, also involve more apparently defined conventions of speech. On the fifth day of her ague, Philip Henry noted that his wife often repeated the same phrase 'sick, sick, never so sick, yet by and by I am better'. Two days later he again reported that she was 'often saying sick, sick'.[48] Such phrases were an outward means by which the sufferer could demonstrate their own adoption of a sick role. That Katherine Henry appeared to deploy the same phrase over a period of days implies that it was, for her at least, a convention. Her use of it may have been a casual, even unconscious, voicing of her status as a sufferer, but may also have been a definite signal to others of her changed condition. Becoming unable to articulate these inner feelings through sickness was also disturbing. In another instance, Henry noted that the loss of speech due to illness in a friend 'was to those about him, very uncomfortable', not least in that it denied the man the chance to repent or display piety.[49] The difficulty lies in knowing how far these comments were noted simply because they appealed to Henry's Puritan convictions of penitence in the face of potential death.

Physical and verbal demonstrations of piety were certainly important to the families of the sick, and tied in with notions of the 'good death'. On 10 August 1682, Katherine Henry was heard by Philip to say 'I repent of all my sins esp. of my unprofitableness ... I know Death cannot hurt me'.[50] For her minister husband, such statements would have been a comforting indication that the soul of the sick was prepared for Heaven.[51] In Monmouthshire, a similar motivation might have prompted John Gwin to record the last words of his wife's mother, 'O Duw kymmer vi' (Oh God take/come for me), 'for which words' wrote Gwin 'and others we received conserninge her, we yeeld all honor glorie and prayse to the lord'.[52] Richard Wunderli and Gerald Broce have contended that Catholics and Protestants in the early modern period shared the view that a person's conduct during sickness, and especially in their last moments, could determine whether they were bound for salvation or damnation.[53] They argue that this was an optimistic way of offering salvation to all in an age of religious upheaval.[54] The message of resurrection for the chosen was strongly reinforced by the presence of ministers or priests at the bedsdes of the sick and dying.[55] In general, the 'good death' took place in the presence of family members who each had a role to perform, and the sick person was likewise expected to display piety and humility in the face of possible death.[56] By the early modern period, the tradition of 'ars moriendi' (the 'art of dying') conduct books was also well established.[57] These reminded people of the need for good conduct during the final sickness, and were designed to guide the dying through the difficult and vitally important last moments on earth. Such books were certainly available in Welsh by the end of the seventeenth century, such as Thomas Williams's translation of William Sherlock's *Practical Discourse Concerning Death*, which sought to remind people always to live in expectation and preparation for death, and which was still in print a century later.[58]

Especially amongst the middle and upper levels of Welsh society during this period, there was a change in the nature of religious understandings of disease causation, and a shift towards a more secular view of sickness and cure. It has been argued that, as religious conceptions of the causation of illness waned towards the later seventeenth century, people began to concentrate more on the actual workings of their bodies.[59] Therefore, in one sense, disease became both cause and effect. There is no doubt that, for many people, religion certainly still coloured people's attitudes, and the clergy continued to extol the virtues of piety and humility in the face of sickness. While it was Puritanism that had fuelled Philip Henry's concerns over conduct during sickness, the growth of Methodism in eighteenth-century Wales provided a similar impetus for men like John Harries, minister of Mynydd Bach and Abergorlech in Carmarthenshire, to observe the behaviour of their parishioners.[60] Eighteenth-century Welsh Methodism certainly contained strong echoes of Puritan notions of disease causation. In 1747, Howell Davies wrote to the Methodist minister Howell Harris that 'I am still here very low under the Lord's Rod' mirroring Philip Henry's comments of nearly a century before.[61] Nevertheless, in the diary of Anglesey parson Owen Davies, for example, it is noticeable that God, while still sometimes entreated to spare or repair the sufferer, is not actually invoked as a causal factor in any one of Davies's noted sickness episodes.[62]

But, there was another side to sickness self-fashioning, and it could be argued that the increasing use of the written word and, in particular, the letter brought forth new opportunities for the construction of suffering. Literacy allowed people to present themselves in a wholly different, and controlled, way. It offered opportunities to elaborate on the personal 'feelings' of illness, and even to construct an individual sickness 'persona'. Letters were a common source of medical discourse between family, friends and practitioners throughout the early modern period, but the eighteenth century clearly brought about changes in the ways in which sufferers depicted themselves on paper. This was a new 'epistolary' sick role, a narrative story with characterisation, plot and drama, and there is evidence to show that some parts of Welsh society embraced it wholeheartedly. Sickness and symptoms were always at the forefront of early modern correspondence. It was common for letters to family or friends to open with some reference to the health or past sickness of the recipient, and for medical advice or even remedies to be duly despatched.[63] Equally common was for sufferers to provide descriptions of their symptoms and sickness habits. On one level, health was a natural topic of conversation, an accepted part of the minutiae of daily life. On another, however, such communication almost represented a 'sick role' in itself. Here, the sufferer could make (literally) a public statement about their conditions, while careful management of their own behaviour could be used either to garner sympathy or otherwise demonstrate piety or conformity. This 'epistolary sick role' also coincided with changes in the ways that people viewed and depicted their illnesses, and increasingly so from the end of the seventeenth century.

The status of the sickness sufferer was clearly undergoing changes, not least of which was the apparent embracement of an 'ideal' of sickness, especially amongst the literati of Welsh society. We must therefore be cautious not to assume that this was a uniform experience. But if the seventeenth century saw some people content to rid themselves quickly of their ailments and not submit to the sick role for longer than absolutely necessary, the next half-century appears to have ushered in a new stage in the practice of suffering. The Morris brothers of Anglesey exemplify this new desire to embrace the role of sufferer, and for them it reached almost competitive heights. In December 1760, Lewis Morris noted that he was suffering from 'sudden fits of coughing' which broke his sleep, and also that he continually dosed himself with purges and vomits which bound and then loosened him. He was, he concluded, 'very sick'.[64] A reply from his brother Richard protested the severity of his own cough, but Lewis was not to be outdone. 'You complain of your cough and asthma; I own your cough is heavy, but if you had such an asthma as I have, it would be impossible for you to go to the office or sit there'.[65] This example illustrates a key point; to be sick was, for the Morris brothers, effectively a badge of honour. Here, sickness was something if not wholly desirable, then at least fashionable, since it put the sufferer in almost a heroic light, as they struggled with their symptoms.

Letters allowed the sufferer to go even further in dramatising their sickness, and were clearly fashioned to provoke a response from the reader. A heroic fatalism began to underpin eighteenth-century medical correspondence, and the sick set themselves up as romantic heroes locked in a struggle with their potentially fatal symptoms. A propensity to prepare for death during sickness was certainly nothing new and, given the omnipresence of death in the early modern period, was a natural concern. Philip Henry often prepared himself for death, and reasoned that each sickness might be a final test from God. His notions of mortality were thus refracted through the lens of his Puritan convictions. In Lewis Morris's letters, however, it is noteworthy that mortal sickness had been almost entirely secularised and divorced from connotations of religious causation. On many occasions during their sicknesses, Morris indicated to his brothers that death might be imminent. In 1760, he wrote to his brother Richard that he was 'taken with a most cruel, pleuritic fever about a fortnight ago' and was 'just returned from the shades of death'.[66] A week or two later, he stoically announced that, although 'my materials are decayed, and I suspect my lungs are hurt' he would 'trudge on while I live'.[67] In 1761, he was 'scarce alive' after a fit of palsy 'had like to take away my life'.[68] Lewis in fact lived until 1765. Here, though, there was a strong difference between Morris's sick role and that of someone like Philip Henry, especially in terms of the intended audience. Henry's diary entries often appealed directly to God. When describing his illnesses, Henry sought God's favour and, in some senses, also His appreciation that Henry was continuing to comport himself well through the test of illness. For figures such as Lewis Morris, however, the recipients of the letters were flesh and blood. Favour and appreciation were still being sought, but the persona of the sufferer had now shifted from religious to secular, as he portrayed himself as the embattled victim. There is certainly no doubt that he had been quite ill at times, since other letters to and from his brothers show a great deal of concern at his predicament. In another account of an ague fit in March 1762, Morris wrote that he was 'like to go off' but quick action from his wife in finding a man to open his veins gave him instant relief.[69] He asked his brother Richard to send some papers which he promised to look over 'if I recover'.[70] But how far did Lewis really believe he was going to die? His letter begins and ends with general pieces of news indicating that he was far from having given up on life. In another letter, Lewis began what he again seemingly considered might be his last 'if coughing and giddiness will give me leave', before proceeding to write several hundred words, and concluding that he was, in actuality, 'pretty well except [for] cough and giddyness'.[71] Within this one letter was effectively a full story which began with the writer at death's door, and ended with optimism for his recovery. Literate narrativisation of the sickness episode, then, was a new and key element in self-representation.

While seventeenth-century sickness depictions in letters often mentioned symptoms and often something of the state or condition of the sufferer, the eighteenth-century sufferer presented their sickness effectively as a story, complete with plot, dramatisation and even serialisation. This was a secular 'sick role', where the body was the main player and, in many ways, this brought illness to the fore of eighteenth-century correspondence. 'Epistolary sick role' letters were often, as in the case of the Morris brothers, written either in the midst or at the end of sickness. They were effectively news bulletins, updating the reader on latest developments. They also allowed the sufferer to control their own 'story' and present themselves in the guise of the battered, but resolute victim. People had always been keen to share their symptoms with others in great detail but, indeed, sickness seems almost to have gone from being a regular element within letters to the primary reason for writing. One letter to his brother, from Roger Jones, an attorney of Talgarth, for example, was written for no other reason than to detail his symptoms. Whilst travelling to Hay, Jones was 'taken with a numbness and a sleepiness' and returned home. He was duly bled, cupped and blistered by a local physician and reported that he had taken 'a vast deal of medicines and yet without effect'.[72] He desired his brother to visit him as soon as he was able, to help him make a will and settle his affairs.[73] Here, the sickness episode was again presented in full narrative form, providing the beginning of the symptoms, the results and likely outcome. Clearly, in this case, Jones believed that his life was in danger, but the level of detail also shows that he was keen to present the full facts of his situation. There were even sometimes elements of dark humour in these depictions. In another letter, Jones noted his having taken purges, glisters and opening pills, the only effect of which was to make him a great deal thinner![74] Howell Davies presented a similar narrative in a January 1747 letter. Davies was 'greatly affected with the gravel and consumption . . . which is like to turn into a wind dropsy'.[75] His apparently repeated requests to Griffith Jones, founder member of the SPCK and reputedly also 'a quack in physick' elicited the response that Jones 'refus'd to give me any thing towards my health, said it was too late for him & yt I must apply to some Doctor, wch I have accordingly done, yt I am at present so closely confined'.[76] Here again was a complete story, working from diagnosis to current situation but this time without resolution. Davies was at once the hero and the victim of his ailments.

What were the possible reasons for these changes? Certainly during the later eighteenth century, as Roy Porter has noted, illness was growing more fashionable. Certain types of condition were becoming increasingly popular, and this reflected wider changes in disease classifications and also the appearance of 'new' diseases. Even disease sufferers were not immune to the desire to associate themselves with the new spirit of enlightened science.[77] Glyn Penrhyn Jones noted that gout and apoplexy were increasingly reported amongst the Welsh literati.[78] Given its connections with affluent living, Welsh society figures could be quick to attribute arthritis or joint pain to gout while the Morris brothers, as well as many prominent Methodists, also suffered from what Jones describes as 'fashionable melancholia'.[79] Such changes also reflected a wider desire amongst the Welsh to be seen as part of fashionable society, and to shake off perceptions of rustic backwardness. The adoption of metropolitan manners and fashions was one means by which the Welsh could attempt to demonstrate their parity with England.[80]

But, importantly, it was not only the upper orders for whom literacy could be utilised in self-representation since the poor were often especially skilful in deploying their sicknesses and symptoms as part of their entreaties for financial relief. When John Jones of Llandenny, a poor labourer, fell sick, his wife Mary begged their landlord for excusal from rent payments upon their cottage built on the waste, arguing that, even when well, her husband only earned threepence a day.[81] Mary's case was built upon continued references to both the severity and duration of her husband's sickness. She described how John 'went sick' more than four years previously, and was now 'broken and gone old' and unable to provide for his family. The family's misfortune was apparently compounded by the death of a local benefactor, whose replacement, in Mary's eyes, wanted 'to punish the poor man in spite'.[82] As Thomas Sokoll points out, pauper letters were strategically written and used carefully chosen language in order to balance deference (in the case of request letters) with a presentation of the facts.[83] For the literate poor, letters also allowed opportunities to seek help in situations where face-to-face contact might have been uncomfortable. One such letter survives from an employee, addressed to 'Mrs Lloyd of Penpedust', near Cardigan.

> Madam Lloyd, by submission to your Honour, my little grand Child whome I nurs'd Since he was a year old, Happen to fell sick, this day fortneight, and had been very low, I hope that he begin to recover, he is longing for Rosted meat, that ever he had in my cottage, and I sure that he cannot distinguies between any sort of Rosted meat. If your honour please to send a bit, or order me to wait for it, I will be very glad and in so doing you will add to the obligation of your honest old shoemaker, and your most humble servant, John Jenkin, alias, Little Shoemaker[84]

Jenkin was obviously keen to martial his evidence to elicit a sympathetic response from 'Mrs Lloyd'. This was not a straightforward account of symptoms, but a carefully constructed plea, with the child 'longing' for meat, and 'very low'. The sincerity of the letter is plain, but Jenkin's self-promotion as the 'honest' and 'humble servant' struggling in his role as carer, says much about the ways in which letters could use sickness both to bridge social gaps and manage the self-image of the sufferer. Chapter 8 will look in more detail at the question of self-representation of the poor in context of petitions for poor relief.

Conclusion

Sickness and the 'sick role', therefore, were far from being a uniform experience. There were, instead, a multiplicity of different sickness experiences and behaviours affected and informed by a range of different factors. Likewise, because of this there was not, and indeed could not be, a uniquely Welsh sick role, any more than there was an English one. There was, however, undoubtedly a Welsh sickness experience, one offshoot of which is disease terminologies through the Welsh language. Welsh people understood and perpetuated sickness through their own language even though this was subject to outside influences. Nevertheless, individual sufferers reacted to sickness in different ways, but these reactions were also tempered by a range of Welsh social and religious factors. The decision to even undertake a 'sick role' – if we employ the term uncritically for a moment – was undoubtedly contingent upon the financial situation of the sufferer but, as the above examples have demonstrated, how to approach sickness was a personal choice, and one which many people elected to avoid. Sickness behaviour could likewise be coloured by a range of factors, and also involve a variety of mechanisms, from undertaking bed-rest to the use of verbal conventions to reinforce the 'otherness' of the sufferer. Similarly, sickness could be manipulated in order to present an image to others. The changing patterns of this role can be seen in the growing eighteenth-century fashioning of sickness, reinforced by the use of literacy in controlling self-image. As noted above, however, we must be careful not to assume that this literary sick role was necessarily reflective of wider trends.

Having now dealt in some detail with sickness from the point of view of the sufferer themselves, we now need to cast the net wider and explore the external sickness experience, that of looking after a sick person. Who looked after the sick? What emotional, social and financial effects could this have on individuals, families and communities? The following chapter, therefore, will turn to the important issue of care in early modern Wales.

Notes

1 For some examples see Roy Porter (ed.), *Patients and Practitioners: Lay Perceptions of Medicine in Pre-Industrial Society* (Cambridge: Cambridge University Press, 2002 edition); Margaret Pelling, *The Common Lot: Sickness, Medical Occupations and the Urban Poor in Early Modern England* (London and New York: Longman, 1998); Lucinda McCray Beier, *Sufferers and Healers: The Experience of Illness in Seventeenth Century England* (London and New York: Routledge and Kegan Paul, 1987); Patricia Crawford, *Blood, Bodies and Families in Early Modern England* (Harlow: Pearson, 2004); Margaret Pelling, 'The Women of the Family? Speculation around Early Modern British Physicians', *Social History of Medicine*, 7:3 (1995), pp. 383–401.

2 Mary Fissell, *Patients, Power and the Poor in Eighteenth-Century Bristol* (Cambridge: Cambridge University Press, 2002 edition).

3 Roy Porter, *Quacks: Fakers and Charlatans in Medicine* (Stroud: Tempus, 2003 edition); Dorothy Porter and Roy Porter, *Patient's Progress: Doctors and Doctoring in Eighteenth Century England* (Stanford: Stanford University Press, 1989); Roy Porter, *Bodies Politic: Disease, Death and Doctors in Britain, 1650–1900* (London: Reaktion, 2001).

4 Robert Ralley, 'Medical Economies in Fifteenth-Century England' in Mark S.R. Jenner and Patrick Wallis (eds), *Medicine and the Market in England and its Colonies, c. 1450 – c. 1850* (Basingstoke: Palgrave Macmillan, 2007), p. 37.

5 Byron J. Good, *Medicine, Rationality and Experience: An Anthropological Perspective* (Cambridge: Cambridge University Press, 2007 edition), p. 5.

6 Ibid., p. 5.

7 Ludmilla Jordanova, 'The Social Construction of Medical Knowledge' in Frank Huisman and John Harley Warner (eds), *Locating Medical History: The Stories and Their Meanings* (Baltimore and London: Johns Hopkins University Press, 2006 edition), p. 346.

8 Mary Stainton Rogers, *Explaining Health and Illness: An Exploration of Diversity* (Hemel Hempstead: Harvester Wheatsheaf, 1991), pp. 17–18.

9 Ibid., pp. 24–25.

10 See Bryan S. Turner (ed.), *The Talcott Parsons Reader* (Oxford: Blackwell, 1999), pp. 104–105; Roland Robertson and Bryan S. Turner (eds, *Talcott Parsons: Theorist of Modernity* (London: Sage, 1991), p. 205; John C. Burnham, *What is Medical History?* (Cambridge: Polity Press, 2005), p. 37.

11 Burnham, *What is Medical History?*, p. 38.

12 Dorothy Porter and Roy Porter, *In Sickness and in Health: The British Experience 1650–1850* (London: Fourth Estate, 1988).

13 Lucinda McCray Beier, 'In Sickness and in Health: A Seventeenth Century Family's Experience' in Roy Porter (ed.), *Patients and Practitioners: Lay Perceptions of Medicine in Pre-Industrial Society* (Cambridge: Cambridge University Press, 2002 edition), p. 125.

14 Porter and Porter, *In Sickness*, pp. 188–190.

15 Wayne Wild, *Medicine-by-Post: The Changing Voice of Illness in Eighteenth-Century British Consultation Letters and Literature* (Amsterdam and New York: Rodopi, 2006).

16 Beier, *Sufferers and Healers*, p. 245.

17 Ibid., p. 245.

18 Beier, 'In Sickness and in Health', pp. 124–125.

19 Hugh Owen, 'The Diary of Bulkeley of Dronwy, Anglesey, 1630–1636', *Transactions of the Anglesey Antiquarian Society* (1937), p. 71.

20 Ibid., p. 7.

21 Ibid., p. 43.

22 Ibid., p. 117.

23 Ibid., p. 37.

24 Matthew Henry Lee (ed.), *The Diaries and Letters of Philip Henry, M.A. of Broad Oak, Flintshire A.D. 1631–1696* (London: Kegan Paul, Trench and Co., 1882), pp. 150, 242.

25 Michael Roberts, 'Gender, Work and Socialisation in Wales, c. 1450 – c. 1850' in Sandra Betts (ed.), *Our Daughter's Land: Past and Present* (Cardiff: University of Wales Press, 1996), p. 19.

26 Lee (ed.), *Diaries of Philip Henry*, p. 315.

27 Ibid., p. 315.

28 Allan Chapman, 'Astrological Medicine' in Charles Webster (ed.), *Health, Medicine and Mortality in the Sixteenth Century* (Cambridge: Cambridge University Press, 1979), p. 280.

29 Quoted in Melvin Humphreys, *The Crisis of Community: Montgomeryshire 1680–1815* (Cardiff: University of Wales Press, 1996), p. 59.

30 Ibid., p. 59.

31 Pelling, *The Common Lot*, pp. 82–85; Adrian Teale, 'The Battle against Poverty in North Flintshire, c. 1660–1714', *Flintshire Historical Society Journal*, 31 (1983/84), p. 86.

32 National Library of Wales (hereafter NLW) MS Joan David, LL/1735/109.

33 Lee (ed.), *Diaries of Philip Henry*, p. 56.

34 Ibid., p. 285.

35 Ibid., p. 96.

36 J.B. Williams, *Memoirs of the Life and Character of Mrs Sarah Savage* (London: Holdsworth and Hall, Fourth edition, 1829), p. 57.

37 Lee (ed.), *Diaries of Philip Henry*, p. 224.

38 Ibid., p. 224.

39 Leonard Owen, 'The Letters of an Anglesey Parson, 1712–1732', *Transactions of the Honourable Society of Cymmrodorion*, 1 (1961), p. 89.

40 Jeremy Gregory, 'Homo Religiosus: Masculinity and Religion in the Long Eighteenth Century' in Tim Hitchcock and Michele Cohen (eds), *English Masculinities 1660–1800* (London: Longman, 1999), pp. 88–90.

41 Alexandra Shepard, *Meanings of Manhood in Early Modern England* (Oxford: Oxford University Press, 2003), p. 48.

42 NLW MS 1613A, Misc. Flintshire Notebooks and Diaries, Notebook attr. Thomas Ffoulkes, c. 1724, p. 60.

43 Ibid., p. 60.

44 For discussions on passive resistance and challenges to authority see James C. Scott, *Domination and the Arts of Resistance* (Yale: Yale University Press, 1992).

45 Gwent Record Office, MS D/PA.29.10, Pocketbook of William Davies of Clytha, 1654–1720, p. 8.

46 Ibid., p. 9.

47 See Ralph Houlbrooke, *Death, Religion and the Family in England 1480–1750* (Oxford: Clarendon Press, 2000 edition), esp. chapter 7.

48 Lee (ed.), *Diaries of Philip Henry*, p. 315.

49 Ibid., p. 264.

50 Ibid., p. 315.

51 Houlbrooke, *Death, Religion and the Family*, p. 154; Andrew Wear, 'Puritan Perceptions of Illness in Seventeenth Century England' in Porter (ed.), *Patients and Practitioners*, pp. 64–65.

52 Gwent Record Office, MS D43:4216, Commonplace Book of John Gwin of Llangwm, 17th century, p. 71.

53 Richard Wunderli and Gerald Broce, 'The Final Moment before Death in Early Modern England', *Sixteenth Century Journal*, 20:2 (1989), p. 259.

54 Ibid., p. 267.

55 Houlbrooke, *Death, Religion and the Family*, p. 155.

56 Lucinda McCray Beier, 'The Good Death in Seventeenth Century England' in Ralph Houlbrooke (ed.), *Death, Ritual and Bereavement* (London and New York: Routledge, 1989), p. 45.

57 Wunderli and Broce, 'The Final Moment', p. 263.

58 William Sherlock, *A Practical Discourse Concerning Death* (London: Printed for W. Rogers, 1690); Thomas Williams, *Ymadroddion Bucheddol Ynghylch Marwolaeth o Waith Doctor Sherlock* (London: Printed for Leon Lichfield, 1691); Thomas Williams, *Ymadroddion Bucheddol Ynghylch Marwolaeth o Waith Doctor Sherlock* (Brecon: Printed by E. Evans, 1777).

59 Wear, 'Puritan Perceptions', p. 75.

60 NLW MS 371B, Register of Mynydd Bach Chapel.

61 Gomer Morgan Roberts (ed.), *Selected Trevecka Letters (1747–1794)* (Caernarvon: The Calvinist Methodist Bookroom, 1962), p. 13.

62 Owen, 'Letters of an Anglesey Parson'.

63 Roy Porter, 'The Patient in England c. 1660 – c. 1800' in Andrew Wear (ed.), *Medicine in Society: Historical Essays* (Cambridge: Cambridge University Press, 1998 edition), p. 102.

64 John H. Davies, *The Letters of Lewis, Richard, William and John Morris of Anglesey (Morrisiaid Mon) 1728–1765*, 2 Volumes (Aberystwyth: Privately Published, 1907), Volume 2, pp. 283–284.

65 Ibid., p. 293.

66 Ibid., p. 277.

67 Ibid., p. 281.

68 Ibid., p. 361.

69 Ibid., p. 451.

70 Ibid., p. 451.

71 Ibid., pp. 496–498.

72 NLW, D.T.M. Jones (3) MS 1191, Letter from Roger Jones to the Reverend John Jones, 17 February 1769.

73 Ibid.,

74 NLW, D.T.M. Jones (3) MS 1192, Letter from Roger Jones to John Jones, 5 August 1770.

75 Roberts (ed.), *Trevecka Letters*, p. 13.

76 Ibid., pp. 13–14.

77 Porter, 'The Patient in England', p. 105.

78 Glyn Penrhyn Jones, 'A History of Medicine in Wales in the Eighteenth Century' (Liverpool University: Unpublished MA thesis, 1957), p. 48.

79 Ibid., p. 47.

80 Geraint H. Jenkins, *The Foundations of Modern Wales, 1642–1780* (Oxford: Oxford University Press, 2002 edition), p. 262.

81 NLW, Badminton 1 (Manorial 2) MS 2197, Petition to John Burk from Mary Jones, undated, c. 1700.

82 Ibid.

83 Thomas Sokoll, 'Old Age in Poverty: The Record of Essex Pauper Letters, 1780–1834' in Tim Hitchcock et al. (eds), *Chronicling Poverty: The Voices and Strategies of the English Poor, 1640–1840* (Basingstoke: Macmillan, 1997), p. 131.

84 NLW MS 182-D, Remedy Collection and Miscellanea of 'Madam Lloyd' of Penpedust, undated, 18th century, p. 6.

7

Caring for the sick

As Mary Fissell points out, most early modern healthcare was just that: care.[1] Often, the historiographical emphasis lies so firmly upon sickness and treatment that discussions of care, the actual processes of looking after, and being looked after, fall by the wayside. In early modern Wales, but little is known about healing roles within the family, and especially the importance of gender roles in caring for the sick. Much emphasis is often laid upon the female medical role in the early modern household in both creating and applying medicines. Far less is known, as Fissell also points out, about how far men 'cared' in the early modern household.[2] This chapter will explore the issue of domestic care for the sick, with particular emphasis on gender healing roles within the family unit. It will also highlight the important medical relationships between parents and children, such as that of father and daughter, and foreground the important role of men in collating and recording household medical knowledge. Further, as evidence in Welsh sources demonstrates, care for the sick, and especially for children, was a shared responsibility, and we should not necessarily see women as the sole providers of medical care and treatment within the home.

At all levels of Welsh society, the main arena for sickness was undoubtedly the sufferer's home. There were few formal places of medical care available in Wales beyond the home until the nineteenth century. The lack of large towns in Wales meant that, unlike even provincial English towns such as Bristol, where the infirmary appeared as early as 1736, formalised medical care was not an option for the majority of the population.[3] In fact, it was not until 1814 that Wales had its first formal hospital with the opening of the Swansea dispensing hospital, which later became the infirmary in 1817. Sickness in early modern Wales, therefore, almost always required familial care. But how can this unit be defined? The early modern family has been the subject of much historical debate, and the terminology used has been roundly debated. As Naomi Tadmor has argued in her analysis of familial relationships in early modern England, the term 'family' was generally taken by contemporaries to mean the immediate, nuclear household of a male head and his dependents.[4] In this way, the 'family' might include house-hold servants who lived in, but not necessarily extended kin or close relatives who lived elsewhere.[5] This interpretation seems to fit with evidence from large parts of Wales, such as in Montgomeryshire, where 81% of the total number of households in Bishop Lloyd's 1680s proto-census consisted of a head and spouse, with between one and three children.[6] The average household size in Wales has been put at around 4.4 members, generally smaller than the English average, although some incidental evidence for Flintshire parishes suggests the average family size in poor Welsh households may have been as low as 3.15.[7] The family could, equally, however, encompass wider kin and blood relatives.[8] Kinship net-works could be predicated on a number of principles, from wider family such as cousins, nephews and nieces, matrilineal and patrilineal relatives by descent, to relatives by law, such as step-children and sons/daughters-in-law, but friends and other relations.[9] For the time being, however, we will concentrate upon the domestic, nuclear family.

In the early modern period, physicking the family was, at least culturally, part of the domestic duties of women, and they were expected to have a basic knowledge of herbs and medical preparations.[10] The important role of women in the care process has long been stressed, and female medical care was doubtless part of the wider household economy which included care of the household as much as care of children and the sick. Early modern healthcare involved large amounts of time devoted to the physical needsof the sufferer, such as preparation of medicines, maintenance of the fire and laundry, all traditionally female domes-tic tasks. Many early modern remedies were likewise extremely labour-intensive, often requiring many stages of preparation and continuous monitoring. Women were certainly regarded as legitimate sources of domestic medical authority, and, in areas such as midwifery, their authority as experts on the female body, birth cycles and such matters as bastardy was noted.[11] In English poor law records, it was women who were called upon to act as nurses, carers, laundresses, watchers of the sick and so on.[12] Female practitioners, however defined, also certainly existed in large numbers, and recent work has shown the extent to which they were often participant in 'orthodox' medicine, with a range of publications tai-lored towards specifically female practice.[13] Broadly, then, women 'cared' and were largely expected to do so. This was certainly the case in Wales, as Michael Roberts has pointed out, since the female role as mother and carer was also no less deeply embedded within Welsh culture, and was reinforced through popular legends and stories from the early modern period through to the nineteenth century.[14] Welsh women, moreover, were confident in being able to invoke their 'natural' caring role, and sometimes did so in cases of child custody. Garthine Walker notes the sixteenth-century example of one Agnes Thomas, who claimed guardianship of her child by drawing upon discourses of her maternal role, and nursing the child 'as in nature she is most bound to do'.[15]

And yet, as historians have recently begun to argue, the extent to which women were solely and uniformly responsible for medicating the household should be questioned.[16] As Elaine Leong has argued, it is easy to overstate the extent to which idealised, published, views of women's domestic duties were accurate at grassroots level, since men had at least as strong an interest in the collection and exchange of medical remedies as did women.[17] In fact, for Wales, it is also worth noting that primary sources are largely quiet about women's caring duties within the family home. Some discussion of women as domestic carers follows below, but Chapter 8 will explore female carers in more detail in context of their wider roles within the community. While the female caring role has been well defined in medical historiography, though, the male domestic medical role has received scant attention. Domestic medicine in Wales, as we shall see, was a shared responsibility. Clearly, at the most basic level, it was the household family who looked after the sick within their own walls but his provision depended greatly on *who* was sick. With these points in mind we turn to the issue of domestic care in early modern Wales.

The household family and the domestic medical environment

Within individual households, people took a pragmatic approach to the sickness of a family member, and care of the sick was clearly a shared responsibility. Sickness disrupted normal familial routines at all levels of Welsh society: it involved complex decision-making, such as options of diagnosis and treatment, and could radically alter the dynamics of power and division of labour within a household. At its most serious, it could threaten self-sufficiency and productivity, and even throw entire families into poverty.[18] For the sufferer, sickness represented a disruption to daily life, and was clearly recognised as a legitimate reason for excusal from work or social duties. In a 1674 petition to the Bishop of St David's, the parishioners of Llandeilo Fawr wrote in support of their curate, John Mathias, accused of not appearing in the Bishop's court, arguing that his 'sickly infirme constitution of body [put him] in a desperate lingering condition, unable to goe or ride'.[19] Likewise, in 1707, John Davies of Trewylan wrote to Thomas Cupper at Chirk Castle, excusing himself from attendance there due to a distemper and jaundice which he feared was 'creeping upon me'.[20] For the rest of the family too, though, disruption to familial routines was inevitable and this could even affect usual social roles. For women, the presence of a sick husband meant more domestic work, laundry and physical attendance, as well as the necessity to mix and administer medicines. The sickness of a male provider might also subvert normal familial roles and place women in the role of breadwinner. Around 1700, Mary Jones of Llandenny, Monmouthshire was pushed into severe financial difficulties when her husband, a labourer, fell sick and was unable to pay rent on their cottage. After four years of looking after her husband, by now 'broken and gone old', and struggling to raise their three children, Mary wrote a desperate letter to a local magistrate, entreating him to help her and 'take pitty on your poor parishoners [and] . . . be as charitable as you can'.[21] Likewise, when John Jones of Gyfylliog died in 1721, his wife Anne was left to raise seven children between the ages of two months and ten years, forcing her upon the mercy of the parish and into an earning role.[22] This situation could also happen in reverse however. Robert Bulkeley of Dronwy was forced to take over some domestic responsibilities, such as ordering and preparing food, when his wife fell ill in January 1631.[23]

To access the actual processes of care, however, is difficult since few Welsh sources yield much detailed information on the subject. No diaries or similar sources provide narratives of sickness episodes which include specific details of care. Far more often, as in the examples noted from probate inventories in Chapter 5, references are made to those who 'cared' or 'looked after' a patient in their sickness, without mention of how that was actually done. In several examples of letters from men which mention the sickness of their wives, there is frustratingly little evidence of physical care, with the majority merely noting the sickness episode.[24] Letters from Magdalen Lloyd in Chirk, Denbighshire, to her cousin Thomas Edwards in 1680 provide brief glimpses of the problems of nursing a difficult patient. Apparently looking after an elderly aunt, Magdalen noted the difficulties in getting the old lady to eat or take medicines, and noted that 'she takes nothing of sustenance'.[25] In an earlier letter, she worried at not having the correct medicines for her aunt's condition, and was forced to send out for more.[26] Overall, however, the problem lies in assessing how much domestic medical preparation was done by the patient themselves when they were able, since correspondence often gives the impression that people self-medicated. The letter of John Davies, noted above, implies that Davies himself took responsibility for his own medication. Having been forced to stay in bed by his sickness, Davies noted that he had '4 times every day these 3 last taken Jesuit's Powder' and 'sent for some things to prevent ye jaundice'.[27] He seems to have taken responsibility both for ordering his own medicines and dosing himself. Other sources do make some fleeting references to help from others. Letters from Roger Jones of Talgarth to his brother during a prolonged bout of sickness show that he was at times reliant upon the care of others. Hindered on the one hand by the fact that his voice was 'almost totally lost' and on the other by having a servant who was 'thick of hearing', Jones called in desperation upon the services of the local innkeeper's wife who 'assisted in giving [him] the Puke'.[28]

As part of the household family, servants too could become domestic patients as well as carers, and the sickness of wage labourers could have serious effects for agricultural employers. In the years of high mortality of the late 1720s, Owen Davies of Llanfechell, Anglesey, wrote to his friend that 'I believe you are not overstocked with hands at Bodewryd & that Thomas depended on their staying. Those goe off for their health sake. It's so most part of the countrey over; hands are not to be had for love or money'.[29] The decision to undertake care for domestic employees was as much economic as it was sympathetic and there is, in fact, much evidence to show that Welsh employers treated their sick servants well. The account book of William Davies of Clytha, Monmouthshire, noted in Chapter 6, provides a number of useful details about his payments to his domestic servants, and this included payments when they were ill. In May 1718, Davies hired William Prosser to his service, at two pounds and four shillings wages. In June 1718, Prosser was unable to work for eleven days through sickness, and Davies noted that he paid him one shilling.[30] Davies, it seems, was a munificent employer, providing for the upkeep and maintenance of his servant, such as one shilling and sixpence 'paid for your stockings' and an unnamed amount 'paid for mending your shoose'.[31] In some cases, it seems that even non-domestic employees were allowed to move in to the family home and be cared for. A note in the 1707 probate inventory of William Cozen of Radyr states that Cozen was 'sick of ye sickness whereof he dy'd in the house of Edmund Rees, Yeoman, where he had lived for severall months then last past'.[32] Cozen was a labourer, not a domestic servant, whom Rees had allowed into his home to recover. Star Chamber records also show that employers sometimes had to pay for the care of servants injured in the course of their work, even if such duties were sometimes illicit. Faction fights in late sixteenth-century Cardiff led to many assaults and injuries, and it was often servants who were sent to do the dirty work. Several witnesses in a 1596 case testified that 'Edward Lewes did send to Cardiff on the day articulate . . . certain money to be employed towards the relief, cure, help and surgery of certain of his servants that then there lay at surgery, sore, hurt and wounded'.[33]

But, in terms of the gender roles of domestic medicine, there are certainly some indications in Welsh sources that while women were generally expected to perform the mechanical aspects of care, and be knowledgeable in the selection and preparation of medicines, some medical authority, at least as regards the acquisition and recording of medical knowledge, as well as some of the practical and economic aspects of medicines for the home, could fall on men. Here, though, caution must be exercised since literacy can skew the picture. Literacy levels across Europe were generally higher for men than women.[34] Literate women were most likely to belong to well-to-do families and, in fact, the correlation between medicine and female literacy can be usefully exemplified in the numbers of surviving English domestic remedy collections authored by women. Jennifer Stine, however, also argues that 'household practices were . . . a source of medical authority' and she places the collection of remedies firmly within the context of female power roles within the home.[35] Until fairly recently, the orthodox view of domestic remedy collections has tended to foreground the female role in assembling bodies of medical knowledge, and draw comparisons between the interlinking recipe cultures of medicine and cookery. Given the numbers of surviving collections by women, there are undoubtedly strong arguments for this, and such sources often highlight well the ways in which medicine could fall within the purview of women's domestic roles. There are indeed many examples of Welsh remedy collections which can be at least partially attributed to women.[36] To highlight a few examples, one 'Madam Lloyd' of Penpedust, near Cardigan, was the compiler of one such document in the early eighteenth century, and also appears to have been called upon for her medical services by local people.[37] Catherine Nanney, part of the large Nanney family of north Wales assembled a large collection of medical remedies, while, lower down the social scale, women like the untraced 'Mrs Spyors' of Cardigan were no doubt typical of Welsh housewives who had their own store of both kitchen and medical receipts.[38] On another level, however, the acquisition of medical knowledge could fall just as easily within the remit of paternalistic roles and the patriarchal duty of men to look after their families. As Welsh sources show, many men clearly did take an active part in domestic care.

It could be argued that domestic life was actually more disrupted when women fell ill and men were forced into the caring role. Men such as Robert Bulkeley, noted earlier, took over responsibility for some elements of running the household when their wives fell sick. But when faced with having to 'nurse' a sick wife back to health, men were in an isolated position. Conduct books for women laid special emphasis upon their house-running duties, and many volumes, such as *The English Housewife* or *The Good Huswifes Jewell*, were devoted to educating women in how to dose and treat a variety of conditions.[39] Women had a strong female support network of carers whom, as we shall see in the following chapter, they could call upon for advice and also to share in the caring duties. But although publications such as the *Gentleman's Magazine* devoted pages to new medical discoveries or remedies, there was little for men in terms of practical advice on actually how to care for a sick family member, with conduct literature concentrating mainly upon the moral and patriarchal duties of a male householder.[40] Medical interest for men, therefore, tended to be more towards the acquisition of medical knowledge than, unless forced by contingent circumstances, the application of physical care.

An interest in medicine was increasingly part of the intellectual pursuits of the better off. As Part II of this book has argued, gentry libraries often contained large stocks of medical books, while medical texts were also beginning to appear in the possessions of those much lower down the social scale by the end of the seventeenth century. But a large number of examples attest to the fact that Welsh men also appear to have been active in compiling remedy collections. Part of this can be attributed to the tradition of manuscript copying for personal collections, which most often belonged to men, while several gentry figures also seem to have authored their own remedy collections.[41] Many gentlemen, in particular, kept notes of anecdotes, tales and jokes which they could then quote verbatim.[42] Manuscript commonplace books and notebooks could contain a wide range of information, but the emphasis lay with the potential value of the information for future use.[43] Remedies were therefore just the sort of information which compilers of commonplaces, notebooks and diaries might want to include as a means of text collection for potential usage at a later point. The Brecon gentleman Philip Howell kept just such a document between 1628 and 1638. Amongst a variety of different types of information, Howell noted two remedies to kill worms in hollow teeth, one of which was provided, and apparently proved by, an acquaintance known only as 'RR'. The specificity of these two cures may indicate that Howell was particularly susceptible to tooth complaints and therefore only noted down remedies which he felt were particularly relevant to his case.[44]

Others were less selective and noted down a wide range of receipts to cover a greater number of eventualities. For John Meller of Erddig, Denbighshire, a large collection of remedies tied in with his interest in science and chemical medicines, and his 'Physical Observations' made notes about the effects of certain substances upon his body.[45] Henry, the fifth Baron Herbert of Cherbury kept a large remedy collection while one Sydney Vaughan is the attributed author of a remedy book in the Peniarth collection of the National Library of Wales.[46] This male authorship is even more noticeable in Welsh-language sources and, in fact, no Welsh-language remedy collections seem to have survived that can be definitely attributed to women, although this is far from conclusive. One possible explanation might be that Welsh-language sources often seem to be very deliberate and formal, unlike the sometimes prosaic and ad hoc English-language collections. This may indicate that they fall within the strong tradition of manuscript copying in Welsh, which was again largely a male practice.

In fact, the extent to which men collected remedies ad hoc in notebooks and diaries points strongly towards an active interest in procuring and recording domestic medicines. Here we must be cautious since it is clearly possible that men included medical remedies within their books at the specific behest of their (perhaps illiterate) wives. The numbers of ad hoc remedies appearing within men's non-medical sources, such as diaries, notebooks and miscellanies, however, are telling. In a random sample of ten such sources from the early modern period, all contained medical remedies, and often in large numbers.[47] The form of these remedies, however, also points to a materialistic interest in the actual processes of obtaining remedies. It is noteworthy too that men's sources often record specific details about the price and location of medical ingredients. In 1655, John Gwin visited a Bristol apothecary and made detailed notes about his transactions, even haggling over the price of the goods to obtain them cheaper than a relative who visited a shop further up the street.[48] For future reference he noted the exact location of this apothecary, 'in mary port streete over against the lambe'.[49] This is mirrored elsewhere. The commonplace book of Philip Howell of Brecon contained a remedy for toothache which required the ingredient henbane. Howell noted that the 'Henban[e] seed growes in the lanes or hie waies, for it is a weed that seedeth, the Appoticaries sells it by the Oz @ 6d'.[50] A letter containing a medical remedy addressed to Walter Middleton of Slebech, Carmarthenshire, pointed out that Middleton would not get as much of the medical powder Diascordium for his money in Wales as he would in London, and therefore directed him to purchase more than normally required. Mindful of the advice, Middleton kept the letter for future reference.[51] Responsibility for sourcing and purchasing medicaments could, then, fall within the purview of men as controllers of domestic finances. It may also be possible to read an element of control into such compilations. To collate the information within non-medical volumes introduced an element of ownership, making the owner a point of reference. It may be possible that men wished to retain some measure of control over a traditionally female activity, and that commonplace books and other such sources presented an opportunity to do so.

Apart from the physical aspects of care, we must also consider the importance of authority in terms of the seeking and giving of medical advice. As regards gender roles in the care of children, the importance of familial medicine and domestic care is often tied in with the concept of the physical space of the family dwelling as a place of healing, but it is clear that family medicine was not necessarily delimited by physical proximity.[52] Even when children had moved away, parents continued to take a strong interest in their well-being, providing advice and remedies where necessary. In this way, a strong link remained with the concept of the home as the ultimate repository of knowledge and care. Care of children, and especially infants, however, was clearly a collective responsibility, and both parents undertook the physical and spiritual nurturing of their offspring. In better-off households, maternal care was sometimes supplemented by additional child nurses. Servants were often essential to the smooth running of the household and it is highly likely that they played a key role in support of the primary carer.[53] In the absence of both parents, servants could be greatly involved in the care of children. When Sir Charles Kemeys was away in London, his wife Mary was left to cope with a seriously ill child. A letter written to Kemeys in 1702, shows that Mary was prepared not only to defer some of the caring duties on to a family nanny, but even to consult her on the suitability of medical practitioners.[54] In poorer households the large size of some families meant that child-caring duties may even have been shared between neighbours.

In terms of responsibility for medicating children, however, there is strong evidence in Welsh sources to show that men played a central role in providing medical advice for their offspring, and also that their opinions were often actively sought, especially by older or grown up children. When the daughter-in-law of William Griffith of Trefarthen on Anglesey fell ill in 1640, it was to him, rather than a medical practitioner, that she wrote from her home in Caernarvon to ask for advice. His reply contained detailed descriptions of the medicines she should take as well as directions for general conduct and regimen. Griffith was particularly keen to learn of the effects of his advice, and entreated her to 'lett me heere from you soone iii dayes after howe you doe'.[55] It is reasonable to assume that his was not the only advice sought, since common practice was to obtain the opinions of a wide range of people. It is possible that Griffith had some recognised proficiency in medicine, and that this was the reason for the consultation. His daughter-in-law recognised him as a source of medical authority, and Griffith clearly considered himself sufficiently qualified to answer in some detail. The seeming strength of this paternal medical advice role is reinforced in another unusual source, a letter written from Frances Ridgway to her father Sir William Mawrice of Clenennau in 1620. The circumstances of the letter are unclear, but hint at an earlier estrangement between father and daughter. Frances wrote that she was visited 'with a greate sicknes' leaving her 'in great miserie' and her children in grave danger.[56] In begging for his help, Frances invoked the strength of the paternal bond through the 'tender bowell of fatherly affection' and entreated him to send relief and 'yor fatherly blessing'.[57] Fathers were also not slow to use their social positions in order to try and secure advice or treatment for their offspring, even after they were married. In 1664, John Lloyde of Wigfair wrote to a kinsman in London asking advice on the possibility of having his daughter 'sickly of a long tyme . . . [and] troubled with the Kings Evill . . . to have access to the Kings Royall P[er]sone to have his gracious touch'.[58] As Margaret Pelling has pointed out, the father-daughter relationship has become more prominent in recent historiography, but this often privileges the relationship in terms of daughters caring for sick fathers, especially in the context of Victorian novelistic conventions.[59] It does seem here, however, that the father of the family was viewed as being a source of medical authority, both within and beyond the home.

Absent fathers also continued to take a strong interest in the health of their children. From his office in London, the MP for Pembrokeshire, John Campbell, wrote letters to his son Pryse back on his estate near Carmarthen, dispensing paternal advice as well as keeping track of his son's ailments and maladies. The boy's health took up much space in the letters and, unable to attend his son personally, Campbell could do little more than encourage Pryse to do 'everything the Dr orders' and to 'take his physick like a Man'.[60] Philip Henry also wrote several times to his son Matthew, living in London, offering advice on his symptoms. In May 1686, upon hearing that Matthew was unwell, Henry wrote to chastise him for not resting after being let blood, arguing that it was 'convenient after blood-letting to bee sedate'.[61] On another occasion, noting that Matthew was 'subject to feavors', Henry warned him not to drink small beer or sack, which would overcool his body.[62] Fathers understood and were prepared to take some responsibility for managing the humoral balances of their offspring. They were also confident enough to invoke this knowledge, even for grown up children. Lisa Smith has argued that, increasingly during the eighteenth century, fathers were exhorted to provide medical advice to their offspring, both in terms of a healthy body influencing a healthy mind, but also as part of wider ideas about the importance of a healthy population.[63] Despite their not necessarily being physically present to dispense advice, the importance of the family, and especially of fathers, as points of medical reference is clear from these examples.

But such concern for family health extended beyond the nuclear family and into wider kin, such as nephews and nieces, aunts and uncles, and they too could be regarded as sources of medical authority. This could sometimes occur even when there was great distance between correspondents. Charles Lloyd of Drenewydd wrote several letters to Edward Wynne, Chancellor of Hereford, in 1739, in which he enquired about the health of his 'dear neece', Wynne's wife Anne.[64] Lloyd took particular interest in both the health and treatment of his niece, and seemed to have a detailed knowledge of her symptoms and regular medicines. In one letter he hoped that 'her asses milke will have its usual goode effect' implying that he understood the correct medicines for her constitution.[65] Another series of letters from a different branch of the same family kept the Lloyd sisters Jane and Elizabeth in regular contact with their aunt, 'Madam Wynn', and both their own health, and that of their mother, was a constant topic.[66] We have, in Chapter 4, also encountered remedies from wider kin, with the use of 'My aunts [remedy] for and forth continued swelling above a mouth', amongst documents from the Seys family of Ogmore.[67] In general, however (the above case of Magdalen Lloyd excepted), such letters do not indicate that kin participated to any great extent in the *physical* care of relatives. More attention should be devoted to family medical correspondence, and to the question of kin participation in the sickness experience. At least theoretically, kin were expected to provide relief to poor or needy relations.[68] Consanguineal (blood) kin were obviously a strong source of medical information, but a greater insight is needed into how far these patterns were repeated across other, wider, kinship categories. Medical kin relationships also extended beyond immediate family or relations living nearby. The commonplace book of John Gwin, for example, contains remedies from Gwin's wife's cousin, Walter Cradock, who was therefore not blood-related to Gwin himself.[69] Such communication could be viewed as an attempt by kin to continue to play an active part in familial sickness experiences, the letters acting as a proxy in lieu of physical presence. In fact, given the complexities of the early modern kinship system, and the potentially wide network of kin contacts within individual networks, medical advice and correspondence from wider family can provide a lens through which to view questions such as trust, and the reliability of information gained through familial association.[70]

Medical practitioners

One issue we have yet to deal with is that of medical practitioners. How far were 'doctors' a part of the sickness and care experience in early modern Wales? Clearly, the decision to seek the services of a medical practitioner lay first and foremost with the individual sufferer. As much recent historiography has convincingly shown, the early modern patient exercised a great deal of agency in the types of practitioners they consulted. They assessed the efficacy of remedies, sought multiple opinions and doubtless exercised their own agency in determining the ultimate sources of their care.[71] Much has been written (and continues to be written) about the Welsh doctor, although such depictions usually follow a well-trodden path. In the 1920s, in his unfinished medical history of Wales, David Fraser-Harris wryly commented that 'if one were suddenly asked to say for what the Welsh were noted as a nation, we [would] not answer "contributions to the practice of medicine"'.[72] In the 1970s and 1980s, historians wrote of Welsh 'so-called doctors', different entirely to skilled physicians, cited a 'stagnant and backward-looking profession', and proclaimed its members staunchly opposed to new ideas.[73] The trend continues to this day. In his recent work on witchcraft in Wales, Richard Suggett notes that 'physicians, surgeons, apothecaries and other specialists . . . usually practiced in towns'.[74] Quoting the 1694 complaint of the parishioners of Llandegly in Radnorshire that the parish had 'no doctor of physick, midwife nor surgeon', Suggett concludes that this was 'presumably the rule rather than the exception throughout rural Wales'.[75] Such views are mirrored elsewhere in Welsh medical historiography, where articles about Welsh practitioners tend to rely on a well-worn list of 'usual suspects', from the Physicians of Myddfai to Thomas Wiliems of Trefriw, from Edward Lhuyd to the 'Silurist' Welsh poet and physician Henry Vaughan.[76] Little attention has been paid to 'regular' doctors in Wales, with an apparent assumption that they numbered few and mattered little to the early modern Welsh population.

This paucity of 'orthodox' medical practitioners is generally set against a vibrant and enduring irregular Welsh medical practice, consisting of cunning folk, healers, charmers, conjurors, 'Dewiniaid' (wizards), bonesetters, all in all, in Roy Porter's words, a 'ragtag and bobtail army' of ready healers.[77] Of the widespread popular belief in, and acceptance of, the power of such figures in Wales there can be little doubt. The relative failure of the Protestant Reformation to impact upon the deeply entrenched ancient and pre-Reformation rituals almost certainly aided retention of beliefs in the power of the supernatural, and reinforced the invoking of various physical and metaphysical forces in the service of healing. Moreover, cunning folk and local healers, in constructing their magical charms and blessings, drew upon popularly understood discourses of both Catholicism and Non-conformity, making them at once familiar and trustworthy.[78] The rural and upland environment of much of Wales meant that life in small, close-knit communities was the norm and the community played a strong part in processes of care. Moreover, local healers relied on reputation; they gained power and legitimacy through repeated consultations and deployed a range of tactics to ensure that their own practices remained esoteric and inaccessible to 'ordinary' people.

In a sense, the quantity and quality of existing studies of these types of healers in Wales renders further discussion here largely superfluous. Their survival and popularity have been amply proved, and it is not my intention to downplay the significance of supernatural and magical healing for large sections of the early modern Welsh population. What is proposed, however, is an alternative view. The extent of the access of ordinary people in Wales to 'regular' medicine, and especially in rural areas, has tended to be overlooked or even ignored. As Lisa Tallis has recently argued, the majority of work on unorthodox practice in Wales concentrates merely upon the magical aspects of cunning folk and other such healers. What is often forgotten is the extent to which they were also 'orthodox' practitioners.[79] Should we even, in fact, consider the two as being separate entities? Likewise, as Ian Mortimer's research on the south-west of England has demonstrated, even urban practitioners could work within a wide sphere, serving outlying rural areas as well as their urban bases.[80] In this part of the chapter, I want to re-examine the question of Welsh medical practice by looking anew at the role of Welsh doctors in everyday sickness experiences. As well as utilising magical, or else folkloric, medicine, people in all parts of Wales in fact had access to 'orthodox' medical practitioners in the sense that, as Tallis points out, this 'orthodoxy' was ubiquitous and not limited to towns.[81] On the part of medical practitioners themselves, I will argue that there was a growing desire to be accepted and legitimised, and even a sense of professional pride amongst Welsh practitioners, evidenced in their adoption of professional nomenclature, and most importantly the term 'doctor'. Such figures played an important part in the sick rituals of Welsh people, and we should not see their practices as binary opposites to any sort of 'regular' medicine. Moreover, a new case study of practitioners in Wales has wider import: it asks new questions of the relationship between centres and peripheries, and also between urban and rural, and sheds light on a region far away from the control of the centres of medical licensing and regulation.

So who were these people? How were they trained? What did they do? The first question to address concerns the medical hierarchy in Wales. To stick to the well-trodden model of medical practice for a moment, there was, at least notionally, a tripartite hierarchy of medical practitioners in England, based largely on assumptions of professionalism and training. At the apex of this pyramid were university trained physicians, followed on the lower levels by surgeons and apothecaries, with a homogeneous base level of unlicensed, lay, magical or else irregular healers. Given the lack of a Welsh university, and the distance from medical centres, the traditional view of the Welsh medical hierarchy has been to remove the top of this pyramid, leaving the lower levels of village healers and cunning folk, punctuated by the odd surgeon or urban 'doctor'. There can be no doubt that such figures were widespread and had great popular appeal, not least in their accessibility, reputations and also familiarity. But other types of practitioners also flourished in Wales during this period. Apothecaries were dispersed widely across Wales and could be found in a variety of rural and urban locations. Despite imperatives to become licensed, and a nominal ban on practising, Welsh apothecaries performed an important function, often serving as both doctor and dispensing chemist.[82] However, it is another group of healers, the doctors or physicians, upon whom the remainder of this chapter will concentrate.

Of an elite group of Welsh physicians in any sense there is little evidence, at least in terms of university training or licensing. As we have already noted, the lack of medical training facilities in Wales meant that attainment of a medical degree was contingent upon the applicant leaving Welsh soil and relocating to Oxford or London. Far away from the purview of the London Colleges, unlicensed practice flourished. During the seventeenth century, a number of Welsh practitioners sought Diocesan licences, and the number of applications seems to have increased markedly after 1750.[83] Why were there not more applicants before then? Firstly, it is possible that the lack of pressure from external forces to actually prosecute unlicensed physicians in Wales may have rendered the possession of a licence superfluous. There were, moreover, few instances of actual prosecutions for unlicensed practice in Wales. Some Welsh doctors were even openly disdainful of licensing in general. At the end of the eighteenth century, William Jones of Llangadfan grumbled at the pretensions of those who 'plume themselves on their dignity of being licensed'.[84] As a group, Welsh practitioners sometimes appeared to be jealously protective of their 'Welshness' and took a certain degree of pride in their distance from English physicians. Such was certainly the case when William Wynn of Gwydir was refused treatment by a Welsh practitioner because he had already consulted a London doctor.[85] Yet many others clearly did view the obtaining of a medical licence as a legitimate badge of authority, possibly in an effort to distance themselves from pejorative images of rustic herbalism and align themselves with the world of the medical professional. Perhaps the strongest evidence of this is in the continued use of the word 'doctor' by Welsh physicians. Great numbers of Welsh sources attest to the use of the title 'doctor' and some go even further. The Metaphysical poet Henry Vaughan, for example, was referred to in his will as 'Dr of Physyk' and his gravestone apparently included the letters 'M.D.' despite his apparently never having taken a degree.[86]

A large number of Welsh probates occur for medical practitioners under a range of titles, the use of such titles implying that this is how they were commonly referred to in life. During the early modern period, around thirty inventories exist for those listed as either 'surgeon', 'chyrurgeon' or a variation such as 'barber-surgeon'. Five records occur for men described as 'physitian'. These men were John Fowles of Carmarthen, died 1717, Andrew Barnett of Wootton (Salop), died 1709, Thomas Litleton of Wrexham, died 1668, Philip Rosser of Carmarthen, died 1660 and William Williams of Carmarthen, died 1774.[87] A further sixteen wills can be found for those described as 'doctor' or 'doctor in phisick', as well as variations such as 'medicinal doctor' and 'practicer'.[88] Out of these, three inventories refer to practitioners identified, like Henry Vaughan, as 'M.D.', implying that they had achieved medical degrees.[89] Actually, only one of those listed, John Jones of Carmarthen, appears to have applied for a licence and, given the commonness of the name, whether this is even the same man is not certain. In 1717, a petition was made to the Bishop of St David's to grant a licence to a 'John Jones of Llandisil' (a town in Carmarthenshire) to practice 'physick and surgery' due to a lack of practitioners in that county.[90] Such men apparently represented a body of Welsh practitioners who were clearly known and referred to in 'official' terms, but had not necessarily been university-trained or licensed. Why, then, did they adopt the term 'doctor'? The use of this title by unlicensed practitioners was a well-known and increasing tactic in England, where apothecaries, by the mid-eighteenth century, were beginning to use the title in recognition of the duality of their functional role.[91] But the adoption of English medical nomenclature by Welsh practitioners was also perhaps a deliberate attempt to assume the authority and status which the title of 'doctor' implied, and also appears to predate the appropriation of the title by apothecaries. Welsh practitioners, even if they did not necessarily trouble to go through official channels were, nonetheless, still keen to distinguish themselves from lay practitioners and ally themselves with the medical profession. The fact also that Welsh doctors were seeking to employ English identifiers may also be significant, and adds a further dimension to this process.

One thing which is abundantly clear from Welsh sources is that people at all levels of Welsh society routinely consulted these figures as part of their treatment options. At the upper echelons of Welsh society, elites could afford the luxury of their own private physician. Sir John Wynn of Gwydir employed the Welshman Thomas Wiliems of Trefriw, while other wealthy gentry, such as Sir Thomas Aubrey of Llantrithyd, Glamorganshire, paid relatively large sums to doctors and apothecaries to treat their ailments.[92] Predictably, the opportunity to secure a wealthy patron was not to be missed, and Welsh doctors vied for position to try to gain exclusive practising rights by discrediting their rivals. In Wynn's case, his consultations with another practitioner, Alexander Read, caused friction when Read reacted angrily to comments about his abilities made by Thomas Wiliems, and stated that he 'would be taught by no apothecary'.[93] Likewise, in 1691, John Powell of Carmarthen, a Welsh physician licensed by the Archbishop of Canterbury to practice medicine and surgery within the dioceses of Hereford and Llandaff, also took issue with the instructions of another physician to his patron Sir Edward Mansell of Margam regarding treatment of his afflicted hands.[94] In a letter to John Williams, his friend and an employee of Mansell's at Margam, Powell wrote that he was 'not fully satisfied as to ye use of leeches to Sir Edwards hands', recommended by another practitioner, as he feared that they would 'rather draw ye humours now into ye hands than drain much out of them'.[95]

On the part of medical practitioners, and especially those of more wealthy patrons, there was a vested interest in maintaining a certain degree of esotericism in order to bolster a position of medical authority. This might be necessary to reassure the patient that they were paying for exclusive knowledge which only the practitioner possessed. During the early modern period, medical consultations were generally a two-way transaction where the practitioner was expected merely to confirm the patient's diagnosis rather than actually provide one.[96] In one sense, the use of a more scientific vocabulary represented an attempt by practitioners to exert medical power over the patient by occupying intellectually restricted ground.[97] This did not mean though that practitioners utilised a separate terminology; this would merely have led to confusion. Rather, they tended to embellish their diagnoses and remedies with terms less familiar to the layman. Thus, in receipts for treatments to one 'Capteine Dodds' of Flintshire in 1665 can be found such examples as 'A cordiall bolus' and 'A Decoction of Manna'.[98] These were in essence basic treatments, a 'cordiall bolus' being, according to the medical catalogue of the seventeenth-century doctor Thomas Fuller, a simple paste applied to encourage sweating.[99]

In larger houses, it was also common to hold accounts with individual practitioners or apothecaries for medical services, and surviving receipts give some idea as to both the types of treatments and the costs which could be incurred. In fact, as in England, in many cases, apothecaries and physicians/surgeons were clearly interchangeable. Surviving bills from John Surner, a Denbigh apothecary, to the Yorke family of Erddig, show that the use of practitioners was a regular occurrence. In April 1699, Surner made no less than thirteen separate trips to Erddig, virtually one every other day, and treated three members of the family, his bill amounting to one pound and twelve shillings for twenty-nine different items.[100] Surner's preparations also demonstrate a mix of 'orthodox' and Paracelsian chemical remedies. In amongst unguents, pills and purges, and specific treatments such as 'scaby eyes prepared', Surner also listed items such as 'Chymicaloyle of pill by the glasse', and 'sp[iri]t sol amoniacke' demonstrating his familiarity with various types of treatments.[101] The wealthy Pennant family of Whitford in Flintshire also regularly employed the services of a number of Welsh apothecaries and physicians, such as Robert Lloyd and Foulke Davies of Wrexham, and once again the sources indicate a range of treatments.[102] The amounts spent by the Pennants also range from simple preparations costing a shilling or a few pence, to complete treatments costing several pounds, as occurred in December 1703 when the cost of treating 'Madam Pennant' by Robert Lloyd amounted to more than seven pounds.[103] In another 1703 bill for treatment of 'Mad'm Pennant', several prescriptions relate to attacks of nerves or fits. Lloyd was obviously confident that his receipts of 'An Hysterick Julep' and 'Antihysterick pills' would prove the cure. It is only to be hoped that poor Lady Pennant did not suffer the potential side effects of the 'hysterick julep' which, according to Fuller's descriptions, included sickness and 'abominable fetid belching'![104]

No such receipts for medical services, however, can be found in the Welsh language. Clearly this is inconclusive since it may simply be the case that none have survived. The numbers of English language receipts may also reflect the fact that it was often the wealthier who could afford the services of medical practitioners, and it is in the household accounts of such figures that medical bills and receipts are most often found. Nevertheless, the lack of equivalent sources in Welsh suggests that the language of orthodox medical practice in Wales was in fact English. This eschewal of their native tongue points to the ambitions of Welsh doctors to appear more metropolitan to their aspiring patrons.

Also noteworthy is the extent to which practitioners might be used as a means to 'spring clean' the entire family, as well as ministering to sick individuals. In most examples of surviving bills, preparations for other family members, and sometimes even servants, are listed. When William Taylor visited David Pennant, father of the author and naturalist Thomas Pennant, in 1736 for example, he also provided 'the gargle' for Madam Pennant, and 'a purging draught for Miss Sally' – not one of his children – costing sixpence.[105] This is mirrored elsewhere. In 1743–47, bills from John Jackson, London apothecary, to Lord Herbert, the ninth earl of Pembroke, show that alongside entries for 'My Lord', there were prescriptions for 'Jenny White' and 'William Colly', presumably servants, as well as entries for the treatment of a 'coachman' and 'housemaid', and even a purge for his dog. Between January 1744 and May 1747, the number of individual prescriptions runs to an astonishing 848.[106] In some cases, wealthy families might seek the services of more than one 'elite' physician, especially in cases of prolonged illness. Surviving letters show that the sickly Lady Eleanor Stepney, wife of Sir John Stepney, sixth Baronet Llanelly, was attended by the licensed physician John Powell of Carmarthen, who sent regular receipts for medicaments, as well as Perrot Williams of Haverfordwest, a rising star of Welsh medical practice who in 1723 had reported to the Royal Society about the Welsh practice of inoculation against variola smallpox.[107] Lady Eleanor travelled to Bath to try to restore her health, sadly dying at the young age of thirty-two in 1743.

The seeking of medical opinions by letter was another apparently common practice amongst many sections of Welsh society, and had the added benefit of providing a useable, permanent record of the consultation. Margaret Bridges of Ogmore consulted several medical opinions for her ailments, and kept the detailed receipts amongst her records.[108] The unidentified doctor who wrote to Walter Middleton of Slebech, Carmarthenshire (died c. 1720), included details of the necessary prices and measurements in his receipt, showing Middleton that he would do better to send to London for the ingredients where he would get more for his money.[109] Postal consultations highlight the important role that medical practitioners could play even in domestic networks, since their remedy, once sent, became part of the domestic knowledge economy and, in effect, a proxy consultation of itself. It could be reused at a later date without further recourse to the practitioner and also recycled for the use of others.

Medical practitioners and the lower orders

Even lower down the social scale, it is clear that 'doctors' played a part in sickness routines. The correspondence of Charles Lloyd of Drenewydd and Edward Wynne, noted above, records the role of physicians in the sickness of Lloyd's niece. In one letter Lloyd congratulated Wynne on his choice of practitioner, 'who must be an honest Gent by his use of kitchen physick'. Good, basic medicine could evidently be viewed with equal favour as the ministrations of learned physicians.[110] The mid-seventeenth-century commonplace book of John Gwin of Llangwm contains references to his having consulted a 'Doctor Richard Greadar', unfortunately untraced, but who treated both Gwin and his family with Helmontian and Paracelsian chemical remedies.[111] For those with modest incomes, such consultations might involve a range of healers, and sometimes for the same condition. In 1653, Walter Powell of Llantilio, Monmouthshire, consulted three different practitioners in two months in an attempt to cure his cataracts.[112] As well as regularly consulting a 'Mr Bray', apparently his regular physician, he also consulted a 'D[oct]or Bold', 'Doctor Middleton' and 'D[oct]or Brees'.[113] In using this term, Powell appears to endorse them as 'regular' healers. On another occasion, he noted that his eyes were 'cooched by Anthony Atwood', here not given a title. Thus, in Powell's view, Atwood was perhaps not in the same category and was instead perhaps a lay healer, an occulist specialising in cataracts or even a cunning man.[114]

Reputation was perhaps the single most important aspect in practitioner choice, and it is this which foregrounds the ubiquity of local lay healers. Healers, and cunning folk especially, relied on a veil of secrecy over their medicaments; they needed to retain an air of inaccessibility and esotericism in order to preserve the illusion that they possessed secret or magical knowledge unavailable to the patient.[115] Cunning folk tended to be members of the local community, often performing other trades or functions, and patronage of their services made sense in both financial and social terms inasmuch as they were familiar and accessible. But this same familiarity perhaps made it easier for magical healers to exploit the credulity of local clients, and furnish them with nothing more than placebos, and sometimes even well-known 'regular' medicines subsumed within ritual and magical paraphernalia. A woman accused of bewitching her neighbours with a magic powder in a sixteenth-century trial argued that it was nothing more than burnt alum recommended for her own toothache by a respected physician, and which she had passed on.[116] Even 'regular' practitioners could sometimes be cautious with their remedies, despite the London College of Physicians' boast that, unlike lay healers, their doctors did not hold secret remedies. When Mary Kemeys consulted a 'sea chirurgion with experience beyond sea' regarding her infant daughter's illness, she 'would not venter until he would till us what his medicines were which he did on our promising not to till any one wt ye ingredients were'.[117] In many respects then, and especially in the types of remedies they prescribed, both regular and lay practitioners were merely different branches of the same tree.

When and for what types of conditions did people consult medical practitioners? Here we are at something of a disadvantage, since there are few surviving practitioner records from which to draw conclusions. As such, the 1681 probate accounts of James Preston, a 'Chirurgeon Barber' of Wrexham, are especially important, since they provide a list of monies due to Preston for various cures. On this evidence, Welsh practitioners treated a variety of both minor and serious conditions, and for people across the social spectrum. They also seemingly tailored their fees towards the incomes of the patient, giving even the lower orders access to the services of a 'regular' doctor. It is firstly clear that people sought outside medical attention for conditions which they could not easily treat themselves, or which required some degree of skill to apply. As Ian Mortimer has pointed out, the potential distance between the patient and practitioner certainly affected treatment decisions, and he notes that minor conditions were more likely to be treated 'in house' in cases where a practitioner was some distance from the home, such as remote rural areas.[118] In Preston's records there are several cases of what might be considered routine medical attention, or else the continued treatment of pre-existing medical conditions or wounds. Thus did Hugh Roberts owe money for 'dressing his legg', while another reference related to 'letting bloud and glistering Mr Owens', demonstrating the involvement of practitioners in regular health regimens.[119] Given the commonness of accidental trauma during the early modern period, treatment of accident wounds was clearly another part of the practitioner's remit, and Preston attended injuries relating to falls from a horse, as well as those caused by a physical assault. In terms of specific conditions, the list is less satisfactory, since in many cases the document merely lists 'the cureing of' a particular person. Nevertheless, two references are made to the 'dress of a squinsey' and for 'cureing [William Whittmore] of a squinsey'. Squinsey (otherwise squinancy or quinsy) was a painful inflammation and sometimes abscess of the throat and one which was certainly considered as potentially dangerous, and not only to the patient.[120] In 1657, an Essex minister died of a gangrenous finger after putting it into the mouth of a man suffering from quinsy –the patient had unintentionally bitten him.[121] Another specific condition mentioned is a 'Bustion' appearing on a finger. Although it is difficult to identify, it may well refer to a painful excrescence, running sore or ulcer, which might be difficult to treat at home. Records are also made of non-specific cures for particular parts of the body, such as 'the cure of Sarah Evans Throat' or 'the cure of [Phillip Hughes's] thighe'.[122]

More widely, it does seem clear that Welsh people were prepared to seek outside medical attention for their children. Firstly, in some ways, child illness was more closely interrogated than that of adults for possible evidence of witchcraft. People monitored the health of their children, as they did their own, but symptoms which appeared irregular or suspicious immediately became subject to scrutiny. Many Welsh witchcraft cases, for example, centred upon children and the perceived intervention of witches in cursing or disabling them.[123] But a desire to seek outside intervention in cases of child illness also reflected the acknowledged danger of illness in children. Lawrence Stone's now roundly contested view that parents did not invest emotional capital in their children for fear of losing them is also not borne out by the physical and economic lengths which some parents went to in trying to restore their children to health.[124] The Anglesey diarist Robert Bulkeley, provides good evidence of the use of outside practitioners for his son, Theophilus, over a prolonged recovery period and probably at considerable expense. On 26 November 1634, Bulkeley recorded, 'aboute sunset, the stacke of turves fell upon Theophilus & broke his thigh'.[125] Obviously in great pain, the boy was taken the next morning to two local practitioners, probably bonesetters, 'Jon Pue & Moris Lloyd [who] closed up his thigh'.[126] A month later, however, Theophilus was still clearly receiving treatment, having the same men redress his thigh and, again, in January 1635, Bulkeley noted that he 'pd Moris Lloyd for setting son Theo: bone 2s'.[127] In other cases, as with adults, it is clear that the services and opinions of many different practitioners were sought. In trying to establish whether the symptoms of his daughter were indeed the 'King's Evil', John Lloyde of Wigfair consulted several 'able & p[ro]ficient men in phisick' before turning to the question of treatment.[128] Likewise, the letters of Mary Kemeys to her husband Sir Charles, contain a variety of treatment options for their infant daughter, suffering from fits. Several were considered, even including sending the child to London to be seen by 'yt Lady yt cures fitts'.[129] People like Bulkeley and Kemeys could certainly afford to pay for such treatments, and the lack of evidence for practitioner consultations at a lower social depth is frustrating. But, even on this limited evidence, people seemed prepared to invest much time and expense in their children's health.

What sorts of people consulted these 'doctors'? If we return now to the social status of Preston's patients, the wide variety of social classes who sought the attention of practitioners can be discerned. At the upper social end of Preston's client base were several wealthy patrons. A debt owed by Owen Thelwall is likely to refer to the wealthy local gentleman and Justice of the Peace of this name, who resided in Llwyn-y-Knottie in Gresford.[130] The name 'William Whittmore' also appears in the account, perhaps Sir William Whittmore, MP for Bridgnorth, who died in 1695. Whitmore lived in Apley, Shropshire, but certainly had connections with estates in Denbighshire and Cheshire.[131] Lower down the social scale were local businessmen such as Hugh Roberts 'of the Red Lion' in Wrexham, and in a subsequent entry also listed as being 'of the Swann', making him potentially a fairly prosperous local figure.[132] But, as Joan Lane points out, the practitioner who treated the local gentleman often also treated middling sorts and poor alike.[133] Here we find poorer artisans such as 'John Davies, shoemaker' whose son

was cured by Preston.[134] For many of the remaining names on the list it is difficult to draw conclusions, especially with generic Welsh names such as 'David
Thomas', 'William Griffith' and 'Sarah Evans'. If we take the monies owed as
being representative of the fees charged by Preston, however, then it may also be
possible to aver something of the social classes of his patients from this, since the
evidence seems to point to the tailoring of fees to the individual.[135] In cures for
William Whittmore, three separate treatments are noted. The first refers to 'the
cure by which he was hurt by Mr Carter', perhaps injuries from an assault, but for
which he was charged the relatively large sum of five pounds. For 'ye cure of him
when he fell of his horse' Preston charged one pound, and a further pound 'for
cureing him of a squinsey'.[136] The fact that Whittmore appears to have regularly
consulted Preston, together with the amounts charged, implies fees relative to the
ability of a wealthy gentleman to pay. For 'dressing the leg' of Hugh Roberts, the
public house landlord, Preston charged the lower fee of one pound, with another
treatment costing seven shillings and the supply of a 'searcloth' at one shilling.
It might certainly be argued that Whittmore's needswere potentially greater (we
unfortunately cannot know the extent or seriousness of his injuries requiring
five pounds-worth of medical attention) but, on another level, this could also
be seen as a case of cloth being cut according to measure. In another instance,
Preston charged the same sum of a pound to cure both 'Edward Wills & his
wife'. Overall, eleven out of twenty-four treatments were charged at over one
pound, with 'Capt. Powell' and 'David Thomas', both unfortunately untraced,
being the recipients of cures totalling four and three pounds respectively. At the
other end of the scale, however, some cures were discharged for a few shillings.
For the treatment of his son, the shoemaker John Davies was charged the much
lower sum of three shillings and sixpence, while the lending of fifteen shillings to
Phillip Hughes, at the same time as charging two shillings and sixpence to attend
to his thigh, further hints at a poor man.[137]

It is also clear that people could on occasion act as intermediaries and even
beneficiaries for others, and secure treatment on their behalf. It is certainly possible that this was done sometimes through charitable interest. One record notes
the money owed to Preston by Owen Thelwall 'for ye cure of fool of Bangor,
soe called'. It is possible that, given his status, Thelwall sought to pay for the
compassionate treatment of a potentially mentally ill or disturbed parishioner
through conventions of munificent hospitality, or moral or religious obligation.
In another example, money was due to Preston from 'Mr Ed[war]d: Jones of
Havod y Bwch for ye cure of David George', perhaps a servant or employee. This
beneficence is reinforced by another entry in the debts of Hugh Roberts which
explicitly notes the cure of his maid. Also noteworthy is the way in which female
patients are often recorded in terms of being 'the wife of' a male parishioner,

rather than as patients in their own right.[138] This is supported by another source of a Welsh practitioner, Thomas Griffiths of Mold, whose pocketbook contains a small amount of information about his patients. In one entry, Griffiths records that 'Edward Dickson bro. me acc[ompanied] of his wife and Hannah Cooper the former supposed to be in a Consumption'.[139] The term 'brought' puts the responsibility for initiating the consultation firmly with Edward Dickson, rather than his wife. Such entries may simply reflect the fact that husbands were most likely to be paying for treatment of their wives, and thus appear on accounts and bills for this reason. Nevertheless, the distinction still seems apparent.

Conclusion

The evidence we have discussed here shows the extent to which sickness was very much a social and familial event. The sickness of a family member involved all members of the household, and both men and women participated in the physical care of the patient. While women clearly played a large part in the mechanics of care, the important role of men in both caring and also as sources of medical authority and knowledge should not be downplayed. Whilst it may be difficult to argue for well-defined medical gender roles within the household, the historiographical tendency to remove men from the care process should certainly be questioned. From the evidence here, it is also clear that practitioners played a large part in the Welsh sickness experience. Aside from the undoubted role of a range of lay healers, charmers and cunning folk in everyday medical practice, the importance of Welsh 'doctors', both licensed and unlicensed, I would argue, deserves greater recognition. There are clear signs that Welsh practitioners desired 'legitimacy' and aspired to be viewed as orthodox, and their numbers and spread should raise questions about the almost total dominance of magical and lay practice in Wales.

From the particular we now need to move to the general, and investigate wider structures of care, such as community provision and the Old Poor Law in early modern Wales. Chapter 8 will explore such factors within the important context of neighbourliness and shared community moral and religious obligations towards the sick. As will be argued, the early modern community in Wales played an important and active support role in caring for the sick and, in effect, became what might be regarded as an extended, if temporary, medical family.

Notes

1 See Mary E. Fissell, 'Introduction: Women, Health and Healing in Early Modern Europe', *Bulletin of the History of Medicine*, 82:1 (2008), pp. 11, 13.

2 Ibid., p. 13.

3 Mary E. Fissell, *Patients, Power and the Poor in Eighteenth Century Bristol* (Cambridge: Cambridge University Press, 2002 edition), pp. 74–75.

4 Naomi Tadmor, *Family and Friends in Eighteenth Century England* (Cambridge: Cambridge University Press, 2001), p. 19.

5 Ibid., pp. 22–23.

6 Melvin Humphreys, *The Crisis of Community: Montgomeryshire 1680–1815* (Cardiff: University of Wales Press, 1996), p. 31.

7 Geraint H. Jenkins, *The Foundations of Modern Wales, 1642–1780* (Oxford: Oxford University Press, 2002 edition), p. 91; Adrian Teale, 'The Battle against Poverty in North Flintshire, c. 1660–1714', *Flintshire Historical Society Journal*, 31 (1983/84), p. 79.

8 Will Coster, *Family and Kinship in England 1450–1800* (London: Longman, 2001), p. 6.

9 Ibid., p. 40.

10 Andrew Wear, *Knowledge and Practice in English Medicine, 1550–1680* (Cambridge: Cambridge University Press, 2000), p. 52; Lucinda McCray Beier, 'In Sickness and in Health: A Seventeenth Century Family's Experience' in Roy Porter (ed.), *Patients and Practitioners: Lay Perceptions of Medicine in Pre-Industrial Society* (Cambridge: Cambridge University Press, 2002 edition), p. 118.

11 For a good survey of women's domestic and public roles in a patriarchal culture see Bernard Capp, *When Gossips Meet: Women, Family and the Neighbourhood in Early Modern England* (Oxford: Oxford University Press, 2004).

12 Fissell, 'Introduction: Women, Health and Healing', p. 13.

13 See for example, Margaret Pelling, 'The Women of the Family? Speculation around Early Modern British Physicians', *Social History of Medicine*, 7:3 (1995), pp. 383–401; A.S. Weber, 'Women's Early Modern Medical Almanacs in Historical Context', *English Literary Renaissance*, 33:3 (2003), pp. 358–402.

14 Michael Roberts, 'Gender, Work and Socialisation in Wales c. 1450 – c. 1850' in Sandra Betts (ed.), *Our Daughter's Land: Past and Present* (Cardiff: University of Wales Press, 1996), pp. 22–23.

15 Quoted in Garthine Walker, '"Strange kind of Stealing": Abduction in Early Modern Wales' in Michael Roberts and Simone Clarke (eds), *Women and Gender in Early Modern Wales* (Cardiff: University of Wales Press, 2000), p. 59.

16 Lisa Smith, 'The Relative Duties of a Man: Domestic Medicine in England and France, ca. 1685–1740', *Journal of Family History*, 31:3 (2006), pp. 237–256; Margaret Pelling, *The Common Lot: Sickness, Medical Occupations and the Urban Poor in Early Modern England* (London and New York: Longman, 1998), p. 15, also see discussions pp. 179–202.

17 Elaine Leong, 'Medical Recipe Collections in Seventeenth Century England: Knowledge, Text and Gender' (University of Oxford: Unpublished DPhil Thesis, 2006), pp. 25, 27.

18 Steve Hindle, *On the Parish? The Micro-Politics of Poor Relief in Rural England, c. 1550–1750* (Oxford: Oxford University Press, 2009 edition), p. 48.

19 National Library of Wales (hereafter NLW), Church in Wales, Diocese of

St David's Episcopal (11) MS 1238, Petition of Parishioners of Llandeilo Fawr, Carmarthenshire, regarding ill health of their curate, 25 March 1674.

20 NLW, Chirk Castle (2) MS 4176, Letter from John Davies to Thomas Cupper, 23 April 1707.

21 NLW, Badminton 1 (Manorial 2) MS 2197, Petition from Mary Jones to John Burk esq. Undated, c. 1700.

22 NLW, Chirk Castle (7) MS 1153, Petition to Denbigh Quarter Sessions of Anne Jones of Gyfylliog, 1722.

23 Hugh Owen, 'The Diary of Bulkeley of Dronwy, Anglesey, 1630–1636', *Transactions of the Anglesey Antiquarian Society* (1937), p. 37.

24 See for examples NLW, Chirk Castle (2) MS 2843, Letter from John Davies to Richard Myddelton, 14 April 1747; NLW, Bodewryd (1) MS 552, Letter from Edward Wynne to Charles Lloyd, undated, c. 1739; NLW, Clenennau 2 (A) MS 494, Letter from Lewis Annwyl at Faenol to his father William Lewis Annwyl at Park, 29 April, 1636.

25 NLW, Chirk Castle (3) MS 4648, Letter from Magdalen Lloyd to Thomas Edwards, 30 October 1680.

26 NLW, Chirk Castle (3) MS 1362, Letter from Magdalen Lloyd to Thomas Edwards, 15 October 1680.

27 NLW, Chirk Castle (2) MS 4176, Letter from John Davies to Thomas Cupper, 23 April 1707.

28 NLW, D.T.M. Jones (3) MS 1196, Letter from Roger Jones at Talgarth to Reverend John Jones, 26 July 1771.

29 Leonard Owen, 'The Letters of an Anglesey Parson, 1712–1732', *Transactions of the Honourable Society of Cymmrodorion*, 1 (1961), p. 89.

30 Gwent Record Office, MS D/PA.29.10, Pocketbook of William Davies of Clytha, 1654–1720, p. 8.

31 Ibid., p. 9.

32 NLW MS William Cozen, LL/1707/155.

33 John Hobson Matthews (ed.), *Cardiff Records, Volume One* (Cardiff: Cardiff Corporation, 1898), p. 319.

34 Eryn M. White, 'Women, Religion and Education in Eighteenth-Century Wales' in Roberts and Clarke (eds), *Women and Gender*, p. 218; Geraint H. Jenkins, *Literature, Religion and Society in Wales, 1660–1730* (Cardiff: University of Wales Press, 1978), p. 274.

35 Jennifer K. Stine, 'Opening the Closets: The Discovery of Household Medicine in Early Modern England' (Stanford University: Unpublished PhD Thesis, 1996), p. 13.

36 NLW, Peniarth MS 517D, Medical Receipts of Catherine Nanney, c. 1730; NLW MS 1560C, Medical Remedies attr. Angharad Llwyd, 16th–17th century; NLW MS 182-D, Remedy Collection and Miscellanea of 'Madam Lloyd of Penpedust', undated, 18th century; Cardiff Central Library, MS 2.998, Medical Remedy Collection of 'Mrs Spyors', 1725.

37 NLW MS 182-D, Remedy Collection and Miscellanea of 'Madam Lloyd' of Penpedust, undated, 18th century, p. 6.

38 NLW, Peniarth MS 517D, Medical Remedy Collection owned by Catherine Nanney, c. 1730; Cardiff Central Library, MS 2.998, Medical Remedy Collection of 'Mrs Spyors', 1725.

39 Gervase Markham, *Country Contentments or The English Housewife* (London: Printed for R. Jackson, 1623); G. Steevens, *The Good Huswifes Jewell . . .* (London: Printed for Edward White, 1596).

40 Alexandra Shepard, *Meanings of Manhood in Early Modern England* (Oxford: Oxford University Press, 2003), pp. 70–71; Roy Porter, 'Laymen, Doctors and Medical Knowledge in the Eighteenth Century: The Evidence of the *Gentleman's Magazine*' in Roy Porter (ed.), *Patients and Practitioners: Lay Perceptions of Medicine in Pre-Industrial Society* (Cambridge: Cambridge University Press, 1985), pp. 291–295.

41 For examples see British Library, BM Add. MS 15078, Translation into Welsh by John ap Ifan of 'The Treasury of Health' by Humfrey Llwyd, unknown date; Cardiff Central Library, MS 2.973, Thomas ap Ifan, Meddygyniaeth, 17th century.

42 Adam Fox, *Oral and Literate Culture in England 1500–1700* (Oxford: Oxford University Press, 2000), pp. 39–40.

43 Earle Havens, '"Of Common Places or Memorial Books": An Anonymous Manuscript on Commonplace Books and the Art of Memory in Seventeenth Century England', *Yale University Library Gazette*, 76:3–4 (2002), p. 142.

44 Cardiff Central Library, MS 3.42, Commonplace Book of Philip Howell of Brecon, 1628–38, p. 76.

45 Flintshire Record Office, MS Erddig D/E/2547, John Meller, 'My Own Physical Observations', 1697, pp. 3–18.

46 NLW MS 5309B, Remedies in the hand of Henry, fifth Baron Herbert, undated, c. late 17th century; NLW, Peniarth MS 348(A), Remedy Collection attr. Sydney Vaughan, 1705.

47 Cardiff Central Library, MS 3.42, Commonplace Book of Philip Howell of Brecon, 1628–38; Cardiff Central Library, MS 5.50, Flintshire Miscellany, various dates, c. 1650; Flintshire Record Office, MS D/HE/432, Diary of Dr Thomas Griffiths of Mold, 1726; Gwent Record Office, MS D43:4216, Commonplace Book of John Gwin of Llangwm, 17th century; NLW MS 434B, Miscellaneous Collection of Robert Lloyd, c. 1656; NLW, MS 15-C, Commonplace Book of Michael Hughes of Lligwy/Richard Evans of Llanmerchedd, c. 1730–70; NLW MS 4492D, Notebook of Richard Phillips of Carmarthen, 1701; NLW MS 788B, Barddoniaeth Humphrey Owen, undated, c. 1665; NLW MS 1023B, 'Llyfr Cynghorion', Sermons and Notes of Ellis Owen, 1712; NLW, Peniarth MS 521A, Diaries and Notebooks of Griffith Wynn of Bodfaen, various dates, 17th century;

48 Gwent Record Office, MS D43:4216, Commonplace Book of John Gwin of Llangwm, 17th century, p. 18.

49 Ibid.

50 Cardiff Central Library, MS 3.42, Commonplace book of Philip Howell of Brecon, 1628–38, p. 76.

51 NLW MS 182-D, Bundle 2, No. 8, Letter to 'Walter Myddelton, Slebedge', undated, c. early 18th century.

52 Elaine Leong and Sara Pennell, 'Recipe Collections and the Currency of Medical Knowledge in the Early Modern "Medical Marketplace"' in Mark S.R Jenner and Patrick Wallis, (eds), *Medicine and the Market in England and its Colonies, c. 1450 – c. 1850* (Basingstoke: Palgrave Macmillan, 2007), p. 134.

53 Beier, 'In Sickness and in Health', p. 114.

54 NLW, Kemeys-Tynte (2) MS CA422, Letter from Mary Kemeys to Sir Charles Kemeys, 6 November 1702.

55 NLW, Clenennau 2 (A) 521, Letter from William Griffith of Trefarthen to this daughter-in-law, '15th of 8'ber, 1640'.

56 NLW, Clenennau (1) MS 40, Letter from Frances Ridgway to Sir William Mawrice, 14t March 1620.

57 Ibid.

58 NLW, Wigfair (2) MS 12402E, Letter from John Lloyde to unspecified recipient, 1664.

59 Pelling, 'The Women of the Family?', p. 385.

60 Carmarthenshire Record Office, MSS Cawdor 128, Stackpole Correspondence, Bundle 1, John Campbell to Pryse Campbell, 30 October 1733, 9tNovember 1733, 19 May 1734.

61 Matthew Henry Lee, *The Diaries and Letters of Philip Henry, M.A. of Broad Oak, Flintshire A.D. 1631–1696* (London: Kegan Paul, Trench and Co., 1882), p. 348.

62 Ibid., p. 361.

63 Smith, 'Relative Duties', p. 240.

64 NLW, Bodewryd (1) MS 530, Letter from Charles Lloyd to Edward Wynne, May 1739.

65 Ibid.

66 NLW, Bodewryd (1) MSS 148–51, Letters of Lloyd Family to 'Madam Wynn', various dates, 1715–22.

67 Glamorgan Record Office, MS D/DF V/206, Remedy in Possession of Seys Family, undated, c. late 17th century.

68 Hindle, *On the Parish?*, p. 49.

69 Gwent Record Office, MS D43:4216, Commonplace Book of John Gwin of Llangwm, 17th century, pp. 16–17.

70 For a useful discussion of the problems of accessing and understanding relationships with 'distant kin', see Coster, *Family and Kinship*, pp. 42–44.

71 For examples see Mary Lindemann, *Medicine and Society in Early Modern Europe* (Cambridge: Cambridge University Press, 1999), p. 199; Roy Porter, *Disease, Medicine and Society in England, 1550–1860* (Cambridge: Cambridge University Press, 2002 edition), p. 23; Pelling, *The Common Lot*, p. 30; Fissell, *Patients, Power and the Poor*, p. 35.

72 Wellcome Library, MS 8968, Notes and Drafts for Unfinished Volume, 'The History and Lore of Cymric Medicine' by David Fraser-Harris, c. 1928.

73 W.S.K. Thomas, *Stuart Wales* (Llandysul: Gomer Press, 1988), p. 190; W. Gerallt

Harries, 'Bened Feddyg: A Welsh Medical Practitioner in the Late Medieval Period' in John Cule (ed.), *Wales and Medicine* (Llandysul: Gomer Press, 1975), p. 178.

74 Richard Suggett, *A History of Magic and Witchcraft in Wales* (Stroud: The History Press, 2008), p. 72.

75 Ibid., p. 72.

76 For just some examples, G.C. Davies, 'The Welsh Doctor as a Poet: Henry Vaughan the Silurist' in Cule (ed.), *Wales and Medicine*, pp. 112–118; Glyn Penrhyn Jones, 'Some Aspects of the Medical History of Denbighshire', *Denbighshire Historical Society Transactions*, 8 (1959), esp. pp. 52–58; Morfydd E. Owen, 'The Medical Books of Medieval Wales and the Physicians of Myddfai', *The Carmarthenshire Antiquary*, 31 (1995), pp. 34–45.

77 Roy Porter, *Quacks: Fakers and Charlatans in Medicine* (Stroud: Tempus, 2003 edition), p. 43.

78 Lisa M. Tallis, 'The Conjuror, the Fairy, the Devil and the Preacher: Witchcraft, Popular Magic and Religion in Wales 1700–1905'(University of Wales, Swansea: Unpublished PhD Thesis, 2007), p. 308; Owen Davies, 'Cunning-Folk in England and Wales during the Eighteenth and Nineteenth Centuries', *Rural History*, 8:1 (1997), pp. 91–107; Owen Davies and Lisa Tallis, *Cunning Folk: An Introductory Bibliography* (London: The Folklore Society, 2005); Geraint H. Jenkins, 'Popular Beliefs in Wales from Restoration to Methodism', *Bulletin of the Board of Celtic Studies*, 27:3 (1977), pp. 440–462.

79 Tallis, 'The Conjuror', p. 173.

80 See Ian Mortimer, 'The Rural Medical Marketplace in Southern England, c. 1570–1720' in Mark S.R. Jenner and Patrick Wallis (eds), *Medicine and the Market in England and its Colonies, c. 1450 – c. 1850* (Basingstoke: Palgrave Macmillan, 2007), pp. 69–87.

81 Tallis, 'The Conjurer', p. 173.

82 Dorothy Porter and Roy Porter, *Patient's Progress: Doctors and Doctoring in Eighteenth Century England* (Cambridge: Polity Press, 1989), p. 126.

83 In the century and a half to 1750 there were only around six applications within Wales for licences. Between 1751 and 1790 alone there were eight. See NLW, Church in Wales, Diocese of Llandaff Episcopal Records, Testimonials Relating to Applications for Licences to Practise Medicine, MSS LL/SM/3; LL/SM/4; LL/SM/6; LL/SM/7; LL/SM/13; LL/SM/14; LL/SM/18; NLW, Church in Wales, Diocese of St David's Episcopal (11) MS 194, Testimonial concerning the grant of a licence to Isaac Rees of Llanwortyd, 18 August 1754. NLW, Eaton, Evans and Williams Collection (2A), MS 2843, Licence from Bishop of St David's to John Maddocks to Practise Medicine, 1708; NLW, Nanhoron MS 158, Licence to Practice Medicine granted by Jesus College Oxford to Francis Lloyd, 1737; NLW, Church in Wales, Diocese of St David's Episcopal (11) MS 193, Certificate and Fiat for a Licence of surgery for William Thomas of Llanelwedd, 1699; NLW, Church in Wales, Diocese of St David's Episcopal (11), MS 1196, Petition to license John Jones of Llandysul to practice physick and surgery, 2 September 1717; NLW, Church in Wales, Diocese of St David's Episcopal (11) MS 512, Petition requesting the grant of

a licence to Richard Prichard of Narberth, 9 August 1720; NLW, Church in Wales, Diocese of St David's Episcopal (9) MS SD/CCB/C(G)/1560, Faculty to David Smith of Swansea to practise surgery, 2 July 1683.

84 Quoted in Glyn Penrhyn Jones, 'Folk Medicine in Eighteenth Century Wales', *Folklife*, 7 (1969), p. 62.

85 Wellcome Library, MS 8985, Notes and Drafts for Unfinished Volume, 'The History and Lore of Cymric Medicine' by David Fraser-Harris, c. 1928.

86 NLW MS Henry Vaughan, BR/1695/151; Davies, 'The Welsh Doctor', p. 115.

87 NLW MSS John Fowles, SD/1717/18; Andrew Barnett, SA/1709/125; Thomas Litleton SA/1668/227; Philip Rosser, SD/1660/162; William Williams, B/1774/73.

88 For examples see NLW MSS Thomas Wright, SD/1745/5; John Barker, C/1692/10; John Lawrence, LL/1721/92; William Bold, SA/1725/30.

89 NLW MSS John Jones, SD/1698/17; Paul Tanner LL/1732/6; Robert Meller SD/1707/176.

90 NLW, Church in Wales, Diocese of St David's Episcopal (11) MS 1196, Petition to licence John Jones of Llandysul to practise physick and surgery, 2 September 1717.

91 Penelope J. Corfield, 'From Poison Peddlers to Civic Worthies: The Reputation of the Apothecaries in Georgian England', *Social History of Medicine*, 22:1 (2009), p. 2.

92 J. Gwynfor Jones, *The Wynn Family of Gwydir: Origins, Growth and Development c. 1490–1674* (Aberystwyth: Centre for Educational Studies, 1995), p. 129; Lloyd Bowen (ed.), *Family and Society in Early Stuart Glamorgan: The Household Accounts of Sir Thomas Aubrey of Llantrithyd, c. 1565–1641* (Cardiff: South Wales Records Society, 2006), pp. 58, 95, 114.

93 Jones, 'Folk Medicine', p. 56.

94 See Lambeth Palace Library, 'Directory of Medical Licences Issued by the Archbishop of Canterbury, 1535–1775', available at www.lambethpalacelibrary.org/files/Medical_Licences.pdf, accessed 10 February 2009.

95 NLW, Penrice and Margam (3) MS 1453, Letter from John Powell of Carmarthen to John Williams at Margam, 28 April 1691.

96 Roy Porter and Dorothy Porter, *Patient's Progress: Doctors and Doctoring in Eighteenth Century England* (Stanford: Stanford University Press, 1989), p. 78.

97 Ibid., p. 73.

98 Flintshire Record Office, Gwysaney MS D/GW/3/510, Apothecary Bills of Robert Seale to 'Capteine Dodds', 1665.

99 Thomas Fuller, *Pharmacopoeia Extemporanea: Or A Body of Prescripts in Which Forms of Select Remedies Accommodated to Most Intentions of Cure Usually Occurring in Practice* (London: Printed for Ben J. Walford, 1710), p. 30.

100 Flintshire Record Office, Erddig MS D/E/255, Medical Bills from John Surner of Denbigh to Yorke Family of Erddig, 3 June 1699.

101 Ibid. This is probably sal-amoniac, an ingredient used by Paracelsus in various preparations. See for example, Edward Arthur Waite, *Hermetic and Alchemical Writings of Paracelsus*, 2 Volumes (Whitefish, MT: Kessinger Publishing, 2002), Volume 1, p. 379.

102 Flintshire Record Office, MSS D/NA/636–49, Misc. Pennant Family Papers inc.

Medical Receipts, 1681–1736; Flintshire Record Office, MS D/NA/646, Medical Bills from William Taylor to Thomas Pennant, October 1736.

103 Flintshire Record Office, MSS D/NA/636–49, Misc. Pennant Family Papers inc. Medical Receipts, 1681–1736.

104 Flintshire Record Office, MS D/NA/636–49, Misc. Pennant Family Papers inc. Medical Receipts, 1681–1736; Fuller, *Pharmacopoeia Extemporanea*, p. 247.

105 Flintshire Record Office, MS D/NA/646, Medical Bills from William Taylor to Thomas Pennant, October 1736.

106 NLW, Powis Castle Deeds(3), Bill of Remedies for Lord Herbert, Delivered by John Jackson, 1743–47, unpaginated.

107 See Perrot Williams, 'Part of two letters concerning a method of procuring the Small Pox, used in South Wales, From Perrot Williams, M.D., Physician at Haverfordwest, to Dr Samuel Brady, Physician to the Garrison at Portsmouth', *Philosophical Transactions of the Royal Society of London*, 32:374 (1723), pp. 262–264; NLW, Cilymaenllwyd MSS 174, 181, 186, Letters from Dr John Powell and Dr Perrot Williams to 'Lady Stepney', 1728–31.

108 Glamorgan Record Office, MSS D/DF V/202–5, Medical Letters Addressed to Margaret Bridges, c. 1628.

109 NLW MS 182-D, Bundle 2, No. 8, Letter to 'Walter Myddelton, Slebedge', undated, c. early 18th century.

110 NLW, Bodewryd (1) MS 552, Letter from Charles Lloyd to Edward Wynne, 13 July 1739.

111 Gwent Record Office, MS D43:4216, Commonplace Book of John Gwin of Llangwm, 17th century, pp. 37–39.

112 Joseph, Alfred Bradney (ed.), *The Diary of Walter Powell of Llantilio Crossenny in the County of Monmouth 1603–1654* (Bristol: John Wright and Co., 1907), p. 45.

113 Ibid., pp. 36, 44, 45.

114 Ibid., p. 45. A name search of both the National Library of Wales and National Archives websites has failed to find a likely reference to this person.

115 Davies, 'Cunning Folk in England and Wales, pp. 99–100; see also, Suggett, *Magic and Witchcraft*, p. 87.

116 Suggett, *Magic and Witchcraft*, p. 75.

117 NLW, Kemeys-Tynte (2) MS CA422, Letter from Mary Kemeys to Sir Charles Kemeys, 6 November 1702.

118 Mortimer, 'Rural Medical Marketplace', p. 71.

119 NLW MS James Preston, SA/1681/216.

120 Ibid.

121 Lucinda McCray Beier, *Sufferers and Healers: The Experience of Illness in Seventeenth Century England* (London and New York: Routledge and Kegan Paul, 1987), p. 197.

122 NLW MS James Preston, SA/1681/216.

123 See the examples quoted in Roberts, 'Gender, Work and Socialisation', pp. 21–22.

124 See Coster, *Family and Kinship*, p. 13; Pelling, *The Common Lot*, p. 109.

125 Owen, 'Diary of Bulkeley', p. 133.

126 Ibid., p. 133.

127 Ibid., p. 135.

128 NLW, Wigfair (2) MS 12402E, Letter from John Lloyde of Wigfair relating to the sickness of his daughter, undated, c. 1664.

129 NLW, Kemeys-Tynte (2) CA422, Letter from Mary Kemeys to Sir Charles Kemeys, 6 November 1702.

130 See NLW, Peniarth Estate (21), MSS DF 282–91, Documents relating to sale of Penbedw Manor, Denbighshire, 1675.

131 See NLW, Ruthin MS 1799, Notes on Lands of William Whittmore in Denbigh, undated; NLW Ruthin MS 978, Grant of Water Mills in Ruthin to William Whittmore Esq, 10 February 1614.

132 NLW MS James Preston, SA/1681/216; at the time of writing, both the Swan Inn and the Red Lion Inn in Wrexham still survive, the latter trading continuously since 1492.

133 Joan Lane, *A Social History of Medicine: Health, Healing and Disease in England, 1750–1950* (London and New York: Routledge, 2001), p. 45.

134 NLW MS James Preston, SA/1681/216

135 Lane, *A Social History*, p. 45.

136 NLW MS James Preston, SA/1681/216.

137 Ibid. For bleeding and glistering 'Mr Owens' the again relatively small sum of five shillings was charged.

138 Ibid. For example 'for the cure of Edward Bannister his wife'.

139 Flintshire Record Office, MS D/HE/432, Diary of Dr Thomas Griffiths of Mold, 1726, p. 78.

8

'Neighbourliness' and the medical community

So far we have concentrated on the household family and types of care within the confines of the home. It would be wrong, however, to assume that each household was simply an autonomous unit of care. Early modern society was strongly based around concepts of inclusion and neighbourliness, with strong social expectations of good conduct.[1] People were bound together by mutual obligation and a sense of reciprocal support to mitigate times of hardship.[2] The early modern community was also defined by processes of inclusion and exclusion, with strong notions of identity and belonging.[3] In areas such as Wales, with small, nucleated communities, and a distinct linguistic/cultural identity, this sense of responsibility, inclusion and conformity could be amplified. Welsh localism was particularly strong with, as Philip Jenkins argues, parish loyalties running deep.[4] Also, with the lack of official medical infrastructure in Wales, medical care was *de facto* a community concern since it made sense to pool resources. The parish provided a referral network through which medical information could spread, and Welsh people, as elsewhere, were willing to accept their neighbours as points of reference.[5]

Fundamentally, though, sickness could also act as a catalyst for forging and reinforcing social relationships. Care might involve the admission of outsiders into the family home and, as we shall see, there are examples of the subversion of such relationships by those wishing to profit from this same vulnerability. But physical care of the sick was also part of a shared community obligation. In fact, it could be argued that the sometimes limited operations of the Old Poor Law in Wales served to create a different set of processes from that in many parts of England, through which care and support were organised. In rural areas, this community support was mutually beneficial; it provided a small safety net for the less well off since it often provided for external sources of care. As will be shown, the provision of community and charitable donations often enabled the poor to gain access to 'orthodox' medical care. Thus, in some senses, the parish or local community became not only a medical support unit, but effectively a temporary extended medical 'family' in terms of the offer and acceptance of care. These localised medical kinship families – in anthropological terms falling under the category of 'fictive' or 'spiritual' kin – became involved in the care of the sufferer, but were not necessarily explicit or formalised, and were also temporally limited to the duration of the sickness.[6] Care of the sick involved a range of familial and extra-familial players, and a willingness to help others transcended straightforward moral obligations. Equally, the extent to which outside carers were involved in individual sicknesses also raises questions about micro-political power relationships in early modern medicine. Sickness and care, then, can have further implications for our understanding of the 'family', both in early modern Wales and more widely.

Visiting the sick

Visiting the sick was an important component of neighbourliness and a useful social function. Visiting reinforced social norms of inclusion, and also provided a vehicle for the spread of information and gossip. In fact, visits could even sometimes be a barometer of the status of an individual and showed the extent of their acceptance in their local community. One of the ways in which the eighteenth-century English diarist, Elizabeth Baker, perceived a growing sense of exclusion from the Welsh-speaking community around her, was when the number of visitors to her house rapidly dwindled. Gossip had spread about the finances, and continued absences of her friend and benefactor, the Welsh gentleman Hugh Vaughan, in one of whose properties she lived.[7] As elsewhere, amongst the most frequent visitors to the sick were Welsh ministers and clergy. Visiting formed an important part of their pastoral duties, and their diaries often reveal the extent of their obligations to the sick. The Quaker minister John Kelsall of Dolybran, Montgomeryshire, seldom mentioned his own sickness, but noted his visits to sick parishioners such as 'old Ann Griffiths who was very ill [and] weak'.[8] John Harries, rector of Mynydd Bach and Abergorlech, Carmarthenshire, was another regular sickbed visitor during the 1730s,[9] while the sick of Broad Oak in Flintshire regularly called on Philip Henry to minister to them. In fact, in Henry's case, the number of visits could be substantial. On just one day in March 1661, he made no less than five separate journeys, noting that there were 'many sick [who] desired prayers'.[10] The main purposes of such visits were spiritual, and satisfied both sufferer and minister of their comportment and character. There can be no doubt that the presence of a minister mollified the minds of many sick people, while the clergy, for their part, believed that they might make a difference in either the recovery or 'good death' of the individual.[11] In many cases, though, the clergy played an important healing role. The Welsh lexicographer

Sir Thomas Wiliems of Trefriw was also a renowned physician and proponent of the art of uroscopy, offering his diagnoses without necessarily needing to see the patient.[12] Another Welsh healer, Gwilym Pue, was a Monmouth priest-doctor who published medical essays and ministered to both the medical and spiritual needsof his flock.[13] Clergy healers could sometimes be viewed with suspicion, especially since reformist contemporaries drew the comparison between Catholic prayers and healing charms. Thomas Wiliems was accused of recusancy, despite his obvious use of orthodox methods, rather than religious symbolism and charms, while Pue in fact was a practising Catholic, although his essays *De Sceletyrbbe Vel Stomacae* and *Another Discourse of the Scorbute*, were anything but 'magical'.[14] Conversely, religion was actually to become a great stimulus in reviving the use of herbal simples in healing by Non-conformist clergy. Men such as the Puritan John Williams of Castellmarch, on the Llyn peninsular and, later, the renowned Methodist Griffith Jones of Llanddowror (referred to by a contemporary as 'a quack in physick') were amongst those who equated the use of basic, herbal remedies with the duties of a Christian to relieve the suffering of their brethren.[15]

Clergy visits were loaded with meaning in other ways. On the part of the sufferer, admitting (or indeed inviting) the minister, was a public gesture of conformity, indicating that they were both undertaking their Christian duty, and adhering to expected social norms of sickness conduct. For their part, the minister was seen as fulfilling their obligation to tend to the physical and spiritual well-being of their flock. Throughout the early modern period, visiting the sick was clearly an expected part of the duties of ministers, to such an extent that failure to undertake such visits could have legal consequences. In 1626, the curate of Bunbury in Cheshire, John Swann, was indicted before the consistory court for a list of offences which included not visiting sick women in his village.[16] In 1720, Thomas Wright of Didsbury in Shropshire was similarly accused, but this time of overtly refusing to visit the sick. In testimonies from the friends and family of one Hannah Earnshaw, repeated pleas that Wright should 'visit and pray by the said Hannah' were met with outright refusal 'upwards of six times', Wright arguing that he was unqualified to administer the sacrament to her despite their repeated pleas.[17] This was seen as particularly heinous by the villagers since it denied Hannah the opportunity to receive her religious rites, potentially placing her soul in danger. Wright's refusal to visit her, therefore, was a powerful gesture. The withholding of such services might be self-consciously deployed as a deliberate gesture of dissent. The extent of the offence caused by their actions is reinforced by the fact that complainants against errant curates were members of the local community. Moreover, that such transgressions ever came to be reported in the first place shows the degree to which sickness was closely intertwined with concepts of conformity and procedure, against which transgressions were socially and morally offensive.

But visiting the sick was not merely a matter for the clergy, and it is clear that lay visitors, friends and neighbours, were also morally obliged to undertake such duties. Lay visits were different inasmuch as they were less didactic although still tinged with connotations of neighbourly support and conformity. In fact, this process seems almost to have been formalised and involved a well-rehearsed set of social practices. The diarist Robert Bulkeley of Anglesey was an inveterate visitor of the sick, but there is nothing in his diary to show that he offered anything in terms of medical advice, nor that he was particularly strong in his religious convictions. Between January 1631 and May 1633 Bulkeley recorded thirty separate visits to the sick in his community, and the likelihood is that there were many more unrecorded. On many occasions, it seems that the sole purpose of the visit was simply to 'see', in all senses, the sick person. On 13 April 1632 Bulkeley 'visited Mr Owen being sicke' and again on 31 October he 'rid to visit Elin Edw: being sicke', but he also paid visits to bereaved families.[18] Sometimes, Bulkeley accompanied others on such visits, highlighting the extent to which visiting could be a communal, and even socially cohesive, activity. On one occasion he recorded that both he and his wife attended the sickbed first of his sister Mary and, later the same day, Edward ap Hugh, who was 'very sicke'.[19] At other times, Bulkeley accompanied male companions, although he visited both men and women in his locality.[20] Bulkeley was a relatively well-off member of the community, and his motivations for visiting are not recorded. It is likely that a sense of duty and compassion were strong imperatives. Visiting was probably also tied in with the responsibilities that accompanied an advantageous social position. Other possibilities might be a sense of curiosity relating to the somatics of the sufferer or even a sense of guilt at the misfortune of others while he, himself, was relatively healthy. In all likelihood, such visits were therefore part of a shared moral obligation. They showed support for the sufferer, but also acted as a signal that the visitor was conforming to social expectations by demonstrating Christian neighbourly concern.

Once sickness was announced, news could spread with remarkable speed and the sick person automatically became the subject of community scrutiny.[21] This was important in micro-political terms, since the sufferer simultaneously gained and lost power. As we saw earlier, on the one hand, sickness could be empowering; it conveyed a special status upon the sufferer and no doubt focused attention upon them. It could bring legitimate excusal from household or working duties, as well as inviting physical and moral support. On the other, however, the sick person was in turn expected to conform and subject themselves to the scrutiny and advice of others. This meant careful monitoring of behaviour and speech, and also willingness to submit to treatment. The first stage of the process was diagnosis, and it seems that part of the concern of visitors was quickly to establish both the condition of the patient and the cause of their sickness. This network of news also provided a useful mechanism through which community coping strategies could be organised and deployed. The testimonies of witnesses in a 1686 double poisoning case from Wrexham provide evidence of the potential speed of this process.[22] In January 1686, Richard Foulkes, a gentleman from the town of Wrexham, fell sick with severe vomiting, prompting his wife Jane to set out for a local apothecary. On the way Jane first called upon her friend, Jane Kenrick, asking her to accompany her to the apothecary and then back to her home. By the time the two women arrived back at the house, visitors had already begun to arrive. One was 'an old wooman' who helped Richard Foulkes into the room where Jane Kenrick was waiting, and the other 'one Mary Roberts', a neighbour. In her own testimony, Mary Roberts noted that she visited the house after 'hearing of his sickness'. Describing herself as a neighbour, she was obviously in close proximity to the house, but her comment of 'hearing' of the sickness, rather than being called to the house demonstrates the speed with which news of sickness could spread verbally. Aside from his wife and son, therefore, Foulkes's sickness was attended by at least three other people from his local community within the first few hours. Witness testimonies from the other poisoning in the case, that of Hugh Morys of Wrexham, tell a similar story. While Hugh's father visited his son by chance and found him sick, John Jones of Llansanffraid stated that he came especially after '*hearing* [my emphasis] of Hugh Morys suden sicknes'. Once again, word of illness appeared to spread quickly through social networks, and evidently initialised the process of visiting the sufferer.

What exactly were the purposes of these visits? One clear theme in these examples is that of gaining physical access to the sufferer and assessing or diagnosing their condition. There was certainly a social need to ensure that the sufferer's maladies were legitimate, and sufficiently disabling as to merit their sufferer status. People were clearly expected to undertake some form of work unless physically unable, and those, especially women, who claimed sickness but were deemed capable of work risked censure.[23] In each of the above examples, there are strong discourses both of physically 'seeing' the sufferer and of questioning them about their symptoms. In the case of Richard Foulkes, Mary Roberts asked Foulkes 'how he did' and then 'shee asked him where his payn was'. On one level these were natural or logical questions, but on another, they indicate that people were keen to seek their own diagnosis of the sufferer's complaint. But lay visitors were also actively and routinely consulted for their opinions by the sufferer. On being given the preparation (actually containing ratsbane or arsenic) by his wife in a cup of oatmeal, Foulkes 'felt something to grinde or cracke under his teeth' and immediately showed it to Mary Roberts, clearly indicating that he felt Mary to be sufficiently qualified to comment on what this substance might be, and also confident enough of her medical abilities to use her as a referent. In fact, in suspicious cases, the community was also doubtless anxious to ascertain whether any elements of malice, or even malefice, could be discerned.

Community and kinship care

Visiting the sick, then, was a common and socially cohesive practice. But visiting formed only a part of the community's role in the sickness of its members, and local people, often outside the sufferer's immediate family, were prepared to play a far more active role in medical care. Whilst family and friends were clearly key figures in looking after their own, a range of outside carers could also be involved. For the poor, carers often acted out of charity or mutual benefit, whilst the better off might also employ people to look after them. Indeed, the position of carer often brought financial benefits and, as we shall see later, this was sometimes enough to attract the attention of the unscrupulous. This caring role, however, again demonstrates the extent to which the sufferer was tied in with local networks and custom. People were prepared to accept care from friends, neighbours and others in their village or parish. For the poor, in particular, sickness could place great burdens upon the family, especially since their resources for the provision of care were limited. It does seem, however, that support was often readily available, even if it consisted of little more than keeping company with the sick or dying. A range of Welsh sources contain references to those who looked after people in their sickness, and this could often be a formalised arrangement. More importantly, however, the role of non-familial care, what I shall refer to as 'external care', was largely recognised as a female one, and undertaken by women.

Religious doctrines underlined the necessity for provision for the poor and compassion for fellow men, and even the poor were sometimes encouraged to give to those even less fortunate than themselves.[24] But there were also other more earthly considerations. Care of the sick was closely interwoven with the notion of mutual benefit, with the potential financial reward of caring for others sometimes proving as much a motivation as social or religious obligation. Probate inventories often indicate that possessions were left to those who cared for the dying in their final sickness, and these were often neighbours or relatives. In 1680, Edward Morris of Trelawnyd, troubled with 'a long and tedious sickness' was cared for by his neighbour, William Williams, while Roger Hughes of Cwm, Flintshire, left possessions to his niece who had looked after him in sickness and old age.[25] Rees Jones of Cardiff, a poor man with an inventory value of only one pound, left all his 'household stuff' except for the bed in which he died to John

Bassett and his wife, who 'gave him attendance in his sickness'.[26] But most refer-ences to care involve women, and this could be a potentially lucrative occupation. Indeed, in some cases, the amounts given to female carers were greater than those left to actual relatives. In her nuncupative will, Wenllian Nicholls of Penarth, Glamorgan, instructed that 'to Kath Powell for tending me I do order 9 shillings'. To her sister and daughter, however, Wenllian left only her 'waring cloths and bed cloths' to be divided between them.[27] Provision for carers in wills sometimes reflected Welsh custom. The wearing apparel of a poor woman from Saint Athan was 'given to the woman who attended her in her sickness and dress'd her corpse after her death according to ye custom of ye country'.[28] This is supported by another example from Pembrokeshire, where Elin ferch Lewis left 'all my Ragged apparel for daies wearing as bedd clothes unto Maud William for her paines takeing in attendinge me in my sicknes'.[29] The feminine care role in this context sits astride concepts of female nurturing but also of notions of types of work adjudged acceptable for women. In one sense, caring for the sick was an accepted role for women and one which they performed within a domestic environment. Nevertheless, the earning potential of this external care role also allied it closely with accepted concepts of female roles in domestic service, and thus provided a legitimate means for women to earn money.

In fact, for those who could afford it, women were sometimes employed by the sick under more formal conditions to tend them, and this raises further ques-tions about caring roles. The 1733 probate accounts of Jennet John of Llancarvan include the entry that she 'P[ai]d Anne Merrick for attending her w[hen] sick', the use of the term 'paid' rather than bequeathed, and the appearance of the entry within an account record, suggesting that Merrick was effectively hired by Jennet to look after her.[30] The 1682 inventory of Mary Thomas of Pendoylan also shows that the formal role and title of nurse was adopted by some Welsh women. Thomas refers to a 'Nurse Coxe' and bequeathed the woman (assum-ing it was indeed a woman) 'ten shillings for a ring', one of nine such bequests for the purpose of buying a ring.[31] The term 'nurse' was often attached in the context of childrearing, and it is possible that this bequest was made in recogni-tion of past gratitude in maternity care although this seems unlikely given that Mary was a spinster and made no provision for any children in her will. Several other documents refer to women as 'nurse'. In 1621, Owen Nicholas ap Morgan wrote to his cousin Morice Williams at Hafod Garegog in Montgomeryshire, mentioning 'your nurse Catherin verch William Thomas'.[32] The same woman appears in another letter to Williams from his brother-in-law, relating to money 'your nurse hath in there [sic] hands'.[33] John Owen of Cefn in Caernarvonshire referred to a woman known as 'Ellen the nurse' in a lease document in 1650, while William Awbery, official to the Bishop of St David's, left money to 'Mary David my nurse'.[34] The title of 'nurse' was clearly known in early modern Wales and appears to have signified a definite female function. It might also, however, point to the adoption by women of formal 'medical' nomenclature to identify their status as healers or carers. If so, this may further support arguments made earlier about the importance of the assumption of practitioner and doctor titles in order to garner legitimacy.

Even familial care, though, was sometimes reducible to expectation, if not of recompense or reward, then at least of reciprocity. In 1707, Ann John of Cardiff was sued by her own estranged husband for amounts he had spent in looking after her. Amongst his long list of claims were one shilling for a pound of honey, two penny loaves and one shilling, all relating to 'her Attendance one weeke when shee was sick.[35] Here relationships of care were conducted along clear lines of obligation. While they were married Ann John's husband was emotionally and morally obligated to care for his wife. Upon their separation, however, this obligation was clearly viewed as terminated, and he retrospectively shifted this care role towards one of economics rather than emotion. In this sense, emotional care might effectively be seen as being contingent upon qualification through settled relationships.

It is also clear, however, that the potential rewards of caring for the wealthy sick were not lost on would-be fraudsters. In 1613, Elen Owen, a widow of Fernyll, Salop, conspired with a local gentleman, Pierce Griffith, to attempt to defraud the wealthy landowner John Salisbury of Rug, Merionethshire, who had recently inherited money from the sale of lands. The Chancery decree for the case against Owen takes up the story:

> The said money being known to be in John Salisburie's hands, and he himself growing weak and sickly, Elen Owen, wife of John Owen, gent., deceased, having insinuated herself into familiarity with him by offer to be a nurse to him in his weakness and to employ her best cares for the recovery of his health, sought to make a prey to herself and her accomplices of the whole estate of money, land and goods of the said John Salisburye and to divide the same with her adherents, i.e. John Owen, her husband, Piers Griffith, esq., Thomas Vaughan, John Wyn Salisbury, and Piers Lloyd, and finding that John Salisbury had retired to a little farmhouse called Poole Parke, co. Denbigh, of his own inheritance on purpose there to remain private with little expenses and to attend to the directions given him for the recovery of his health and strength, Elen persuaded him to remove to her husband's house at Fernyll, co. Salop, to live with them, which he did about 2 years before he died. He and her confederate[s] persuaded him to sell other lands of his ancient inheritance to the value of £2000.[36]

Seeing that Salisbury had grown 'weak and sickly', Owen clearly saw the chance to use the guise of a female nurse to gain access first to his confidence, and then to his money. This example raises several issues. Firstly, in moral terms, the notion of a single man moving in with a couple and then, when her husband died, apparently remaining with Ann Owen on her own, was apparently not viewed as extraordinary, especially given the potential for perceptions of impropriety. Female nurses cared for both men and women, and the close proximity and daily contact often required from care could clearly present opportunities for dalliance. Given that Owen lived with Salisbury for more than two years, and there is no hint of either romantic or sexual connotations to the relationship, it is possible that the caring role was viewed as being neutral in sexual terms, making it acceptable for single men and widowed women to cohabit in this way.[37] As regards gender roles and, in particular masculinity, this is also interesting. There was a hazy boundary between private and public spheres in terms of women's roles, and the provision of medical poor relief and care was one area in which women could be seen as achieving parity or even superiority over men.[38] Another possibility may be that sickness was perceived to render the sufferer either unwilling or incapable of sexual contact, again validating the relationship. The fact, secondly, that Salisbury was willing to accept the invitation of the woman to care for him, indicates that the employment of external carers was sufficiently plausible for him not to become suspicious. One of the key elements of patriarchal status was that of householding, and a man's authority was grounded within his ability to own and manage a home.[39] In this sense, the surrender of his house and independence had important implications for Salisbury. Might it be possible that, in doing so, some elements of his patriarchal and masculine status were diminished? Thirdly, that Owen and her co-conspirators chose this method at all implies that the position of carer was seen as a viable potential means of gaining reward, and that they were confident that Owen's care of the man would lead to his persuasion to make provision for her in his will. Finally, though, it should be noted that Owen apparently did appear to look after John Salisbury, seemingly employing her 'best cares for the recovery of his health'. The crime, then, lay in the persuasion, rather than in an inferred lack of due diligence in looking after the man.[40]

Medicine and micro-politics: medical provision and the poor law in early modern Wales

Medical care, especially of the poor, also fell under the auspices of the parish, although this was by no means the only structure. Legally, the parish was bound to make provision for the sick poor, but other systems of relief, such as those of Dissenters, existed alongside. Quakers, for example, often used donations made from monthly and quarterly meetings, rather than by the parish, to provide for the sick.[41] By the latter part of the eighteenth century, provision from 'friendly societies' in Wales was also designed to take pressure off the parish chest.[42] However, Tudor poor law statutes made provision through taxation for the relief of the 'deserving poor', which included cash payments and various other forms of support.[43] The category of 'deserving' was somewhat nebulous, but generally implied that a person, through no fault of their own, had become unable to labour or support themselves. Such categorisations both encapsulated and articulated social values and expectations of moral conduct, and recipients of relief were expected to reciprocate parish generosity by demonstrating civility, sobriety, piety and a willingness to return to a working role at the earliest possible juncture.[44] Sickness was certainly a legitimate reason for parish relief and, in some senses, brought almost an automatic qualification.[45] Nevertheless, relief for the 'undeserving poor', i.e. the indolent, drunken or immoral, was sometimes given with the caveat that it 'remodelled' the sufferer into an active and contributory member of the community.[46]

In England, although not universally, the poor law tax was widely enforced at a parish level by the early seventeenth century.[47] In terms of medical provision, this could lead to the contracting out of medical services to the poor, especially in larger towns such as London and Norwich, and fitted in with wider European trends towards providing single 'parish chests' of funds for local distribution.[48] In some cases, and especially for the poor, the parish as a whole could intervene by proxy in many aspects of medical care, such as paying for sick parishioners to visit orthodox practitioners or visit healing spas.[49] Margaret Pelling's work on early modern Norwich has shown a coherent system of medical poor relief in English towns, based around the employment of practitioners and also the provision of healthcare in institutions.[50] Mary Fissell, too, has demonstrated the important link between the Bristol hospitals in the eighteenth century, and the system of poor relief in the city. Fissell notes that hospitalisation occurred most often in cases of the dual calamities of sickness and poverty. But, the same was not necessarily true for English rural dwellers, since a large proportion of those using city hospitals came from the city itself.[51] What, then, of Wales?

In terms of medical poor relief the situation in Wales was more complex. The orthodox historical view of the Old Poor Law in Wales until recently has been of the limitations of poor relief there, and the impression left is that Welsh parish authorities appear to have been far less diligent in the collection of the poor rate than their English counterparts.[52] In fact, according to some accounts, large parts of Wales did not see poor rates levied regularly until well into the eighteenth century.[53] On such readings, Welsh rural parishes therefore relied far more on outdoor relief, such as ad hoc collections, church and personal donations, and also fund raising activities.[54] A.H. Dodd argued that the extent of moral obligation in Wales, in the form of charitable relief and church collections, actually rendered the levying of formalised poor rates redundant.[55] If true, in terms of medical provision, this has important implications since it emphasises the strong element of localism, both in parish fund collections and distribution, and again reinforces the reciprocity of care within Welsh parishes. Without the rigidity of official poor law collections, Welsh parish authorities could effectively act arbitrarily, placing medical care again firmly within the remit of the community and this, in turn, affects our understanding of the relationships of power in early modern parochial medical relief. Importantly too, Welsh relief for the sick poor could not be linked in with institutional care; there simply were no medical institutions in place. Thus, while poor relief in English towns became increasingly linked with the provision of hospital, indoor relief and official care, the orthodox view is that Welsh care was often forced to remain firmly within the context of local and private spheres.

As recent work has also begun to show, however, this picture may not be universally accurate. Richard Allen, in his study of Monmouthshire poor law records, has convincingly demonstrated that some parts of Wales in fact had well-organised administration and regular collections of poor relief, and this included a great deal of provision for the sick.[56] But equally, even where official levies of poor rates were absent this did not mean that provision for the sick poor was inferior compared to English parishes, nor that it was inadequate. As the rest of this chapter will demonstrate, evidence from other parts of Wales tends to support Allen's arguments for comprehensive and pragmatic local structures of care. The general paucity of evidence for poor law collections in Wales before 1700 means that the findings of this part of the chapter should not be writ large across the whole of the country. Nevertheless, it is clear that Welsh communities could intervene in a wide variety of ways to provide for their sick parishioners, including both economic and pastoral support, provision of external carers, and also a variety of treatment options. In fact, the evidence points to a well-ordered system of care provision for the sick in at least some parts of Wales, both urban and rural.

Poor law records for pre-eighteenth-century Wales are scarce, and it is difficult to make generalisations from the limited records available. Also, poor relief provision could vary across different regions, and even sometimes from parish to parish, again making generalisations difficult.[57] Nevertheless, it is clear that many areas of Wales did carry out detailed assessments of their poor and levied parishioners according to the poor law statutes. In 1684, the parish authorities in Cundy hamlet in the parish of Llangynwyd, Glamorganshire, rated those eligible for poor law collections in the hamlet, valuing their contributions at seven pounds and nine shillings.[58] The parishioners of Llantrisant parish in Montgomeryshire were similarly rated in 1686 at a value of two and a half pence in the pound, while similar records exist for Abertanat, Shropshire in 1716, Llanstephan, near Carmarthen, in 1731, Margam in 1725 and Llanvihangel, Monmouthshire, in 1753.[59] It may be no coincidence that each of these areas were either proximally close to England or, like Margam and Llanstephan, on the coastal margins of Wales, although they were still a significant part of Welsh society and culture.

Payments to the poor were based on a number of criteria which, although varying by degree from parish to parish, usually fell within the same general parameters. Money was often paid to those in temporary distress through loss of income, changing family circumstances or other limiting factors. The elderly were regular recipients of relief, as were parents of small children left unable to maintain or provide for them, perhaps through the loss of a partner. Aside from strict religious or charitable motivations, the desire to help the sick was also based on more practical considerations, such as returning the sufferer to a productive or useful state within the community.[60] In terms of the amounts raised, it seems that Welsh parishes tended towards lower payments than their English counterparts. In north Wales, payments had not risen above a general rate of between four and seven pence in the pound even as late as the mid-eighteenth century.[61] As Joan Kent and Steve King have noted in their study of rural poor relief, however, by far the most generous amounts of relief were allocated to the sick.[62] In English parishes, they note, sickness was one of the most common reasons for the granting of casual relief, and this could range from ad hoc payments to cover loss of income, through to provision of medical care and services, and, where sometimes necessary, provision for a decent burial.[63] Welsh parish authorities were no less supportive of their sick poor and could intervene in a variety of different ways.

Some of the most frequent payments were those made to the 'deserving poor' (i.e. those rendered in need of help through no fault of their own) on the basis of contingencies, such as accidents, loss of income of a breadwinner or sudden illness.[64] Thus, in the early eighteenth century, did the churchwardens of Towyn in Merionethshire, donate the contents of the church offertory to an elderly woman who 'wounded herself very much with falling down the church gallery stairs Xmas day last'.[65] On other occasions, overseers might note a blanket sum for the treatment of the sick, such as George Richard and Walter Rees, overseers of Llanmaes parish in Glamorgan in 1637 and 1638, who set aside monies 'for the reliefe of the sicke' and also paid three shillings and fourpence 'to the maymed Souldiers at 2 sevrall times'.[66] This was somewhat amplified in ports and towns, where local authorities saw greater numbers of visitors through trade, and also of itinerant poor searching for work, or opportunities to beg. The minute books of Beaumaris Corporation reveal a range of payments from 'bringing a lame soldier to Portaethwy' to 'looking after a boy found almost dead in the street'.[67]

Alternatively, overseers and churchwardens provided ad hoc payments to those suffering from specific conditions, as did the wardens of Henllan parish in 1760, providing seven shillings and sixpence to David Davies and his family 'having been sick of a fever'.[68] Specific charity briefs might also be issued via the parish church to exhort local people to give money to an individual in particular need.[69] In October 1656, the people of Llanfydd in Pembrokeshire were entreated to 'bestow their benevolence' upon John Owen, 'a poore ould man borne and breed in the parish of Llanfydd being grievously troubled with a disease . . . that he is not able to travel and seeke or get his bodily foode & sustenance by reason it is broken out in several places of his body, the quantity of seven or eight places'.[70] In asking 'all good and charitable people out of charitie to commiserate his distressed state', the petitioner argued that 'in soedoing, god will reward them'.[71] Here, emphasis was laid upon not only the vulnerability of the man, but also the moral and Christian responsibility of the parish to care for its own. As Ole Peter Grell has argued, religious affiliation also played a strong part in how people viewed their charitable duties towards the sick, while the Reformation was a strong driver of imperatives for poor relief.[72] Wales was a country upon which the Reformation sat lightly, and retained many elements of pre-Reformation practice and symbolism; we should be careful in recognising that doctrinal differences were not rigid. Yet, the provision of poor relief in Wales seems more allied with Protestant 'love my neighbour' notions of Christian duty for its own sake, than it does with Catholic concepts of rewards in Heaven for good works on Earth.[73]

How did charity affect the individual agency of the sufferer? One of the strongest themes in early modern medical historiography is that of the power and choice of the early modern patient. According to the orthodox view, the individual sufferer exercised a range of choices about their own treatment, deriving opinions from various sources and employing treatment options as they saw fit. Little work has been done, however, to explore the shifts in such choices which could occur once a sufferer was forced onto the charity of others. Once an individual sufferer was 'on the parish', much of their agency was immediately and significantly diminished and transferred to the individual overseers on one hand, and in some ways the collective community on the other. Petitions for relief by the sick poor employed submissive terminology to emphasise the extent to which they were at the mercy of the overseers, and made much of their 'weakness'. In 1691, Elizabeth Harper petitioned the Radnorshire Quarter Sessions for relief after her husband absented, leaving her with 'a great charge of children, one being weak & sick of the King's Evil'. Elizabeth herself was 'weak and sickly'.[74] Elinor Bedward's petition described her as 'a poor woman aged 85 and upwards, very weak and lame', while Peeter [sic] Williams was 'miserably poor and like to perish'.[75] Such terms were doubtless aimed at maximising chances of relief, through carefully constructed strategies and discourses of vulnerability.[76] The fact that illiterate paupers often relied on others to act as amanuenses further serves to highlight the potential for deliberate, and perhaps collaborative, constructions of such documents.[77] However, the parish became the final arbiter on diagnosis of the sufferer, and the extent and severity of both apparent and reported symptoms could be treated with suspicion. It might, for example, seek evidence that sickness was genuine before granting relief. In one case from Llanfyllin, Montgomeryshire, there appears to have been some suspicion about the validity of a claim, and payment to Catherine Thomas 'an old maid troubled with the falling sickness *as is alledged* [my emphasis]'.[78] Payment was withheld, since her condition was alleged rather than proved. In terms of treatment, too, the parish held all the cards. Reliance on poor relief removed the element of choice from the sufferer in terms of which practitioner to use, since this was subject to the choice of the overseers or parish authorities. In Carmarthenshire in 1770, churchwardens granted a sum of money towards the healing of a parishioner's leg 'to whatever surgeon we can agree'.[79] Here, the sick man was a passive figure in his own restoration, with little room for his personal preference in practitioner. In such cases, the employment of regular practitioners was more an arrangement of convenience for the parish, and economically motivated, rather than governed by the usual processes of assessing the efficacy or renown of the practitioner by the patient.

But this is not to say that parish authorities paid no heed to the records or reputations of medical practitioners, and this is very clear in records of applications for diocesan medical licences. Where the individual sick poor relief recipient lost agency, the collective community held much sway in determining rights to practice within their own purview. Common practice in applications was the inclusion of a testimonial, often from local clergy or even fellow parishioners, to attest to both the skill and rectitude of the potential licensee. In this way, the community itself could be seen as endorsing their own practitioner. In the case of the midwife Elizabeth Anwyl, reports of her success in the parish of Llandenog, Merionethshire, were supported by personal references, such as a note from 'W Wynne', professing her to be 'the most understanding woman, and skilful in the art of midwifery in this neighbourhood & parish'.[80] David Davis of Llangurig was adjudged by three local clergymen to be 'a very usefull person in our neighbourhood [who] has performed several cures in surgery'.[81] In both cases, the unit of measurement is the 'neighbourhood', and thus by extension it was the collective community that rendered the practitioner legitimate. In a further example, the rectors of Penmorfa, Criccieth and Llanfihangel-y-Pennant, Caernarvonshire, were at pains to stress that the applicant Robert Roberts of Llanfihangel had not only 'given great satisfaction and done considerable cures' but also 'attends the divine service of the Parish church' and 'doth live conformable to the rules and practice of a good Christian'.[82] As well as the strong religious element, the community was again central to this application, and particular emphasis seemed to be laid on the fact that Roberts was fit 'to practice in his neighbourhood'.[83] In essence, it was this same 'neighbourhood' who policed and legitimised his application. It is also clear that those who practised healing charitably were also encouraged within communities. In 1726, a letter to the Bishop of Hereford asked for the discharge of an old, poor woman arraigned for practising surgery without a licence. Ledbury churchwardens Robert Biddulph and John Skipp argued that the woman had 'sometime ago cured a pauper of our parish ... without any prospect of reward', prompting the churchwardens to reward her with five shillings.[84] Conversely, however, as Ian Mortimer has pointed out, the involvement of the parish in such applications also represented a measure of social control. By supporting applications for medical licences, the parish could regulate the types of healers able to practice within its boundaries, and thus keep quacks and itinerant healers at bay.[85] As such, the question of whether this parish authority was a latent power is open to debate. Churchwardens and overseers were compelled to make decisions on behalf of those whose poverty rendered them helpless. Likewise, it has been argued that the poor were active participants in a great deal of decision-making, especially relating to their own situations, even turning poverty to their advantage at times.[86] As evidenced above, communities could intervene positively to protect or support members if they perceived that a wrong had been done. But they could also utilise their powers in order to protect their own interests, or exert a degree of control.

Parish and institutional care

The provision of care to the sick, and especially the infirm and long-term sick, was a large and pressing problem. We have already encountered the social roles of the family and community as ad hoc carers, and also the employment of carers by individual sufferers to look after them. In many cases, however, the provision of carers became the responsibility of the parish, and it was sometimes incumbent upon churchwardens and overseers of the poor to invoke familial and kinship obligations on a more formal basis. As Steve Hindle has noted, although in theory the family were expected to care for their own, the need to provide structures of care often required direct intervention by the parish, and the creation of 'complex residential arrangements' beyond immediate family and kin.[87] To be sure, the family were the first port of call for the provision of care, but this arrangement could be formalised. To give just one example, in 1767, the overseers

of Mitchel Troy in Monmouthshire paid the daughter of Mary Watkins, an elderly widow, to care for her over a period of nineteen weeks.[88] But care could also
come from other sources, such as friends or willing members of the community.
In late seventeenth-century Flintshire, Edward Moris of Trealwyd was cared for
by a local resident, while the Vestry of Llantrisant in Glamorgan resolved to pay
one shilling and sixpence to 'Ann Griffith . . . to take care of Martha Morgan.[89]
In some cases, parish authorities even paid individuals with sufficient houseroom
to take in more than one sick person at a time, and this was sometimes a long-
term arrangement. In Towyn, north Wales, one Humphrey David of Tu-Mawr
was paid three shillings and fourpence a week for the 'diet and nursing' of poor
parishioners Jonett Edward, Elin Humphrey and Jonett William.[90] It was clearly
not extraordinary for a man to be responsible for the 'nursing' of (in this case
three) women and records indicate that he was still performing the same services
to the parish a decade later.[91]

The employment of external carers, and especially women, also raises questions about socially acceptable roles within a parochial society. In England, the
poor were often paid to undertake 'tending' roles, providing general medical care
from domestic work to attending to the physical needsof the sufferer.[92] Such
employment represented a means of finding a 'use' for the poor, serving the dual
purpose of providing care for the sick, and some measure of social responsibility
and participation on the part of the carer. Moreover, it also raises the question
of 'usefulness' in context of the specialist services which female carers might be
seen as possessing. In this sense, the financial rewards of caring might be seen as
empowering such women, allowing them to garner local reputation and prestige
as well as money. Specific payments for treatment of individuals in fact formed a
strong part of community intervention, and the parish could pay for the services
of a range of healers. As in English parishes, there are many examples of the sending of parishioners for specific treatments, and this might include their being sent
outside the parish if required, while some parishes undertook the regular employment of the same practitioner.[93] As Joan Lane points out, the types of healers
employed by parish authorities varied widely according to need, and they would
commonly employ local bonesetters and empiric practitioners.[94] Such was the
case with the churchwardens of Llangynllo in Radnorshire who, upon the death
of a poor woman on the parish, paid three shillings 'to the bonesetter for her' and
nearly two pounds to 'Mary Jones for Tending her'.[95] In another example, ten
shillings were paid by Flintshire churchwardens in 1713 for the cure of a local man,
and also another described as 'crook'd' after breaking his thigh.[96] In a number
of cases, women were also employed specifically as practitioners. Richard Allen
notes two examples from Monmouthshire records including one Mary Watkins
of Abergavenny, paid twenty shillings 'for the cure of Richard Edmunds hands

& for ye cure of Abigail Howell's face', and another known as 'Katherine the aquavita woman'.[97] There is also some evidence, however, that relations between parochial authorities and practitioners were not always harmonious. William Speed was a medical practitioner employed by the parish of Wepre, Flintshire in 1731. The following year he wrote angrily to Joseph Moreton, overseer of the poor in Wepre, complaining that, after more than thirty visits to a sick parishioner, 'attended with a large flux of humour', he had yet to be paid. Speed noted that 'Ive had so much trouble with ye patient wich thay [the Wepre overseers] are no Strangers to' and 'if Ime not paid in a short time ye law shal take its course'.[98]

As well as providing for the services of medical practitioners, there is some evidence to show that charitable donation was used in the construction of several small proto-hospitals around Wales, although their significance in terms of medical provision should not be overestimated. Little is known of these buildings, of their function and extent of healing in the communities they served. Often, they were relatively short-lived, and few records show how formalised they were as places of healing. John Cule has noted several of these 'hospitals', mostly in north Wales, founded or surviving in the early modern period, and often as a direct result of gentry bequests.[99] The problem lies in assessing the extent of the medical role of these buildings, since the word 'hospital' appears to sometimes have been coterminous with 'almshouse'. Almshouses in Denbigh and Ruthin served a dual purpose as places of healing, while Sir John Wynn of Gwydir founded a hospital and school at Llanrwst in the early seventeenth century, which was still active in 1683, and possibly still as late as 1788.[100] Bishops' returns note the existence of 'hospitalls' in Bangor, Penmynydd and Beaumaris, all in north Wales, while an eighteenth-century letter designating Anne Wynne of Bodewryd (Plas Einion) as 'guardian of the Hospitall' probably refers to either Ruthin or Clun hospital in Shropshire.[101] There is incidental evidence for other small hospitals that may have existed periodically in other parts of Wales, but again nothing to confirm medical usage. In 1614, Sir Walter Montague left money for a hospital near Chepstow, Monmouthshire, for 'poor persons' from the parishes of Llanmartin and Penycoed, while a 1721 deed ordered the setting up of 'Game's' hospital in Brecon, 'for the relief of poor and impotent people'.[102] Another bequest by Sir Charles Jones of Lincoln's Inn, Middlesex, set aside money for the building of 'a hospital . . . near the town of pullhely' [Pwllheli] in Caernarvonshire in 1640.[103] In many cases, such buildings were probably little more than 'lying-in' houses for the poor, and offered little in the way of medical support, beyond kitchen physick and occasionally the services of a local practitioner. As noted earlier, there is no evidence for the regimented provision of medical poor relief in Wales until the nineteenth century.

Poor relief in Llanfyllin: A case study

As I have noted, Welsh sources are scarce, but one outstanding document, a set of accounts for poor relief administration, does survive. Providing detailed records of payments to the sick in late seventeenth-century Montgomeryshire, this document can yield much information about the provision of relief to the sick poor in an early modern Welsh parish.

In 1674, Humfrey Evan of Rhyscog and Edward Griffith of Garwhyell, nominated overseers of the poor for the parish of Llanfyllin, were charged by the local justices to administer funds for 'providing of necessary relieffe' to the poor of the parish, including those 'such as be lame & impotent amongst you'.[104] Llanfyllin at this time was a relatively small town of around 110 households, but also one containing some fairly prosperous merchants and a number of shopkeepers, including an apothecary.[105] In the mid-seventeenth century, local authorities had re-applied for borough status, arguing that the presence of bustling markets and fairs, together with the town's commercial potential, justified its reinstatement.[106] A total of 48 parishioners received relief from the parish in 1674, and the total expenditure was just short of seventeen pounds, a not insubstantial sum for a small parish such as Llanfyllin. Indeed, this amount is especially noteworthy given that, for the years 1671–74, a full 57% of Montgomeryshire households were considered too poor to pay hearth tax.[107] But what can these accounts reveal about support to the sick in the parish? A full transcription of these payments is given in Appendix B.

Out of a total of 45 payments where the reasons for relief are given, eighteen (40%) were made on the basis of sickness or treatment either for an individual or a member of their family. Fourteen of the 45 (31%) were to elderly people, including those who were both sick and old. A number of other miscellaneous payments were made on matters of maintenance, either to parents or children, such as the putting out of children to apprenticeship. Turning to those payments made to the sick poor, a number of quite striking factors can be discerned. The first is the apparently substantial increase in the numbers of sick poor provided for in 1674 over the previous year. We must be slightly cautious since the documents do not reveal the numbers of sick poor from the 1673 list who no longer required relief during the following year. Nevertheless, a total of 7 parishioners received sick relief who had also so the previous year, but a further 22 new cases were added in 1674 – a quite marked increase. Without the ability to compare these data with other years in the parish, it is difficult to generalise. Analysis of the parish records for the years 1666–77 does not provide much evidence of a significant mortality peak, although the five years before 1674 did contain several years of mortality above the apparent trend, likely increasing pressure on the most vulnerable. It might also be noted that the document falls within a period of fluctuating mortality in the parish highlighting the extra pressure which could fall on parish authorities in times of increased sickness or mortality.[108]

In terms of the range of ailments referred to within the document, most payments were given to those simply categorised as 'sick' or 'sickly', with no further indication of their conditions. In some cases, however, specific conditions are mentioned, such as 'falling sickness', 'distracted fits' and, notably, 'Kings Evill'. Here, payments were seemingly incremental and contingent upon degrees of severity. Where children were involved, amounts seem likely to have been increased, while those who were 'bedrid' apparently attracted a greater sum of relief. The amounts given to those categorised as 'sick', fall generally within the range of between two and six shillings, depending on other circumstances, whereas both cases where patients are specified as being physically bedridden show an increase in payments to eight shillings. Whilst not substantial, this increase could reflect the greater burden of caring for one confined to their chamber. Those with specific conditions also appear to have garnered larger sums, although we must be cautious not to overstate this. Margaret John, the 'poore maid troubled with distracted fits' was paid the relatively large sum of ten shillings, while the two women rendered lame by sore or injured legs were paid the lower amount of between four and six shillings. Conversely, the payment provided to Oliver Griffith, afflicted with the tuberculous neck condition of scrofula or the King's Evil, an unsightly and doubtless uncomfortable, but not disabling condition, was paid only two shillings and sixpence, so this again points to payment by degrees of actual disablement, rather than physical discomfort.

The gender dispersal of the payments also bears analysis. In early modern England, women represented the majority of recipients of poor relief. This was linked to factors such as women's domestic roles and financial hardships of raising children, especially when male workers became incapacitated. The itinerancy of the male workforce may play a part in skewing the picture from parish to parish, as might the propensity for women to outlive men, making payments to elderly women more frequent.[109] In the Llanfyllin records, the spread of payments overall actually seems to be fairly even between adult men and women. But, in terms of specific payments to the sick, the overwhelming majority of payments (fourteen out of fifteen made to adults) were given to women. In fact, of the two payments to males, one was a child of ten years old, and the other the man stricken with King's Evil. This is unusual and bears further investigation. We can firstly try to estimate the approximate age of these women, and there are some basic signposts within the list itself as to their time of life, also backed up by the fact that the list usually makes explicit reference to parishioners who are old or infirm. In some cases, actual ages are given but, in others, it is possible to approximate given the presence of small children, indicating women who are of, or near, child-bearing age. Based on the information on the list, it seems that twelve out of the fourteen were not considered as elderly or old. One, Elen Robert John, is indeed described as being 'of middle age but infirme', perhaps preternaturally old or afflicted before her time. These sick women, for the most part, therefore seem to be if not young, then at least not elderly. Secondly, of this group, only three can confidently be asserted as being either widowed or left in sole charge of children. Such misfortunes could often affect those on the lowest rungs of the social ladder, leaving them in need of emergency, ad hoc relief.[110] What causes might lie behind this disproportionate number of sick women? The most obvious answer is coincidence, and it may simply be that there were more sick women in the parish than men for those particular years. Especially in the 1674 additions to the record, several women appear to have been suffering from specific complaints, increasing the burden on the parish. Were parish authorities in Llanfyllin more likely to grant sick relief to women than men? We must be careful in reading too much into these figures, but it is not inconceivable that men were discouraged from seeking the help of the parish in times of sickness, possibly even suggesting social pressure for a swift return to productivity upon male breadwinners.

Finally, as well as providing details of payments to the sick themselves, the Llanfyllin records are also explicit in two cases of payments for treatment, pre-sumably by local practitioners. Although no specific details are provided, the sums paid are very similar in both cases, and also that both recipients of the care appear to be children. It is possible that the parish employed a single doctor who charged a relatively fixed sum for his services. This is reinforced by the large disparity in the amounts paid specifically for 'cureing' compared to payments made directly to sufferers.

Conclusion

This chapter has emphasised the extent to which the early modern Welsh com-munity played an active, participant role in the sickness experience of its mem-bers. Firstly, visiting the sick was an important social means both of conforming to moral and religious expectations, and of further disseminating, and indeed acquiring, medical knowledge. The evidence presented shows in particular the close relationship between religion and medical care, and the constituent roles performed both by the sufferer and by those in attendance. Welsh communi-ties took an active interest in the health of their family, friends and neighbours. Secondly, the lengths to which some Welsh parish authorities were clearly pre-pared to go in order to support the sick poor fully support Richard Allen's arguments based on Monmouthshire sources for comprehensive, if not always fully regulated, welfare provision in parts of Wales. We must, however, also be cautious not to overemphasise the extent to which these were necessarily peculiarly Welsh characteristics. Such payments were commonplace across Europe and fitted in with wider themes of neighbourliness and mutual obligation. A broader study of Welsh poor relief is needed to compare factors such as the amounts and frequency of payments with other areas. Likewise, we should be careful of not creating a rural caricature where everyone coexisted in bucolic harmony, and where 'official' help was not needed. As Adrian Teale points out, times of extreme hardship and necessity overrode the reliance on gift and charity and brought the imposition of forced collections.[111] Nevertheless, the regularity and range of options deployed by Welsh parishes, and over such a long period, does point to a strong sense of responsibility for the sick poor. Given the closeness of Welsh communities, and strong ties to the 'local', it is unsurprising that ad hoc payments were apparently the predominant form of provision for the Welsh sick poor through most of the early modern period. This should not, however, be taken as justification for a system that was in any way simple, ineffectual or inadequate.

Notes

1 J.A. Sharpe, *Early Modern England: A Social History 1550–1760* (London: Hodder, 1997 edition), p. 96.

2 Keith Wrightson, *English Society 1580–1680* (London and New York: Routledge, 2003 edition), p. 59.

3 Phil Withington and Alexandra Shepard, 'Introduction: Communities in Early Modern England' in Alexandra Shepard and Phil Withington (eds), *Communities in Early Modern England* (Manchester: Manchester University Press, 2000), p. 6.

4 Philip Jenkins, 'A New History of Wales', *Historical Journal*, 32:2 (1989), p. 390.

5 Wrightson, *English Society*, p. 48.

6 Ibid., p. 40.

7 Simone Clarke, 'Visions of Community: Elizabeth Baker and Late Eighteenth-Century Merioneth' in Michael Roberts and Simone Clarke (eds), *Women and Gender in Early Modern Wales* (Cardiff: University of Wales Press, 2000), p. 240.

8 National Library of Wales (hereafter NLW) MS 2699B, Quaker Diary of John Kelsall of Dolybran, 1722–34, p. 25.

9 NLW MS 371B, Register of Mynydd Bach Chapel, c. 1736, pp. 59–64.

10 Matthew Henry Lee (ed.), *The Diaries and Letters of Philip Henry, M.A. of Broad Oak, Flintshire A.D. 1631–1696* (London: Kegan Paul, Trench and Co., 1882), p. 80.

11 Lucinda McCray Beier, *Sufferers and Healers: The Experience of Illness in Seventeenth Century England* (London and New York: Routledge and Kegan Paul, 1987), pp. 246–247.

12 Richard Suggett, *A History of Magic and Witchcraft in Wales* (Stroud: The History Press, 2008), pp. 72–73.

13 Glyn Penrhyn Jones, 'Some Aspects of the Medical History of Caernarvonshire', *Caernarvonshire Historical Society Transactions*, 23 (1962), p. 73.

14 Suggett, *Magic and Witchcraft*, p. 74.

15 Jones, 'Some Aspects', p. 73; Gomer Morgan Roberts (ed.), *Selected Trevecka Letters (1747–1794)* (Caernarvon: The Calvinist Methodist Bookroom, 1962), pp. 13–14.

16 Chester and Cheshire Archives, MS EDC 5, Bunbury 51, Consistory Court Records, 1626, Richard Brocke and John Swann; See also, Donald A. Spaeth, *The Church in an Age of Danger: Parsons and Parishioners, 1660–1740* (Cambridge: Cambridge University Press, 2001).

17 Chester and Cheshire Archives, MS EDC 5, Didsbury 13, Consistory Court Records, 1720, Thomas Wright.

18 Hugh Owen, 'The Diary of Bulkeley of Dronwy, Anglesey, 1630–1636', *Transactions of the Anglesey Antiquarian Society* (1937), pp. 68, 82, 87, 96. See also the discussion on visiting in England in Roy and Dorothy Porter, *In Sickness and in Health: The British Experience 1650–1850* (London: Fourth Estate, 1988), pp. 194–196 and Beier, *Sufferers and Healers*, p. 248.

19 Owen, 'Diary of Bulkeley', p. 90.

20 Ibid., pp. 37, 41, 47, 72.

21 Porter and Porter, *In Sickness*, pp. 192–193.

22 All the references for this example are taken from the testimonies of witnesses in NLW, Denbighshire Great Sessions Gaol Files MS 4/33/3, Trial of Jane Foulkes and Lettice Lloyd, March 1686, Documents 29–41. I thank Sharon Howard of the University of Wales, Aberystwyth for originally alerting me to the source.

23 Margaret Pelling, *The Common Lot: Sickness, Medical Occupations and the Urban Poor in Early Modern England* (London and New York: Longman, 1998), pp. 142–143.

24 Adrian Teale, 'The Battle against Poverty in North Flintshire, c. 1660–1714', *Flintshire Historical Society Journal*, 31 (1983/84), p. 87.

25 Ibid., pp. 86–87.

26 NLW MS Rees Jones, LL/1680/18.

27 NLW MS Wenllian Nicholls, LL/1722/136.

28 NLW MS Joan David, LL/1735/109.

29 Quoted in Gerald Morgan, 'Bottom of the Heap: Identifying the Poor in West Wales Records', *Llafur*, 7:1 (1996), p. 24.

30 NLW MS Jennet John, LL/1733/57.

31 NLW MS Mary Thomas, LL/1682/152.

32 NLW, Dolfriog MS 43, Letter from Owen Nicholas ap Morgan to Morice Williams, 15 September 1621.

33 NLW, Dolfriog MS 231, Letter from Owen Poole to Morice Williams, undated.

34 NLW, Dolfriog MS 131, Lease for Lands signed by John Owen and Owen Owen, 10 March 1650; NLW, Edwinsford (2) MS 475, 'Letters Testimonial of William Awbery', 22 December 1632.

35 John Hobson Matthews (ed.), *Cardiff Records, Volume Two* (Cardiff: Cardiff Corporation, 1898), p. 287.

36 NLW, MS Bachymbyd 720, 'Inspeximus of a decree in Chancery between William Salisbury, esq. complainant, and Pierce Griffith, esq., and Elen Owen Widow, and others, Defendants', 22 May 1613.

37 The ages of Owen and Salisbury at the time of the case are unknown, so it is not possible to comment on whether issues of impropriety were bypassed if they were elderly.

38 Diane Willen, 'Women in the Public Sphere in Early Modern England: The Case of the Urban Working Poor', *Sixteenth Century Journal*, 19:4 (1988), pp. 559–575.

39 Alexandra Shepard, *Meanings of Manhood in Early Modern England* (Oxford: Oxford University Press, 2003), p. 206.

40 Ibid., p. 206.

41 Adrian Davies, *The Quakers in English Society, 1655–1725* (Oxford: Oxford University Press, 2000), p. 204; Bill Stevenson, 'The Status of Post-Restoration Dissenters, 1660–1725' in Margaret Spufford (ed.), *The World of Rural Dissenters, 1520–1725* (Cambridge: Cambridge University Press, 1995), p. 359.

42 David Howell, *The Rural Poor in Eighteenth Century Wales* (Cardiff: University of Wales Press, 2000), p. 82.

43 Paul Slack, *The English Poor Law, 1531–1782* (Cambridge: Cambridge University Press, 1995), pp. 9–13; Steve Hindle, 'Civility, Honesty and the Identification of the Deserving Poor in Seventeenth-Century England' in Henry French and Jonathan Barry (eds), *Identity and Agency in England, 1500–1800* (Basingstoke: Palgrave Macmillan, 2004), p. 38.

44 Hindle, 'Civility', pp. 38, 40.

45 Pelling, *The Common Lot*, pp. 64, 81.

46 Ibid., pp. 65, 81.

47 Ibid., p. 18.

48 Andrew Wear, *Knowledge and Practice in English Medicine, 1550–1680* (Cambridge: Cambridge University Press, 2000), p. 19.

49 Roy Porter, 'The Patient in England c. 1660 – c.1800' in Andrew Wear (ed.), *Medicine in Society: Historical Essays* (Cambridge: Cambridge University Press, 1998 edition), p. 94; Slack, *English Poor Law*, pp. 18, 49.

50 Pelling, *The Common Lot*, pp. 79–102.

51 Mary Fissell, *Patients, Power and the Poor in Eighteenth Century Bristol* (Cambridge: Cambridge University Press, 2002 edition), pp. 94–97.

52 See Howell, *The Rural Poor*, p. 95; Geraint H. Jenkins, *The Foundations of Modern Wales, 1642–1780* (Oxford: Oxford University Press, 2002 edition), pp. 168–169.

53 Slack, *English Poor Law*, p. 18.

54 Jenkins, *Foundations*, pp. 168–169.

55 A.H. Dodd, 'The Old Poor Law in North Wales', *Archaeologia Cambrensis*, 81:6 (1926), p. 112.

56 Richard C. Allen, 'The Administration of Poor Relief' in Ralph Griffiths et al.

(eds) *Gwent County History Volume 3: The Making of Monmouthshire 1536–1780* (Cardiff: University of Wales Press, 2009), pp. 272–284. I would like to thank Dr Allen for his generous help and advice on this chapter, and also for allowing me access to his work on poor relief in Monmouthshire.

57 Ibid., p. 18.

58 NLW, Penrice and Margam (3) MS 1439, List of Persons Rated for Poor Rate in Hamlet of Cundy, 29 April 1684.

59 NLW, Frederick Holland MS 32, Assessment for Poor Relief in Llantrisant, 16 June 1686; NLW, Brogyntyn (2) MS EAE2/2, Poor Relief Accounts for Parish of Abertanat, 1716; NLW, George Ayre Evans MS 73, Assessment of Poor Relief for Parish of Llanstephan, 1731; NLW, Penrice and Margam (3) MS 1511, List of People Assessed for Poor Rate in Margam, 1725; NLW, Tredegar (11) Box 157/62, Assessment for Poor Relief in Parish of Llanvihangel, 29 January 1753.

60 Pelling, *The Common Lot*, pp. 65, 81, 86.

61 Dodd, 'The Old Poor Law', p. 112.

62 Joan Kent and Steve King, 'Changing Patterns of Poor Relief in Some English Rural Parishes', *Rural History*, 14:2 (2003), p. 131.

63 Ibid., p. 129.

64 Steven King, *Poverty and Welfare in England 1700–1850: A Regional Perspective* (Manchester: Manchester University Press, 2000), p. 20.

65 Henry Thomas, 'An Old Vestry Book', *Journal of the Merioneth Historical and Record Society*, 2 (1953–56), p. 44.

66 Glamorgan Record Office, MSS D/DN240/1, D/DN240/2, Overseers accounts for Llanmaes, 1637 and 1638.

67 Hugh Owen, 'The Corporation of Beaumaris Minute Book (1694–1723)', *Transactions of the Anglesey Antiquarian Society* (1932), pp. 76–77.

68 Quoted in Howell, *The Rural Poor*, p. 103.

69 Steve Hindle, *On the Parish? The Micro-Politics of Poor Relief in Rural England, c. 1550–1750* (Oxford: Oxford University Press, 2009 edition), p. 59.

70 NLW MS 434B, Miscellany attributed to 'Robert Lloyd', c. 1660, p. 106.

71 Ibid., p. 106.

72 Ole Peter Grell, 'The Protestant Imperative of Christian Care and Neighbourly Love' in Ole Peter Grell and Andrew Cunningham (eds), *Health Care and Poor Relief in Protestant Europe 1500–1700* (London and New York: Routledge, 1997), p. 45.

73 Ibid., pp. 50–51.

74 Evan D. Jones, 'Gleanings from the Radnorshire Files of Great Sessions Papers, 1691–1699', *Radnorshire Society Transactions*, 13 (1943), p. 28.

75 Ibid., pp. 12, 28, 31.

76 Thomas Sokoll, 'Old Age in Poverty: The Record of Essex Pauper Letters, 1780–1834' in Tim Hitchcock et al. (eds), *Chronicling Poverty: The Voices and Strategies of the English Poor, 1640–1840* (Basingstoke: Macmillan, 1997), p. 131.

77 Ibid., p. 130; See also Alexandra Shepard, 'Poverty, Labour and the Language of Self-Description in Early Modern England', *Past and Present*, 201:1 (2008), pp. 51–95.

78 NLW, Harrison & Sons MS 1, Parcel/Item no. 9, 1673–6, Administration of Poor Relief in Llanfyllin, Montgomeryshire.

79 D.L. Baker-Jones, 'Notes on the Social Life of Carmarthenshire during the Eighteenth Century', *Transactions of the Honourable Society of Cymmrodorion*, 2 (1963), p. 275.

80 NLW, Church in Wales, Diocese of Bangor Episcopal 1 MS B/SM/1, Testimonial to the skill of Elizabeth Anwyl of Llandenog, in midwifery, 1753

81 NLW, Church in Wales, Diocese of Bangor Episcopal 1 MS B/SM/2, Testimonial to the skill of David Davis of Llangurig, in surgery, 1749.

82 NLW, Church in Wales, Diocese of Bangor Episcopal 1 MS B/SM/8, Testimonial to the skill of Robert Roberts of Llanfihangel-y-Pennant, in surgery, 1751.

83 Ibid.

84 NLW, Bodewryd (2) MS 380, Letter to Bishop of Hereford regarding practising of physic without a licence, 14 March 1726.

85 Ian Mortimer, 'Diocesan Licensing and Medical Practitioners in South-West England, 1660–1780', *Medical History*, 48:1 (2004), p. 66.

86 For example see Sarah Lloyd, '"Agents in their own Concerns?" Charity and the Economy of Makeshifts in Eighteenth Century Britain', in Steven King and Allanah Tomkins (eds), *The Poor in England 1700–1850* (Manchester: Manchester University Press, 2003), pp. 100–136.

87 Hindle, *On the Parish?*, pp. 49–50.

88 Allen, 'Administration of Poor Relief', p. 279.

89 Teale, 'Battle against Poverty', p. 86; Raymond K.J. Grant, *On the Parish* (Cardiff: Glamorgan Archive Service, 1988), p. 23.

90 Thomas, 'An Old Vestry Book', p. 43.

91 Ibid., p. 43.

92 Hindle, *On the Parish?*, p. 63.

93 Howell, *The Rural Poor*, p. 103.

94 Joan Lane, *A Social History of Medicine: Health, Healing and Disease in England, 1750–1950* (London and New York: Routledge, 2001), p. 45.

95 Rev. D. Stedman Davis and Rev. A. Mason, 'Llangynllo', *Radnorshire Society Transactions*, 12 (1942), p. 69.

96 Teale, 'Battle against Poverty', p. 91; See also Stedman and Mason, 'Llangynllo', p. 69.

97 Allen, 'Administration of Poor Relief', p. 273; See also Owen, 'Corporation of Beaumaris', p. 84, with a sum of money paid to 'Mr Green' for 'dressing Henry Morgan's hand, having bruised ye same by carrying Timber to ye heinous [a ship docked in Beaumaris]'.

98 Flintshire Record Office, MS P/45/1/205, Miscellaneous Medical Bills from 'Will. Speed', 1732.

99 John Cule, 'Some Early Hospitals in Wales and the Border', *National Library of Wales Journal*, 20:2 (1977), p. 100.

100 Ibid., p. 116. There is a reference to a 'Jesus Hospital . . . built by Sir John Wynne' in

a 1788 petition to Sir Richard Wynne by the parishioners of Llanrwst, to gain permission to erect a chapel for the 'warden and poor people' of the hospital to attend. (NLW, Harold T. Elwes MS 666).

101 Cule 'Some Early Hospitals', p. 118; NLW, Bodewryd (1) MS 370, Letter from Benjamin Conway to 'Madam Wynn' regarding churchwardens and Cwrt Mostyn's charity to the poor, 8 February 1731.

102 NLW, Tredegar (1) MS 1172, Letter from Edward Griffiths to Octavius Morgan, 10 August 1858; NLW, Maybery (3) MS 4279, Foundation deed for use of land in Llanvaes, Breconshire, c. 1721.

103 NLW, Llanfair and Brynodol (2) MS D1027, Probate of Charles Jones of Lincoln's Inn, November 1640

104 NLW, Harrison & Sons MS 1, Parcel/Item no. 9, 1673–76, Administration of Poor Relief in Llanfyllin, Montgomeryshire.

105 Melvin Humphreys, *The Crisis of Community: Montgomeryshire 1680–1815* (Cardiff: University of Wales Press, 1996), pp. 25, 26, 48.

106 David Jenkins, 'A Late Seventeenth Century Llanfyllin Shopkeeper: The Will and Inventory of Cadwalader Jones', *Montgomeryshire Collections*, 69 (1981), pp. 48, 50.

107 Howell, *The Rural Poor*, p. 95.

108 Powys County Archives Office, Microfiche MP125, Llanfyllin Parish Registers, 1665–1677. For comparison, the burial numbers are: 1665, 24; 1666, 27; 1667, 36; 1668, 52; 1669, 50; 1670, 46; 1671, 38; 1672, 52; 1673, 35; 1674, 40; 1675, 49; 1676, 31; 1677, 35.

109 For a fuller discussion of these points see Willen, 'Women in the Public Sphere', esp. pp. 561–564.

110 Howell, *The Rural Poor*, p. 99.

111 Teale, 'Battle against Poverty', p. 92.

9

Conclusion

This book has sought to restore a balance to the medical history of Wales, by highlighting the many ways in which Welsh people both engaged with, and participated in, wider networks of medical knowledge and practice. At the beginning of this book, we encountered existing works on early modern Welsh medicine which downplayed or ignored the important role of factors such as geographical location, language, literacy and medical commerce. Many, either tacitly or explicitly, portrayed a country dominated by depictions of folkloric medicine; a country largely divorced from wider networks of knowledge and a country whose people, by dint of their unique language, had little or no access to the printed medical word. Welsh medical practice, according to the orthodox view, seemingly consisted mainly of cunning folk, white witches, magical healers and charmers. We now see, by contrast, a country which far from being remote, insular and even marginalised, was actually fully participant in all aspects of early modern medical culture.

Importantly, though, the discussions within this book demonstrate for the first time how far Welsh medical history can be used as a prism through which to view early modern society in Wales more generally and, in turn, its relationship with England and beyond. Welsh history in general has often been reticent in acknowledging the scope and extent of Wales's interaction with its near neighbour, often serving to create an artificial insularity, but the importance of this relationship is undeniable. The signal role of religious beliefs in shaping attitudes towards sickness has been highlighted, and this draws upon wider themes of popular religion and questions of spirituality and magic in Wales. Literacy was a vital component in the acquisition and spread of medical knowledge, and the growing use of books reflects the increasing import of the printed word in Wales, and the complex relationship between oral and literate, English and Welsh cultures. Likewise, the increasing use of correspondence networks as vehicles for the transmission of knowledge can be viewed as part of the same process. Questions of language are always central to studies of Wales, and the medical terminology of

Wales again points to the influence of the English language, reflective both of the increasing market for English books, and of exposure to incoming and itinerant traders in market towns. Analysis of neglected areas of Welsh history such as the Old Poor Law in the context of medicine, has also contributed to debates about the effectiveness of poor relief in Wales, and highlighted areas for new studies.

But, a central aim of this book has been to address broader questions in medical history and not be limited by the geographical borders of Wales. It is here that I believe that substantial contributions have also been made. It would, for example, have been far easier to merely tick off a checklist of themes from the past twenty or so years of medical historiography and drag Welsh medical history 'up to date' by its collars. But this would achieve little beyond bringing Wales to a state of parity with the rest of British and European historiography at best. Instead, Wales has been used as a testbed for wider questions about early modern medical culture. Questioning the concept and usage of the 'sick role', we ask new questions about 'being' sick in the early modern period, and the manifold different factors which could impinge on the actual, lived experience of sickness. Exploring domestic medical care, we have entered debates about concepts of the household family and, in particular, raised questions about gender roles in the context of both medical care and knowledge. Analysis of the extent of medical material culture in rural Wales has implications for other, similar areas and shows that people in rural areas in fact had access to a wide range of medical goods and services. In exploring medical literature, and the ways in which published remedies could enter the vernacular, we can again speculate more freely about the access of illiterate people to the printed word.

In order for Welsh medical history to have a future, it must locate itself not as a separate enclave, but rather as a vital sub-discipline within wider British and European medical culture. Welsh medicine did not exist in isolation and it cannot be understood in isolation. This being the case, it is worrying to note the almost total failure on the part of historians to link Wales with mainstream medical historiography in the past, particularly important given the growing recent attention towards regional medical histories. Addressing this – as this book has attempted to do – is crucial to prevent Wales becoming just another marginal or dead-end topic. This concluding chapter will therefore serve two purposes. It will firstly summarise the main findings of this book, before turning to the important question of the future direction of Welsh medical history.

A new 'story' of medicine in early modern Wales

Until now, the prevailing model of medicine in seventeenth- and eighteenth-century Wales has been one-track, that of a country continually being pulled

backwards to the traditions, culture and religion of its past. Welsh medical practice has been viewed as 'stagnant and backward-looking', its exponents stub-
bornly refusing to adopt or adapt to new methods.[1] It is also remarkable, if
not also deeply concerning, how little these depictions have altered in the past
century or so. The early twentieth-century view of the first academic historian
of Welsh medical history, David Fraser-Harris, that 'wherever science fails to
penetrate there superstition flourishes' certainly appears to be mirrored in Pamela
Michael's recent survey of Welsh medicine in which she seems to see folklore
and, in particular, the Physicians of Myddfai as being essentially indicative of the
medical mores of Wales, virtually until the late eighteenth century.[2] But, as this
book has shown, the true picture was far more complex.

Firstly, there is a great necessity to view medical culture in Wales far more
inclusively than have previous studies. Welsh people clearly conceptualised diseases and their bodies in humoral terms. There was no separate, uniquely Welsh,
'system' of the body, and wider beliefs in the properties of a range of plant,
animal and symbolic healing practices differed from other parts of Britain and
the rest of Europe only in matters of degree. The continual need to seek difference or uniqueness, in this sense the 'Welshness' in Welsh medicine, actually
obscures the wider picture which is that of participation, and not exclusion.
We must, for example, understand the extent to which Wales was, in fact, part
of international networks of knowledge and trade. As much evidence in this
book has shown, Welsh people, even in upland, rural areas had access to a range
of medical goods and services. While individual homes might not have held
great stores of medicines or equipment, Welsh village shops demonstrate that, as
well as basic provisions and essential ingredients, retailers sold exotic herbs and
spices, directly linking Wales to the increasingly global medical trade. Likewise,
throughout the early modern period, English books were in increasing demand
from Wales, and were available from a variety of sources. This included popular
medical advice books, remedy collections and almanacs, containing a wealth of
medical information. Further, although there is not extensive evidence as yet, it
is clear that English and foreign traders certainly entered parts of Wales, a prime
case in point being the Italian mountebank doctor noted earlier in Philip Henry's
diary, and took advantage of Wales's many fairs and markets to ply their trade.
Given such examples, we need to revise views of Wales as intractable or impen-
etrable to outside influence.

Secondly, we need to understand the important role of Welsh communities
in shaping the access to, and spread of, medical knowledge. True, the presence of
small communities and an indigenous language clearly fostered a strong emphasis
on localism, community and neighbourliness in Wales. With no Welsh printing
press until 1718, and low levels of literacy, Welsh oral culture was predominant

in terms of perpetuating, disseminating and sustaining medical beliefs allied closely with the importance of local references and local healers. It is clear that Welsh communities were 'knowledge banks' from which sufferers could draw. Friends, family, neighbours and wider kin all provided ready sources of medical authority. Social gatherings, festivals, fairs and markets yielded opportunities for information gathering, while Welsh oral culture, such as poetry, verse and proverbial wisdom, did much to promulgate medical ideas in the Welsh vernacular. All such aspects might certainly be taken as reinforcing an innate Welsh conservatism and reluctance to adopt or assimilate new ideas, especially since they emphasise factors *within* Wales. Nevertheless, this same oral culture was vital in disseminating knowledge derived from English-language print. Medical remedies were shared and switched back and forth between verbal and written sources. Literate Welsh people, forced by the lack of Welsh publications to purchase English books, were not proprietorial with this knowledge, and it thus began to enter the Welsh oral vernacular. From here, it could return to the written form in remedy collections, and go through further linguistic removes. Perhaps the best indication of the impact of English printed texts can be seen in changes to Welsh-language medical terminology, parts of which show increasing evidence of Anglicisation. In this way, though, both literate and illiterate Welsh people had a great deal of potential access to medical information from England and, through translations of foreign works, to wider European and global medical culture. This also ties in strongly with the relationship between rural and urban in Wales. Although Welsh towns were small, they played a significant role as centres of trade for outlying rural areas. Moreover, certain areas of Wales had strong links with English towns, such as Bristol, Chester and Ludlow, while coastal and port towns traded both nationally and internationally. Although much emphasis has been laid on the poor roads, difficult terrain and poor opportunities for transport within Wales, the people of Wales did show a remarkable mobility, and were not necessarily either physically or intellectually tied to their parishes.

The influential role of local communities is reinforced in issues of care. With no medical institutions, such as the Bristol and Norwich infirmaries, and a perception of a lax system of poor law provision, it would be easy to dismiss local care provision in Wales as inadequate and reliant upon religious and charitable relief. But, Welsh communities were capable of providing a flexible, adaptable and comprehensive care structure, which included emergency relief, employment of carers and practitioners, and even the option to send patients elsewhere for 'better' treatment options if they were available. Moreover, and in agreement with the findings of Richard Allen's assessment of poor relief in Monmouthshire, we should even question the lack of 'official' provision, since parishes in many parts of Wales did in fact raise formal collections. There is a similar dismissiveness in previous depictions of Welsh 'doctors'. Much emphasis on the apparent lack of 'orthodox' practitioners in Wales has tended to give weight to the predominance of 'irregular' practitioners, such as charmers and cunning folk. As Chapter 7 demonstrates, however, there were increasing numbers of Welsh practitioners who apparently sought to distance themselves from accusations of rustic ineptitude or backwardness, and ally themselves firmly with the licensed medical faculty. Although many Welsh practitioners did not actually seek or achieve licences, the adoption of professional medical nomenclature – and especially the English term 'doctor' – demonstrates a desire to assume an air of professionalism. From the early eighteenth century, evidence does, in fact, also show an increasing aspiration towards the legitimacy of a licence, belying depictions of backwardness or reluctance to adapt. The large numbers of such 'doctors' in Welsh sources, together with the large body of apothecaries located across Wales, demonstrate that Welsh people had a range of available alternatives to cunning folk and charmers. Importantly, though, I emphasise alternatives, and not replacements, since the case for the ubiquity and patronage of 'irregular' healers in Wales has been well made.

Religion is another area to which we can add an alternative side to the 'story'. The somewhat unique religious background in Wales, most notably its retention of pre-Reformation beliefs through a combination of poor clergy and relative lack of zeal in punishing recusancy, tends to reinforce depictions of Welsh inertia and has been seen as providing a fertile environment for beliefs in supernatural and magical healing to flourish. But, Non-conformity, Protestantism, Puritanism, Methodism, all had a part to play in stimulating and introducing new medical ideas to Wales, and influenced personal approaches to health and sickness. It is likely that the introduction and location of Paracelsian and Helmontian chemical medicine in Wales was greatly influenced by its popularity amongst Protestant reformers and Puritans, reinforced by its appearance in areas of strong Non-conformist sympathies. Later, in the eighteenth century, Methodism gave rise to alterations in both attitudes towards sickness, and sickness behaviour itself, as sufferers sought to provide tangible proof of their readiness to enter Heaven. Rather, therefore, than acting as a rein on 'progress', religion could in fact directly stimulate change.

And so we return to the question of the 'story' of Welsh medical history in the early modern period. Can we now revise previous depictions of medicine in Wales, whilst still reconciling the importance of the strong folkloric tradition? I believe that we can. Most importantly, medicine in early modern Wales was infused with a fascinating set of paradoxes, tensions and questions. Wales as a whole was a distinct geographical region, but also one of internal variations of upland and lowland, urban and rural. In medical terms, this could impact in a number of ways, from the types of diseases prevalent in given areas, to local attitudes and traditions affecting individual diseases, to the availability of practitioners and the ease of obtaining medical goods. Wales was a country with no medical training facilities, hospitals or universities, and yet possessed a large body of medical practitioners of various kinds, including the licensed and those who could easily be described as 'orthodox', and whose services were readily taken up by large numbers of the Welsh population. Welsh people spoke Welsh, and many of them only Welsh, but the increasing influence of English-language medical terminology was beginning to be felt. Likewise, although the majority of people in Wales could not read, medical information derived from books was able to spread widely across all parts of Wales through the strong Welsh oral culture. We therefore arrive back at the paradox which underpins Welsh medical history: Wales, in medical terms, was a country pulling simultaneously in two directions. On one hand its rural traditions, medical legends and folklore, oral culture and localism pulled it strongly back towards its past. On the other, however, a growing engagement with orthodox medical print culture, first in English and later in Welsh, the availability of medico-material culture and the trade in medical goods and services, both within and from outside Wales, all served to pull Wales out of its apparent isolation, and into the much broader context of early modern British and European medicine. It is this, previously untold, but vitally important, aspect of medicine in early modern Wales, which this book has put forth.

The future of Welsh medical history

In order to conclude, it is worthwhile addressing the potential of medical history in Wales to occupy a position of importance in the growing context of regional medical histories, and there are so many ways in which new Welsh studies could be used to lead, rather than simply provide incremental additions to historiography. It might even be argued that Wales has been something of a 'problem child' of medical history, at least in terms of the early modern period. This is evidenced both by the relative lack of existing studies, and by the domination of the single theme of medical folklore. Extremely problematic has been the lack of any significant body of work, or any semblance of historical debate, which means that it has not been possible to sustain or even achieve any momentum. While themes such as the early modern patient, the family, gender, the form and role of remedies, globalisation and even postmodernism have emerged and been debated, medical history for this period in Wales remains firmly allied with nineteenth-century antiquarianism.

Conclusion

How, then, can this trend be reversed? If this situation is to be changed, it is firstly vital that other historians now take up the baton and begin to question in far greater detail the role of early modern Wales in the wider medical world. At the time of writing there is no centre for Welsh medical history, and a new impetus to bring together a critical mass of historians, and not only Welsh historians, is badly needed. Issues such as medical practice and practitioners in Wales are in great need of revision, and especially the role of more specialist healers such as bonesetters and midwives. The question of licensing in Wales is particularly salient, since Welsh practitioners appeared to have increasingly espoused the legitimacy of a licence during the eighteenth century.

It is vital to integrate studies of Wales into wider historiographical trends, and promote the ways in which new studies can in fact inform and provide models for other areas. As I have attempted to demonstrate within this work, many aspects of Welsh medical history span topics of broader utility than just within the country's borders and so, in this way, Wales could in fact lead from the front. In many ways, Wales is perfectly placed to answer questions posed by recent historical studies. As a distinct region of the British Isles, the dynamics of such issues as information spread, cultural dissemination and social and economic networks into and within Wales address wider questions such as the relations between outlying rural areas and urban centres, and the extent of 'trickle-down' culture between centres and peripheries, both of which are extremely relevant for our understanding not only of early modern Britain, but equally of broader European society. A wider study of probate inventory data across Wales would not only contribute much to our understanding of material culture in Wales, but also question the participation of smaller, rural countries in an increasingly global medical market – another recent historiographical issue onto which more attention must be focused. We still know little about the mechanisms through which medical goods and services were advertised in Wales. Understanding the availability and extent of medical advertising, especially given the issues of language in Wales, raises questions of cultural and economic emulation between European centres and outlying rural and provincial areas. In light of recent renewed interest in the patient experience, the large surviving body of correspondence in Wales would make a fascinating basis for a study of sickness self-fashioning, and the ways in which sufferers represented themselves. Likewise, attempts for a greater appreciation of the processes and mechanics of care, both domestically and within the context of the community, could be enriched by including Wales within a broader skein of regional studies. Ultimately, then, what is most needed is a new direction in Welsh medical history, and a concerted effort in both the undertaking and promoting of new research. It is to be hoped that this book will serve as the beginning, and not the end of this journey.

Notes

1 W. Gerallt Harries, 'Bened Feddyg: A Welsh Medical Practitioner in the Late Medieval Period' in John Cule (ed.), *Wales and Medicine* (Llandysul: Gomer Press, 1975), p. 178.

2 Wellcome Library, MS 8245, Notes and Drafts for Unfinished Volume The History and Lore of Cymric Medicine' by David Fraser-Harris, c. 1928, Draft for Chapter VI, p. 1; Pamela Michael and Charles Webster (eds), *Health and Society in Twentieth Century Wales* (Cardiff: University of Wales Press, 2006), pp. 6–8.

Appendix A

Selection of Welsh disease terms with English translations[1]

Welsh disease/affliction term	English disease/affliction term
'Bol, a Colic a Gwynt Ynddo'	Colic and wind in the stomach
'Brath Ki'	Dog bite
'Brath Neidr'	Adder Bite
'Crachar ben'	Scabs in/on the head
'Crangk'	Cancer
'Y Cryd'	Ague/Shivering
'Clefyt o Vwyn'	Internal disease
'Chwydu'	Vomiting
'Danoedd'	Toothache
'Distempr'	Distemper
'Dolur Pen'	Headache
'Dolwyr/Dolur'	Pain
'Dropsi'	Dropsy
'Fflewm/Fflem'	Phlegm
'Y Frech Goch'	Lit: the red pox/measles
'Y Frech Wen'	Lit: the white pox/smallpox
'Gowt'	Gout
'Gwaetlin'	Haemorrhaging
'Gwayw'	Pain
'Gwresog'	Fever
'Haint Dygwyd'	Epilepsy
'Maniw'	Tumour
'Manwyn'	Scrofula (King's Evil)
'Marw Gig'	Proud flesh e.g. lump or boil
'Meddawt'	Drunkenness
'Pâs/Pesswch'	Cough
'Piso Gwaed'	Lit: 'pissing blood'
'Pla Gwyn'	Consumption

Appendix A

'Pryfed'	Worms
'Tostedd'	Stone
'Wastio'	Wasted
'Ysbinagl'	Quinsy

Note

1 Welsh examples taken from British Library, Add. MS 15045, Anon., 'Caer Rhun no. 16'
– Miscellaneous medical notes and remedies in Welsh, 16th century; British Library,
Add. MS 14913, Welsh medical remedies and treatises copied from texts of Physicians
of Myddfai, c. 16th/17th century; Cardiff Central Library, MS 2.973, Thomas ap Ifan,
Meddyginiaeth, 17th century; Ida B. Jones, 'Havod 16: A Mediaeval Welsh Medical
Treatise', *Études Celtiques*, 8 (1958-59); Wellcome Library, MS 417, 'Llyfr o feddyginia-
eth a physigwriaeth' (book of remedies and medicine c. 1600).

Appendix B

Poor relief in Llanfyllin, showing payments made to parishioners in 1673 and 1674, and stated reasons for relief[1]

Name	Description	1673 rate	1674 rate
Mary David	'Her husband left her wth one child, of about 7 yeares old & shee a sickly woman'	5s	7s
John Owen Gwyneth	'hee hath a wife & 5 smale children'	3s	3s
Elizabeth Jones, spinster	Discharged for not being an inhabitant of Llanfyllin parish	n/a	n/a
Griffith David ap Evan		2s	2s
Gaenor, late wife of Evan David	'Shee had the yeare 1673 three small children sickly & one of them very simple, therefore that yeare had ten shillings but this yeare 1674 but two liveing, the simple child about 12 yeares of age & one other about 9 yeares old'	10s	5s
Elen Robert John	'A person of middle age but infirme'	2s	2s
Mary Bulkeley	'Shee is the base daughter of John Reynold Bulkeley of about 20 yeares of age but sickly'	2s	2s
Cadwaladr David	'Haveing 8 smale children'	4s	10s

Name	Description	1673 rate	1674 rate
Joseph, the son of William the Smith	'Hee is about 9 yeares old'	6s	3s
Catherine the wife of John Reynold Bulkeley	'a sickly bedrid woman'	2s	8s
Jane Morris	'an old woman'	2s	2s
David the son of Richard ap Robert of Globwell	'hee is about 9 yeares old'	1s 6d	1s 6d
Lowry the daughter of the said Richard ap Robt	'lame of a sore legg'	n/a	6s
Dorothy the daughter of Humfrey ap Evan	'shee is about the age of 21 yeares & hath a sore legg'	2s 6d	4s
Catherine Meredith of Globwell, widow	'an old woman of about sixty yeares of age'	3s	3s
Owen the sonne of Edward John & Catherine Poole	'hee is about 18 yeares old but a simple person, his mother a pedlar who hath two other younger children'	2s 6d	2s 6d
Robert the sonne of Richard Bulkeley, dec'd	'towards the putting of him [as] an apprentice 2li, with John Kyffin haveing promised to add 10s to it…'	2s 6d	£2
Mary the daughter of Edward Saie	'shee is about 7 yeares of age…'. Amount of relief reduced due to repeated begging.	£1	10s
Evan the sonne of Cadder ap Evan	'A child of about 10 yeares of age & sickly'	3s	3s
Jane verch John Dailinor, widow	'an old woman of Llanfyllin'	2s 6d	2s 6d
Jane the widow of Rees William, a tinker dec'd	'shee hath several smale children not able to get theire liveing'	3s	3s

Name	Description	1673 rate	1674 rate
Margarett verch Evan	'shee is about sixty yeares of age'	3s	3s
Margarett the widow of Thomas Morgan	'shee is sick & bedrid very often'	3s	8s
Lowry John	'shee hath 3 smale children . . .'	5s	5s
Catherine Ffrancis	'an old woman'	5s	5s
Evan ap Hugh & his wife	'old persons'	3s	3s
Richard the son of Wm ap Evan	'a fatherless & motherless child of about 12 yeares of age'	3s	3s 6d
	TO BE ADDED [sic]		
John Mathew		n/a	2s
Catherine verch Tho:	'shee is taken with the falling sickness'	n/a	5s
Jane the wife of blind David of Globroll	'shee is a sickly woman having many smale children'	n/a	5s
Lowry the wife of Evan Cadder	'she is an old woman'	n/a	2s 6d
John Humfrey	'a poor labourer now old & not able to gett his liveing'	n/a	4s
Ann the widow of David ap Evan of Globroll	'shee & her children being lately sicke'	n/a	8s
Howell ap Humfrey	'an old man'	n/a	4s
Hugh, a son of Edward Parry	'an infand of about 9 yres old, his parents being poor & haveinge many other children'	n/a	2s
Oliver Griffith	'about 20 yeares of age, but sicke of the K[ing]s Evill	n/a	2s 6d
Elizabeth David ap Ellis	'an old maide & sickly'	n/a	5s
The 3 children of Thomas Lewis, Smith, dec'd	'the eldest of them not above 10 yeares of age'	n/a	6s

Name	Description	1673 rate	1674 rate
Elizabeth the late wife of Hugh ap Richard	'an old impotent woman'	n/a	2s 6d
'Cadd: the smiths children'		n/a	6s
James Realand's wife		n/a	5s
Margaret ye daughter of Rich: Evans	'towards the cureing of her sight'	n/a	£2
The 3 children of Mark Tylsley	'towards the cureing of one of the said children'	n/a	£2 5s
Robert son of Rich: Edwards	'abt 7 yeares of age'	n/a	2s
The children of John Evan	'being @ one 7 yeares of age & the other abt 3 yeares old'	n/a	5s
Cadd Poole	'an old impotent man'	n/a	5s
Catherine the daughter of William Thomas	'an old Maid troubled with the falling sickness as is alledged'	n/a	No figure given
Margaret the Daughter of Evan John	'a poore maid troubled with distracted fits'	n/a	10s
Elizabeth the wife of Edward ap Evan Foulke	'an old woman aged 80 yeares & upwards, her husband also being poore & old & not able to Mayntayne her'	n/a	5s
		TOTAL	£16 18s 4d

Note

1   All quotes and amounts taken directly from NLW, Harrison & Sons MS 1, Parcel/ Item no. 9, 1673–76, Administration of Poor Relief in Llanfyllin, Montgomeryshire.

Select bibliography

Primary sources

Manuscript

Bodleian Library, Oxford
MSS Eng. Misc. C. 266–7, Anon., Medical Remedy Books, Cheshire, c. 1753–56
MSS Welsh e. 7–9, Medical Remedies in English and Welsh, 17th and 18th century

British Library
BM Additional MSS
BM Add. MS 14894, Poetry of the Wonders of Wales and Misc. including remedies
BM Add. MS 14900, Anon., 'Llyfr Byr Llangadwaladr', Miscellaneous sermons and remedies, 18th century
BM Add. MS14907, Misc. collection of Lewis Morris of Anglesey
BM Add. MS 14913, Anon./Various, Welsh Language Medical Remedy Collection, c. 16th/17th century
BM Add. MS 15021, Misc. Welsh Manuscripts, autograph of 'Owen Jones'
BM Add. MS 15045, Anon., 'Caer Rhun', Medical Remedies attr. Physicians of Myddfai
BM Add. MS 15049, Anon., Welsh Language Medical Remedy Collection, 17th century
BM Add. MS 15078, Welsh Translation by John ap Ifan of 'The Treasury of Health' by Humfrey Llwyd
Other MSS
BM Sloane MS 398, Medical Receipt Book of Hugo Glynne, MD, of Chester, c. 1555
BL MS C.112.f9, Collection of Medical Advertisements, 17th century
BL MS 551.a.32, Collection of Medical Advertisements, 17th and 18th century

Cardiff Central Library
Phillipps MS 25367, Anon., Medical Recipe Book, c. 1600
MS 1.463, Anon., 'Prethegau' and Commonplace Book
MS 1.475, Anon., Memoranda Including Medical Recipes
MS 2.126, Medical Book attr. Sansom Jones of Bettws, c. 1600
MS 2.157, Diary of Roger Jenkins, c. 1765

Select bibliography

MS 2.209, Anon., Treatise of Urine, 1682
MS 2.281, Medical Recipe Collection attr. David Jones of Llangan
MS 2.622, Anon., Medical Recipes, c. 1700
MS 2.627, Anon., Miscellaneous, including medical recipes
MS 2.632, Anon., Medical Recipe Collection, c. 1600
MS 2.655, Anon., Medical Recipe Collection, 1781
MS 2.973, Thomas ap Ifan, Meddyginiaeth
MS 2.998, Medical Remedy Collection of 'Mrs Spyors', 1725
MS 3.212, Cadwaladr Davies, 'Piser Sioned', undated
MS 3.42, Commonplace Book of Philip Howell of Brecon, 1628–38
MS 4.171, Commonplace Book of Sir Peter Mytton
MS 4.198, Letters and Papers of Walter Powell of Llantilio
MS 4.30, 'Collectanea Wallica', Miscellany, various dates

Carmarthenshire Record Office
MS Castell Gorfod Add. 96, Anon., Medical Remedies attr. to Anne Skinner
MSS Cawdor 128, Bundles 1–4, Letters of Campbell Family of Stackpole Court, 1733–36

Chester and Cheshire Archives
MS EDC 5, Bunbury 51, Consistory Court Records, 1626, Case against Richard Brocke and John Swann
MS EDC 5, Didsbury 13, Consistory Court Records, 1720, Case against Thomas Wright

Flintshire Record Office
Birch MSS
Birch MS D/BC/2796, J. and Nath. Branke, Funeral Expenses including Medical Bills
Erddig Papers
MS Erddig D/E/1147, Letters of Valentina Malyn and Ann Mason, 13 April 1697
MS Erddig D/E/1203, Medical Remedy Collection
MS Erddig D/E/2547, John Meller, 'My Own Physical Observations', 1697
Gwysaney Papers
Gwysaney MS D/GW/3/510, Apothecary Bills of Robert Seale to 'Capteine Dodds', 1665 and Miscellany
Gwysaney MS D/GW/2115, Anon., Recipe for Powder to Cure Blindness
Other MSS
MS D/E/1296, John Meller's letters to Wrexham overseers, 1729
MS D/HE/432, Diary of Dr Thomas Griffiths of Mold, 18th century
MSS D/NA/636–49, Misc. Pennant Family Papers inc. Medical Receipts, 1681–1736

Glamorgan Record Office
Miscellaneous MSS
MS D/D/Xla, Anon., Medical Remedy Collection, 17th century
MS D/DD/53, Deed relating to 'Thomas Matthew' of Glamorgan, 1613

Select bibliography

MSS D/DF V/202–6, Medical receipts and directions to Seys Family of Boverton, Llantwit Major

MSS D/DN240/1, D/DN240/2, Overseers accounts for Llanmaes, 1637 and 1638

Quarter Sessions Records
Glamorgan Quarter Sessions Records, Roll V, Neath, 15 July 1729, M. 39
Glamorgan Quarter Sessions Records, Roll VI, Cardiff, 7 October 1729, M.22

Gwent Record Office
MS D43:4216, Commonplace Book of John Gwin of Llangwm
MS D43:5496, Letter from H.W. to Sir Charles Kemeys at Ruperra
MSS D143.5, D591.6, Misc. Leases of Walter Roberts of Abergavenny
MS D/PA/29.10, Pocketbook of William Davies of Clytha, 1654–1720

National Library of Wales, Aberystwyth
Probate Records
Church in Wales, Diocese of Bangor Probate Records, B/, BR/
Church in Wales, Diocese of Llandaff Probate Records, LL/
Church in Wales, Diocese of St Asaph Probate Records, SA/
Church in Wales, Diocese of St David's Probate Records, SD/

Diocesan Records
Church in Wales, Diocese of Bangor Episcopal 1 MS B/SM/1, Testimonial to the skill of Elizabeth Anwyl of Llandenog, in midwifery, 1753
Church in Wales, Diocese of Bangor Episcopal 1 MS B/SM/2, Testimonial to the skill of David Davis of Llangurig, in surgery, 1749
Church in Wales, Diocese of Bangor Episcopal 1 MS B/SM/8, Testimonial to the skill of Robert Roberts of Llanfihangel-y-Pennant, in surgery, 1751
Church in Wales, Diocese of Llandaff Episcopal 5 MS LL/CC/G 1096, Case against Morgan Jenkin of Porthkerry for practising physic without a licence, 1752
Church in Wales, Diocese of Llandaff Episcopal 6 MS LL/CC/C(G) 939, Deposition against Bloom Williams of Cardiff, unlicensed surgeon, 1764
Church in Wales, Diocese of St David's Episcopal (9) MS SD/CCB/C(G)/1560, Faculty to David Smith of Swansea to practise surgery, 2 July 1683
Church in Wales, Diocese of St David's Episcopal (11) MS 193, Certificate and Fiat for a licence of surgery for William Thomas of Llanelwedd co. Radnor, 1699
Church in Wales, Diocese of St David's Episcopal (11) MS 194, Testimonial concerning the grant of a licence for surgery to Isaac Rees of Llanwortyd, 18 August 1754
Church in Wales, Diocese of St David's Episcopal (11) MS 512, Petition to the Bishop of St David's, requesting the grant of a licence to Richard Prichard of Narberth to practise surgery, 9 August 1720
Church in Wales, Diocese of St David's Episcopal (11) MS 1194, Reference attesting to skill of Benjamin Powell of Gwenthwr in surgery, undated

Select bibliography

Church in Wales, Diocese of St David's Episcopal (11) MS SD/LET/1809, In support of the application of Samuel Exton to practice surgery

Church in Wales, Diocese of St David's Episcopal (11) MS 1196, Petition to license John Jones of Llandysul to practise physick and surgery, 2 September 1717

NLW MSS

NLW MS C.2, Manuscript book of Bened Feddyg

NLW MS 15-C, Commonplace Book of Michael Hughes of Lligwy/Richard Evans of Llanmerchedd, c. 1730–70

NLW MS 182-D, Remedy Collection and Miscellanea of 'Madam Lloyd' of Penpedust, undated, 18th century

NLW MS 434B, Miscellany of 'Robert Lloyd', c. 1660

NLW MS 836D, 'Piser Alice Uch Rees' Miscellany, 1718–42

NLW MS 2558D, Translations of Medical Works by Thos. Willis MD, undated, 17th century

NLW MS 2576B, Letter giving account of medical superstitions in Wales, relating to Thomas Pennant's tour, July 1755

NLW MS 2699B, Quaker Diary of John Kelsall of Dolybran, 1722–34

NLW MS 4492D, Richard Phillips, Misc. including legal precedents, undated, c. 17th/18th century

NLW MS 4599E, Tradesman's book of John Ireland of Cardiff, c. 1790

NLW MS 5309B, Remedy Collection attr. to Henry, fifth Baron Herbert of Cherbury, undated, c. late 17th century

NLW MS 5932A, Anon., Medical Remedies and Miscellany, c. 1635

NLW MS 11457C, Collection of Morrall Family Papers, various dates, 17th and 18th century

NLW MS 13146A, Misc. collection of Edward Williams ('Iolo Morgannwg'), various dates

NLW MS 23069, Medical Notes made by Richard Pughes of Machynlleth, 1754

Bachymbyd

Bachymbyd MS 720, 'Inspeximus of a decree in Chancery between William Salisbury, esq. complainant, and Pierce Griffith, esq., and Elen Owen Widow, and others, Defendants', 22 May 1613

Badminton 1 (Manorial 2)

Badminton 1 (Manorial 2) MS 2197, Petition by Mary Jones of Llandenny to 'John Burke' to be excused rent due to sickness, undated, c. 1700

Bodewryd

Bodewryd MS 96A, Commonplace Book of Anne Penrhos

Bodewryd (1) MSS 148–51, Letters of Lloyd Family of Ruthin to 'Madam Wynn', various dates, 1715–22

Bodewryd (1) MS 370, Letter from Benjamin Conway to 'Madam Wynn' regarding churchwardens and Cwrt Mostyn's charity to the poor, 8 February 1731

Select bibliography

Bodewryd (1), MSS 530, 550, 551, Letters from Charles Lloyd of Drenewydd to Edward Wynne, May 1739
Bodewryd (2) MS 380, Letter to Bishop of Hereford regarding practising of physic without a licence, 14 March 1726

Brogyntyn
Brogyntyn (2) MS EAE2/2, Poor Relief Accounts for Parish of Abertanat, 1716

Chirk Castle
Chirk Castle (2) MS 2843, Letter from John Davies to Richard Myddelton, 14 April 1747
Chirk Castle (2) MS 4176, Letter from John Davies to Thomas Cupper, 23 April 1707
Chirk Castle (3) MS 1362, Letter from Magdalen Lloyd to Thomas Edwards, 15 October 1680
Chirk Castle (3) MS 4648, Letter from Magdalen Lloyd to Thomas Edwards, 30 October 1680
Chirk Castle (3) MS 4652, Letter from George Myddelton to Thomas Wynne, May 1708

Cilybebyll
Cilybebyll (2) MS 522, Richard Davies and William Walker, Miscellaneous legal bonds, December 1667

Clenennau
Clenennau (1) MS 40, Letter from Frances Ridgway to Sir William Mawrice, 14 March 1620
Clenennau 2 (A) MS 494, Letter from Lewis Annwyl at Faenol to his father William Lewis Annwyl at Park, 29 April 1636
Clenennau 2 (A) MS 521, Letter from William Griffith of Trefarthen to his daughter-in-law re: purges, 1640

Coed Coch
Coed Coch (1), MS 482, Richard Wynn of Ruthin, Apothecary, Deed of Sale, 1684
Crosse of Shaw Hill
Crosse of Shaw Hill MS 749, Samuel Bowdler, Margaret Lloyd, Misc. Lease, November 1665

Cwrtmawr
Cwrtmawr, MSS 97, 672, Notebooks of John and Henry Harries
Cwrtmawr 1(A) MS 38B, Notes and Manuscript of Thomas Nicklas of Conwy including folklore and medicine, c. 18th century
Cwrtmawr 2(A) MS 254A, Tithe book of Llangynyw, c. 1646–76
Cwrtmawr (2) MS 491B, Medical Remedies of Thomas Lewis/Evan Thomas, 18th century
Cwrtmawr (3) MS 638A, Anon., 18th-century Miscellany in Welsh/English

Select bibliography

D.T.M. Jones

D.T.M. Jones (3) MSS 1130, 1160, 1185, 1191, 1192, 1194, 1196, Letters of Jones family of Talgarth, c. 1770–90

Denbighshire Great Sessions

Denbighshire Great Sessions Gaol Files MS 4/33/3, Trial of Jane Foulkes and Lettice Lloyd, March 1686

Dolfriog

Dolfriog MS 43, Letter from Owen Nicholas ap Morgan to Morice Williams, 15 September 1621

Dolfriog MS 131, Lease for Lands signed by John Owen and Owen Owen, 10 March 1650

Dolfriog MS231, Letter from Owen Poole to Morice Williams, undated

Edwinsford

Edwinsford (2) MS 475, 'Letters Testimonial of William Awbery', 22 December 1632

Frederick Holland MSS

Frederick Holland MS 32, Assessment for Poor Relief in Llantrisant, 16 June 1686

George Ayre Evans

George Ayre Evans MS 73, Assessment of Poor Relief for Parish of Llanstephan, 1731

Harrison & Sons

Harrison and Sons MS 1, Parcel/Item no. 9, 1673–76, Administration of Poor Relief in Llanfyllin, Montgomeryshire

Kemeys-Tynte

Kemys-Tynte MSS c.92–3, Misc. letters including apothecary bills

Kemeys-Tynte (2) MS CA422, Letter from Mary Kemeys to Sir Charles Kemeys, 6 November 1702

Llanfair and Brynodol

Llanfair and Brynodol (2) MS D1027, Probate of Charles Jones of Lincoln's Inn, November 1640

Maybery

Maybery (3) MS 4279, Foundation deed for use of land in Llanvaes, Breconshire, c. 1721

Peniarth

Peniarth MS 348 (A), Remedy Collection attr. Sydney Vaughan, 1705

Peniarth MS 517D, Medical Remedy Collection owned by Catherine Nanney of Merioneth, c. 1730

Select bibliography

Peniarth MS 521A, Diaries and Notebooks of Griffith Wynn of Bodfaen, 1668
Peniarth Estate (2), MSS A1, A2, A5, Estate Administration Accounts including alma-
    nacks and medical remedies

Penrice and Margam

Penrice and Margam (3) MS 1439, List of Persons Rated for Poor Rate in Hamlet of
    Cundy, 29 April 1684
Penrice and Margam (3) MS 1453, Letter from John Powell of Carmarthen to John
    Williams at Margam, 28 April, 1691
Penrice and Margam (3) MS 1511, List of People Assessed for Poor Rate in Margam, 1725

Tredegar

Tredegar (1) MS 1172, Letter from Edward Griffiths to Octavius Morgan, 10 August 1858
Tredegar (11) Box 157/62, Assessment for Poor Relief in Parish of Llanvihangel, 29
    January 1753

Wigfair

Wigfair (2) MS 12402E, John Lloyde, Letter regarding treatment of the 'King's Evil' for
    his daughter, undated, c. 1664

Wynn of Gwydir

Wynn of Gwydir (1) MS 102, Letter from Sir John Wynn of Gwydir detailing his
    symptoms, c. 1585

Pembrokeshire Record Office
MS HDX/88/1, Anon., Medical Receipts headed '1698 Receipts'
MS HDX/175/1, Anon., Remedy Collection, 17th century
MS HDX/214, Anon., Remedy Collection, 17th century
MS HDX/382/1, George Hartman, A Collection of Choice Approved and Experienced
    Remedies for the Cure of Most Diseases, 1707
MS HDX/4/41, Notebook of Anne Phelps of Witheybush
MS HDX/4/51, Anon., Remedy Book, 19th century
MS H'West Boro 574, Misc. Physicians Accounts relating to the plague, 17th century

Powys County Archives Office
Microfiche MP125, Llanfyllin Parish Registers, 1665–77

West Glamorgan Archives
MS D/D RE 1/261, Misc. Letters and Legal Forms of Mansell Family of Margam, c. 1680
MS D/DZ123/1, Notebook of John Morgan of Palleg, c. 1728–68

Wellcome Library, London
MS 417, 'Llyfr o fedheginiaeth a physygwriaeth' (book of remedies and medicine
    c. 1600)

Select bibliography

MSS 8236–55 and 8968–89, David Fraser-Harris, Research Notes and Drafts for Unfinished Volume, 'The History and Lore of Cymric Medicine', c. 1928

Printed

Anon., *The Life and Mysterious Transactions of Richard Morris Esq. better known by the name of Dick Spot, The Conjuror* (London: T. Maiden, 1799)

Anon., *The Philosophical Transactions Abridged* (London: Hames and Martin, 1734–56)

A.T., *Practitioner in Physicke: A Rich Storehouse and Treasury for the Diseased* . . . (London: Printed for Thomas Purfot and Ralph Blower, 1596)

Best, Michael R. (ed.), *The English Housewife by Gervase Markham* (Quebec: McGill-Queen's University Press, 2003 edition)

Bowen, Lloyd (ed.), *Family and Society in Early Stuart Glamorgan: The Household Accounts of Sir Thomas Aubrey of Llantrithyd, c. 1565–1641* (Cardiff: South Wales Records Society, 2006)

Bradney, Joseph Alfred (ed.), *The Diary of Walter Powell of LlantilioCrossenny in the County of Monmouth, Gentleman, 1603–1654* (Bristol: John Wright & Co., 1907)

Brome, Alexander, *Rump or an exact collection of the choycest poems and songs relayting to the late times by the most eminent wits from 1639 to anno 1661* (London: Printed for Henry Brome, 1662)

Bruce, John et al. (eds), *Calendar of State Papers, Domestic series of the Reign of Charles I: Preserved in the State Paper Department of Her Majesty's Public Record Office*, 26 Volumes (London: H.M.S.O., 1858–97)

Bromwich, Rachel, *Dafydd ap Gwilym: A Selection of Poems* (Llandysul: Gomer Press, 1982)

Chandler, John (ed.), *Travels Through Stuart Britain: The Adventures of John Taylor, the Water Poet* (Stroud: Sutton Publishing, 1999)

Charras, Moses, *The Royal Pharmacopea, Galenical and Chymicall* . . . (London: Printed for John Starkey, 1678)

Culpeper, Nicholas, *Herbal, neu Lysieu-Lyfr. Y RhanGyntaf* . . . *Wedi eu Casglu Allan o Waith N. Culpeper* . . . *Gan D.T. Jones* (Caernarfon: L.E. Jones, 1816)

Davies, John H., *The Letters of Lewis, Richard, William and John Morris of Anglesey (Morrisiaid Mon) 1728–1765*, 2 Volumes (Aberystwyth: Privately Published, 1907)

Denning, R.T.W. (ed.), *The Diary of William Thomas of Michaelston-Super-Ely near St Fagans, Glamorgan* (Cardiff: South Wales Record Society, 1995)

Dineley, Thomas, *The Account of the Official Progress of His Grace Henry the First Duke of Beaufort* . . . *Through Wales in 1684* (London: Blades, Facsimile edition 1888)

E.B., *A Trip to North Wales: Being a Description of That Country and People* (London: 1701)

Edwards, Edward, *The Analysis of Chyrurgery* . . . (London: Printed by Thomas Harper, 1636)

Edwards, Edward, *The Cure of All Sorts of Fevers* (London: T. Harper, 1638)

Edwards, Edward, *The Whole Art of Chyrurgery* (London: Thomas Harper, 1639)

Fuller, Thomas, *Pharmacopoeia Extemporanea: Or A Body of Prescripts in Which Forms of Select Remedies Accommodated to Most Intentions of Cure Usually Occurring in Practice* (London: Printed for Ben J. Walford, 1710)

Gentleman's Magazine (January 1733)

Gerard, John, *The herball or Generall historie of plantes* . . . (London: Printed by Adam Islip,

Select bibliography

Joice Norton and Richard Whitakers, 1663)

Johnson, Robert, *Praxis Medicinae Reformata or The Practice of Physick Reformed* (London: Printed for Brabazon Aylmer, 1700)

Johnston, J.A. (ed.), *Probate Inventories of Lincoln Citizens 1661–1714* (Lincoln: Lincoln Record Society, 1991)

Jones, John, *De Morbis Hibernorum* . . . (London: S. Keble, 1697)

Jones, Thomas, *The British Language in its Lustre or A Copious Dictionary of Welsh and English* (London: Printed and sold by Mr Lawrence Baskervile, 1668)

Jones, Thomas, *Carolau a Dyriau Duwiol* . . . (Shrewsbury: Ac are Werth gan Thomas Jones, 1668)

J.T., *A Collection of Welch Travels and Memoirs of Wales* (Dublin: Printed for J. Torbuck and E. Rider, 1743)

Lee, Matthew Henry (ed.), *The Diaries and Letters of Philip Henry, M.A. of Broad Oak, Flintshire, A.D. 1631–1696* (London: Kegan Paul, Trench and Co., 1882)

Lewis, E.A. (ed.), *Welsh Port Books 1550–1603* (London: Honourable Society of Cymmrodorion, 1927)

Llwyd, Humfrey, *The Treasury of Health containing many profitable medicines, gathered out of Hippocrates, Galen, and Aucien, by one Petrus Hyspanius & translated into English by Humfrie Lloyd* (London: Printed by Thomas East, 1585)

Moulton, Thomas, *The Mirror or Glasse of Health, Necessary and Needefull for Every Person to Looke in* . . . (London: Printed by Hugh Jackson, 1580)

National Library of Wales, *Civil War and Commonwealth Tracts etc* (Aberystwyth: National Library of Wales, 1911)

Pechey, John, *The Storehouse of Physical Practice* . . . (London: Printed for Henry Bonwicke, 1695)

R.B., *The Natural History of the Principality of Wales* . . . (London: Printed for Nath. Crouch at the Bell, Cheapside, 1695)

Recorde, Robert, *The Judgement of Urines* (London: Printed and to be sold by Peter Parker, 1679)

Recorde, Robert, *The Urinal of Physick* (London: Printed by Reynold Wolfe, 1548)

Sherlock, William, *A Practical Discourse Concerning Death* (London: Printed for W. Rogers, 1690)

Stanton Roberts, E. (ed.), *Llysieulyfr Meddyginiaethol a Briodolir I William Salesbury* (Liverpool: Hugh Evans, 1916)

Thomas, D.R., *Y Cwtta Cyfarwydd: 'The Chronicle' written by the famous clarke Peter Roberts, Notary Public, From the Years 1607–1646* (London: Whiting and Co., 1883)

Vaughan, Henry Halford, *Welsh Proverbs with English Translations* (London: Kegan Paul and Trench, 1889)

Williams, J.B., *Memoirs of the Life and Character of Mrs Sarah Savage* (London: Holdsworth and Hall, Fourth edition 1829)

Williams, John, *Faunula Grustensis: Being an outline of the natural contents of the parish of Llanrwst* (Llanrwst: John Jones, 1830)

Williams, Perrot 'Part of two letters concerning a method of procuring the Small Pox, used in South Wales . . . ', *Philosophical Transactions of the Royal Society of London*, 32:374 (1723), pp. 262–264

Williams, Thomas, *Ymadroddion Bucheddol Ynghylch Marwolaeth o Waith Doctor Sherlock* (London: Printed for Leon Lichfield, 1691)

Willis, Thomas, *The London Practice of Physick or, The Whole Practical parts of Physick contained in the works of Doctor Willis* (London: Printed for Thomas Basset, 1685)

W.M., *The Queen's Closet Opened: Prestigious Medicines* (London: Printed for Nathaniel Brooke, 1659)

Wood, Thomas, *The Registers of Glasbury, Breconshire, 1660–1836* (London: Privately Printed for the Parish Register Society, 1904)

Wyndham, Henry Penruddock, *A Gentleman's Tour Through Monmouthshire and Wales in the Months of June and July 1774* (London: Printed for T. Evans, 1781)

Secondary Sources

Books

Arkell, Tom, Evans, Nesta and Goose, Nigel (eds), *When Death Do Us Part: Understanding and Interpreting the Probate Records of Early Modern England* (London: Leopard's Head Press, 2004 edition)

Baber, Colin and Lancaster, John (eds), *Healthcare in Wales: An Historical Miscellany* (Cardiff: University Hospital of Wales League of Friends, 2000)

Ballinger, John (ed.), *Calendar of Wynn (of Gwydir) Papers 1515–1690* (Cardiff: National Library of Wales, 1924–26)

Barry, Jonathan and Jones, Colin (eds), *Medicine and Charity before the Welfare State* (London: Routledge, 1994)

Bartley, J.O., Teague, *Shenkin and Sawney, Being an Historical Study of the Earliest Irish, Welsh and Scottish Characters in English Plays* (Cork: Cork University Press, 1954)

Beier, Lucinda McCray, *Sufferers and Healers: The Experience of Illness in Seventeenth Century England* (London and New York: Routledge and Kegan Paul, 1987)

Beith, Mary, *Healing Threads: Traditional Medicines of the Highlands and Islands* (Edinburgh: Birlinn, 1995)

Berg, Maxine and Eger, Elizabeth (eds), *Luxury in the Eighteenth Century: Debates, Desires and Delectable Goods* (Basingstoke: Palgrave Macmillan, 2003)

Boon, George C., *Welsh Tokens of the Seventeenth Century* (Cardiff: National Museum of Wales, 1973)

Borsay, Anne (ed.), *Medicine in Wales c.1800–2000: Public Service or Private Commodity?* (Cardiff: University of Wales Press, 2003)

Bowen, Peter, *Shopkeepers and Tradesmen in Cardiff and the Vale, 1633–1857* (Cardiff: Peter Bowen, 2004)

Brewer, John and Porter, Roy (eds), *Consumption and the World of Goods* (London and New York: Routledge, 1993)

Burnham, John C., *What is Medical History?* (Cambridge: Polity Press, 2005)

Select bibliography

Burr, Vivien, *Social Constructionism* (London and New York: Routledge, 2005 edition)

Bynum, W.F. and Porter, Roy (eds), *The Companion Encyclopaedia of the History of Medicine*, 2 Volumes (London and New York: Routledge, 1996)

Capp, Bernard, *English Almanacs 1500–1800: Astrology and the Popular Press* (New York: Cornell, 1979)

Capp, Bernard, *When Gossips Meet: Women, Family and the Neighbourhood in Early Modern England* (Oxford: Oxford University Press, 2004)

Charles, B.G., *Calendar of the Records of the Borough of Haverfordwest 1539–1660* (Cardiff: University of Wales Press, 1967)

Cockayne, Emily, *Hubbub: Noise, Filth and Stench in England* (Yale: Yale University Press, 2007)

Cooter, Roger and Luckin, Bill (eds), *Accidents in History* (Amsterdam, Atlanta, GA: Rodopi, 1997)

Coster, Will, *Family and Kinship in England 1450–1800* (London: Longman, 2001)

Crawford, Patricia, *Blood, Bodies and Families in Early Modern England* (Harlow: Pearson, 2004)

Creighton, Charles, *A History of Epidemics in Britain*, 2 Volumes (London: Frank Cass & Co., 1965 edition)

Cressy, David, *Birth, Marriage and Death* (Oxford: Oxford University Press, 1997)

Cule, John, *Wales and Medicine: A Source List for Printed Books and Papers Showing the History of Medicine in Relation to Wales and Welshmen* (Aberystwyth: Privately Printed, 1980)

Cule, John (ed.), *Wales and Medicine* (Llandysul: Gomer Press, 1975)

Cunningham, Andrew and French, Roger (eds), *The Medical Enlightenment of the Eighteenth Century* (Cambridge: Cambridge University Press, 1999)

Cunningham, Andrew and Grell, Ole Peter (eds), *Healthcare and Poor Relief in Northern Europe, 1500–1700* (London: Routledge, 1997)

Curth, Louise Hill, *English Almanacs: Astrology and Popular Medicine, 1550–1700* (Manchester: Manchester University Press, 2007)

Curth, Louise Hill (ed.), *From Physick to Pharmacology: Five Hundred Years of British Drug Retailing* (Aldershot: Ashgate, 2006)

Davies, Adrian, *The Quakers in English Society, 1655–1725* (Oxford: Oxford University Press, 2000)

Davies, Owen and Tallis, Lisa, *Cunning Folk: An Introductory Bibliography* (London: The Folklore Society, 2005)

Davies, R.R., Griffiths, Ralph A., Jones, Ieuan Gwynedd and Morgan, Kenneth O. (eds), *Welsh Society and Nationhood* (Cardiff: University of Wales Press, 1984)

Davies, R.R. and Jenkins, Geraint H., *From Medieval to Modern Wales* (Cardiff: University of Wales Press, 2004)

Debus, Allen (ed.), *Science, Medicine and Society in the Renaissance* (London: Heinemann, 1972)

Dingwall, Helen M., *A History of Scottish Medicine: Themes and Influences* (Edinburgh: Edinburgh University Press, 2003)

Dingwall, Helen M., *Physicians, Surgeons and Apothecaries: Medicine in Seventeenth-Century Edinburgh* (East Linton: Tuckwell Press, 1995)

Select bibliography

Dobson, Mary J., *Contours of Death and Disease in Early Modern England* (Cambridge: Cambridge University Press, 2002 edition)

Dunn, Diana (ed.), *War and Society in Medieval and Early Modern Britain* (Liverpool: Liverpool University Press, 2000)

Dyfnallt Owen, G., *Elizabethan Wales: The Social Scene* (Cardiff: University of Wales Press, 1967)

Edgar, Iwan Rhys, *Llysieulyfr Salesbury* (Cardiff: University of Wales Press, 1997)

Elmer, Peter (ed.), *The Healing Arts: Health, Disease and Society in Europe 1500–1800* (Manchester: Manchester University Press, 2004)

Erler, Mary C., *Gendering the Master Narrative: Women and Power in the Middle Ages* (Ithaca: Cornell University Press, 2003)

Fairs, Geoffrey L., *A History of the Hay: The Story of Hay-on-Wye* (Chichester: Phillimore, 1972)

Fissell, Mary E., *Patients, Power and the Poor in Eighteenth Century Bristol* (Cambridge: Cambridge University Press, 2002 edition)

Fissell, Mary E., *Vernacular Bodies: The Politics of Reproduction in Early Modern England* (Oxford: Oxford University Press, 2004)

Fox, Adam, *Oral and Literate Culture in England 1500–1700* (Oxford: Oxford University Press, 2000)

Fox, Adam and Woolf, Daniel (eds), *The Spoken Word: Oral Culture in Britain, 1500–1850* (Manchester: Manchester University Press, 2002)

Fox, Cyril and Lord Raglan, *Monmouthshire Houses Part III: The Renaissance* (Cardiff: National Museum of Wales, 1954)

Foyster, Elizabeth A., *Manhood in Early Modern England: Honour, Sex and Marriage* (London and New York: Longman, 1999)

French, Henry and Barry, Jonathan (eds), *Identity and Agency in England, 1500–1800* (Basingstoke: Palgrave Macmillan, 2004)

French, Roger and Wear, Andrew (eds), *British Medicine in an Age of Reform* (London and New York: Routledge, 1991)

Gentilcore, David, *Healers and Healing in Early Modern Italy* (Manchester: Manchester University Press, 1998)

Gittings, Clare, *Death, Burial and the Individual in Early Modern England* (London: Routledge, 1988)

Good, Byron J., *Medicine, Rationality and Experience: An Anthropological Perspective* (Cambridge: Cambridge University Press, 2007 edition)

Gowing, Laura, *Common Bodies: Women, Touch and Power in Seventeenth-Century England* (London and New Haven: Yale University Press, 2003)

Grant, Raymond K.J., *On the Parish* (Cardiff: Glamorgan Archive Service, 1988)

Grell, Ole Peter, Cunningham, Andrew and Roeck, Bernd (eds), *Health Care and Poor Relief in 18th and 19th Century Southern Europe* (Burlington: Ashgate, 2005)

Grell, Ole Peter and Cunningham, Andrew (eds), *Health Care and Poor Relief in Protestant Europe 1500–1700* (London and New York: Routledge, 1997)

Grell, Ole Peter and Cunningham, Andrew (eds), *Medicine and the Reformation* (London and New York: Routledge, 1993)

Select bibliography

Grell, Ole Peter and Cunningham, Andrew (eds), *Religio Medici: Medicine and Religion in Seventeenth-Century England* (Aldershot: Scolar Press, 1996)

Griffiths, Ralph, Gray, Madeleine and Morgan, Prys (eds), *Gwent County History Volume 3: The Making of Monmouthshire 1536–1780* (Cardiff: University of Wales Press, 2009)

Gwyndaf, Robin, *Welsh Folk Tales* (Cardiff: National Museums and Galleries of Wales, 1999)

Heal, Felicity and Holmes, Clive, *The Gentry in England and Wales 1500–1700* (Basingstoke: Palgrave, 1994)

Hindle, Steve, *On the Parish? The Micro-Politics of Poor Relief in Rural England, c. 1550–1750* (Oxford: Oxford University Press, 2009 edition)

Hitchcock, Tim and Cohen, Michele (eds), *English Masculinities 1660–1800* (London: Longman, 1999)

Hitchcock, Tim, King, Peter and Sharpe, Pamela (eds), *Chronicling Poverty: The Voices and Strategies of the English Poor, 1640–1840* (Basingstoke: Macmillan, 1997)

Houlbrooke, Ralph, *Death, Religion and the Family in England 1480–1750* (Oxford: Clarendon Press, 2000 edition)

Houlbrooke, Ralph (ed.), *Death, Ritual and Bereavement* (London and New York: Routledge, 1989)

Howe, G. Melvyn, *People, Environment, Disease and Death: A Medical Geography of Britain Throughout the Ages* (Cardiff: University of Wales Press, 1997)

Howell, David, *The Rural Poor in Eighteenth Century Wales* (Cardiff: University of Wales Press, 2000)

Howells, B.E. (ed.), *A Calendar of Letters Relating to North Wales 1533–circa 1700* (Cardiff: University of Wales Press, 1967)

Howse, W.H., *Radnorshire* (Hereford: Radnorshire Society, 1973)

Isaac, Peter and McKay, Barry (eds), *The Mighty Engine: The Printing Press and its Impact* (Winchester: St Paul's Bibliographies, 2000)

Jenkins, Geraint H., *A Concise History of Wales* (Cambridge: Cambridge University Press, 2007)

Jenkins, Geraint H., *The Foundations of Modern Wales, 1642–1780* (Oxford: Oxford University Press, 2002 edition)

Jenkins, Geraint H., *Literature, Religion and Society in Wales, 1660–1730* (Cardiff: University of Wales Press, 1978)

Jenkins, Philip, *A History of Modern Wales 1536–1990* (London and New York: Longman, 1992)

Jenner, Mark S.R. and Wallis, Patrick (eds), *Medicine and the Market in England and its Colonies c. 1450 – c. 1850* (Basingstoke: Palgrave Macmillan, 2007)

Jones, Emrys (ed.), *The Welsh in London 1500–2000* (Cardiff: University of Wales Press, 2000)

Jones, Gareth Elwyn and Smith, Dai (eds), *The People of Wales* (Llandysul: Gomer Press, 2000 edition)

Jones, Glyn Penrhyn, *Newyn a Haint yng Nghymru* (Caernarfon: Llyfrfa'r Methodistiaid Calfinaidd, 1962)

Select bibliography

Jones, J. Gwynfor, *Early Modern Wales c. 1525–1640* (Basingstoke: Macmillan Press, 1994)

Jones, J. Gwynfor, *The Wynn Family of Gwydir: Origins, Growth and Development* c. *1490–1674* (Aberystwyth: Centre for Educational Studies, 1995)

Jones, Philip Henry and Rees, Eiluned (eds), *A Nation and its Books: A History of the Book in Wales* (Aberystwyth: National Library of Wales, 1998)

King, Steven, *Poverty and Welfare in England 1700–1850: A Regional Perspective* (Manchester: Manchester University Press, 2000)

King, Steven and Tomkins, Alannah (eds), *The Poor in England 1700–1850* (Manchester: Manchester University Press, 2003)

Lane, Joan, *A Social History of Medicine: Health, Healing and Disease in England, 1750–1950* (London and New York: Routledge, 2001)

Lemire, Beverley, *The Business of Everyday Life* (Manchester: Manchester University Press, 2005)

Lindemann, Mary, *Medicine and Society in Early Modern Europe* (Cambridge: Cambridge University Press, 1999)

Lodwick, Joyce and Lodwick, Victor, *The Story of Carmarthen* (Carmarthen: St Peter's Press, 1994)

Lord, Peter, *Words With Pictures: Welsh Images and Images of Wales in the Popular Press, 1640–1860* (Aberystwyth: Planet, 1995)

Love, Harold, *Scribal Publication in Seventeenth Century England* (Oxford: Oxford University Press, 1993)

Mackay, Charles, *Extraordinary Popular Delusions and the Madness of Crowds* (Ware: Wordsworth, 1995 edition)

McNeill, William H., *Plagues and Peoples* (Oxford: Basil Blackwell, 1977)

Michael, Pamela, *Care and Treatment of the Mentally Ill in North Wales 1800–2000* (Cardiff: University of Wales Press, 2003)

Michael, Pamela and Webster, Charles (eds), *Health and Society in Twentieth Century Wales* (Cardiff: University of Wales Press, 2006)

Miles, Dilwyn, *A History of the Town and County of Haverfordwest* (Llandysul: Gomer Press, 1999)

Morgan, Kenneth O., *Rebirth of a Nation: A History of Modern Wales* (Oxford: Oxford University Press, 1981)

Morgan, Prys (ed.), *Wales: An Illustrated History* (Stroud: Tempus, 2005)

Morris, Owen, *The 'CHYMICK BOOKES' of Sir Owen Wynne of Gwydir: An Annotated Catalogue* (Cambridge: LP Publications, 1997)

Mortimer, Ian, *The Dying and the Doctors: The Medical Revolution in Seventeenth-Century England* (Woodbridge: Boydell Press/The Royal Historical Society, 2009)

Mui, Hoh-Cheung and Mui, Lorna H., *Shops and Shopkeeping in Eighteenth-Century England* (London: Routledge, 1989)

Myddelton, W.S., *Chirk Castle Accounts 1666–1753* (Manchester: Manchester University Press, 1931)

Nagy, Doreen G., *Popular Medicine in Seventeenth Century England* (Bowling Green, OH: Bowling Green State University Popular Press, 1988)

Select bibliography

Newman, William R., *Gehennical Fire: The Lives of George Starkey* (Chicago and London: University of Chicago Press, 1994)

Overton, Mark, Dean, Darren, Whittle, Jane and Hann, Andrew (eds), *Production and Consumption in English Households, 1600–1750* (London and New York: Routledge, 2004)

Owen, Elias, *Welsh Folk-Lore: A Collection of the Folk Tales and Legends of North Wales* (Felinfach: Llanerch, 1996 facsimile reprint of 1896 edition)

Owen, Trefor M., *Welsh Folk Customs* (Llandysul: Gomer Press, 1959)

Oxley, Geoffrey, *Poor Relief in England and Wales 1601–1834* (London: David and Charles, 1974)

Palmer, Roy, *The Folklore of Old Monmouthshire* (Woonton Almeley, Herefordshire: Logaston Press, 2004 edition)

Park, Katherine, *Doctors and Medicine in Early Renaissance Florence* (Princeton: Princeton University Press, 1985)

Parker, Keith, *A History of Presteigne* (Woonton Almeley, Herefordshire: Logaston Press, 1997)

Parker, Keith, *Radnorshire from Civil War to Restoration* (Woonton Almeley, Herefordshire: Logaston Press, 2000)

Parry-Williams, T.H., *The English Element in Welsh: A Study of English Loan-Words in Welsh* (London: Honourable Society of Cymmrodorion, 1923)

Peate, Iorweth, *The Welsh House: A Study in Folk Culture* (Liverpool: Brython Press, 1944)

Pelling, Margaret, *The Common Lot: Sickness, Medical Occupations and the Urban Poor in Early Modern England* (London and New York: Longman, 1998)

Pelling, Margaret and Smith, Richard M. (eds), *Life, Death and the Elderly: Historical Perspectives* (London and New York: Routledge, 1991)

Porter, Roy, *Bodies Politic: Disease, Death and Doctors in Britain, 1650–1900* (London: Reaktion, 2001)

Porter, Roy, *The Greatest Benefit to Mankind: A Medical History of Humanity from Antiquity to the Present* (London: Fontana, 1999 edition)

Porter, Roy, *Quacks: Fakers and Charlatans in Medicine* (Stroud: Tempus, 2003 edition)

Porter, Roy (ed.), *The Cambridge History of Medicine* (Cambridge: Cambridge University Press, 2006)

Porter, Roy (ed.), *Patients and Practitioners: Lay Perceptions of Medicine in Pre-Industrial Society* (Cambridge: Cambridge University Press, 2002 edition)

Porter, Dorothy and Porter, Roy, *In Sickness and in Health: The British Experience 1650–1850* (London: Fourth Estate, 1988)

Porter, Dorothy and Porter, Roy, *Patient's Progress: Doctors and Doctoring in Eighteenth Century England* (Stanford: Stanford University Press, 1989)

Porter, Roy and Wear, Andrew (eds), *Problems and Methods in the History of Medicine* (London: Croom Helm, 1987)

Powell, Christabel, *Walter Powell's Gwent: An Architectural Biography of a 17th Century Diarist* (Risca: Starling Press 1985)

Price, Michael (ed.), *The Account Book for the Borough of Swansea, Wales: A Study in Local Administration during the Civil War and Interregnum* (Lampeter: Edwin Mellen Press, 1990)

Select bibliography

Pughe, John (ed.), *The Physicians of Myddfai: Translated and with an Introduction by John Pughe* (Felinfach: Llanerch Publishers, Facsimile edition 1993)

Raach, John H., *A Directory of English Country Physicians* (London: Dawsons of Pall Mall, 1962)

Rabb, Theodore and Rotberg, Robert (eds), *The New History: The 1980s and Beyond* (Princeton: Princeton University Press, 1982)

Riley, James C., *Sickness, Recovery and Death* (Basingstoke: Macmillan, 1989)

Roberts, Gomer Morgan (ed.), *Selected Trevecka Letters (1747–1794)* (Caernarvon: The Calvinist Methodist Bookroom, 1962)

Roberts, Michael and Clarke, Simone (eds), *Women and Gender in Early Modern Wales* (Cardiff: University of Wales Press, 2000)

Roberts, T.R., *The Proverbs of Wales: A Selection of Welsh Proverbs with English Translations* (London: Francis Griffiths, 1909)

Robertson, Roland and Turner, Bryan S. (eds), *Talcott Parsons: Theorist of Modernity* (London: Sage, 1991)

Ross, Anne, *Folklore of Wales* (Stroud: Tempus Publishing, 2001)

Scott, James C., *Domination and the Arts of Resistance* (Yale: Yale University Press, 1992)

Scott, James C., *Weapons of the Weak: Everyday Forms of Peasant Resistance* (New Haven and London: Yale University Press, 1985)

Shepard, Alexandra, *Meanings of Manhood in Early Modern England* (Oxford: Oxford University Press, 2003)

Shepard, Alexandra and Withington, Phil (eds), *Communities in Early Modern England* (Manchester: Manchester University Press, 2000)

Shuttleton, David, *Smallpox and the Literary Imagination, 1660–1820* (Cambridge: Cambridge University Press, 2007)

Sikes, Wirt, *British Goblins: Welsh Folklore, Fairy Mythology, Legends and Traditions* (Doylestown, PA: Wildside Press, Facsimile edition 2002)

Simpson, Jacqueline, *The Folklore of the Welsh Border* (Stroud: Tempus, 2003 edition)

Siraisi, Nancy, *Medieval and Early Renaissance Medicine: An Introduction to Knowledge and Practice* (Chicago: University of Chicago Press, 1990)

Slack, Paul, *The English Poor Law, 1531–1782* (Cambridge: Cambridge University Press, 1995)

Slack, Paul, *The Impact of Plague in Tudor and Stuart England* (London: Routledge and Kegan Paul, 1985)

Smith, W.J., *Herbert Correspondence* (Cardiff: University of Wales Press, 1968)

Soulsby, Ian, *The Towns of Medieval Wales* (Chichester: Phillimore and Co., 1983)

Spufford, Margaret (ed.), *The World of Rural Dissenters, 1520–1725* (Cambridge: Cambridge University Press, 1995)

Stainton Rogers, Mary, *Explaining Health and Illness: An Exploration of Diversity* (Hemel Hempstead: Harvester Wheatsheaf, 1991)

Stobart, Jon, Hann, Andrew and Morgan, Victoria, *Spaces of Consumption: Leisure and Shopping in the English Town, c. 1680–1830* (London and New York: Routledge, 2007)

Stoyle, Mark, *West Britons: Cornish Identities and the Early Modern British State* (Exeter: University of Exeter Press, 2002)

Select bibliography

Suggett, Richard, *A History of Magic and Witchcraft in Wales* (Stroud: The History Press, 2008)

Tadmor, Naomi, *Family and Friends in Eighteenth Century England* (Cambridge: CambridgeUniversity Press, 2001)

Thirsk, Joan (ed.), *The Agrarian History of England and Wales Vol. VIII: 1640–1750, Agrarian Change* (Cambridge: Cambridge University Press, 1985)

Thomas, Hugh, *A History of Wales 1485–1660* (Cardiff: University of Wales Press, 1972)

Thomas, Keith, *Religion and the Decline of Magic* (London: Penguin, 1991 edition)

Thomas, W.S.K., *Stuart Wales* (Llandysul: Gomer Press, 1988)

Trevelyan, Marie, *Folk-Lore and Folk-Stories of Wales* (London: E. Stock, 1909)

Turner, Bryan S., *The Body and Society: Explorations in Social Theory* (London: Sage, 1996)

Turner, Bryan S. (ed.), *The Talcott Parsons Reader* (Oxford: Blackwell, 1999)

Waite, Edward Arthur, *Hermetic and Alchemical Writings of Paracelsus*, 2 Volumes (Whitefish, MT: Kessinger Publishing, 2002)

Walker, Garthine (ed.), *Writing Early Modern History* (Oxford: Oxford University Press, 2005)

Walter, John and Schofield, Roger (eds), *Famine, Disease and the Social Order in Early Modern Society* (Cambridge: Cambridge University Press, 1991 edition)

Waters, Ivor, *Chepstow Parish Records* (Newport: Chepstow Society and Monmouthshire branch of the Historical Association, 1955)

Wear, Andrew, *Knowledge and Practice in English Medicine, 1550–1680* (Cambridge: Cambridge University Press, 2000)

Wear, Andrew (ed.), *Medicine in Society: Historical Essays* (Cambridge: Cambridge University Press, 1998 edition)

Weatherill, Lorna, *Consumer Behaviour and Material Culture in Britain 1660–1760* (London and New York: Routledge, 1998 edition)

Webster, Charles (ed.), *Health, Medicine and Mortality in the Sixteenth Century* (Cambridge: Cambridge University Press, 1979)

Wild, Wayne, *Medicine-By-Post: The Changing Voice of Illness in Eighteenth-Century British Consultation Letters and Literature* (Amsterdam and New York: Rodopi, 2006)

Wilkins, Charles, *The History of the Literature of Wales from the Year 1300 to the Year 1650* (Cardiff: Daniel Owen and Co., 1884)

Williams, Glanmor, *The General and Common Sort of People 1540–1640* (Exeter: University of Exeter Press, 1977)

Williams, Glanmor, *Renewal and Reformation Wales c. 1415–1642* (Oxford: Oxford University Press, 2002 edition)

Williams, Glanmor, *Wales and the Reformation* (Cardiff: University of Wales Press, 1967)

Williams, Glanmor, *The Welsh and their Religion* (Cardiff: University of Wales Press, 1991)

Williams, Glanmor (ed.), *Glamorgan County History, Vol. IV: Early Modern Glamorgan* (Cardiff: Glamorgan County History Trust, 1974)

Williams, Gwyn, *An Introduction to Welsh Poetry* (London: Faber and Faber, 1964)

Williams, John, *Faunula Grustensis: Being an Outline of the Natural Contents of the Parish of Llanrwst* (Llanrwst: John Jones, 1830)

Select bibliography

Witmore, Michael, *Culture of Accidents: Unexpected Knowledges in Early Modern England* (Stanford: Stanford University Press, 2001)

Wood, Andy, *Riot, Rebellion and Popular Politics in Early Modern England* (Basingstoke: Palgrave, 2002)

Woolley, Benjamin, *The Herbalist: Nicholas Culpeper and the Fight for Medical Freedom* (London: Harper Collins, 2004)

Wrightson, Keith, *Earthly Necessities: Economic Lives in Early Modern Britain, 1470–1750* (London: Penguin, 2002 edition)

Wrightson, Keith, *English Society 1580–1680* (London and New York: Routledge, 2003 edition)

Chapters in edited collections

Allen, Richard C., 'The Administration of Poor Relief' in Griffiths, Ralph, Gray, Madeleine and Morgan, Prys (eds) *Gwent County History Volume 3: The Making of Monmouthshire 1536–1780* (Cardiff: University of Wales Press, 2009), pp. 272–284

Arkell, Tom 'Interpreting Probate Inventories' in Arkell, Tom, Evans, Nesta and Goose, Nigel (eds), *When Death Do Us Part: Understanding and Interpreting the Probate Records of Early Modern England* (London: Leopard's Head Press, 2004 edition), pp. 72–102

Barry, Jonathan, 'Piety and the Patient: Medicine and Religion in Eighteenth Century Bristol' in Porter, Roy (ed.), *Patients and Practitioners: Lay Perceptions of Medicine in Pre-Industrial Society* (Cambridge: Cambridge University Press, 2002 edition), pp. 145–176

Beier, Lucinda McCray, 'The Good Death in Seventeenth Century England' in Houlbrooke, Ralph (ed.), *Death, Ritual and Bereavement* (London and New York: Routledge, 1989), pp. 43–61

Beier, Lucinda McCray, 'In Sickness and in Health: A Seventeenth Century Family's Experience' in Porter, Roy (ed.), *Patients and Practitioners: Lay Perceptions of Medicine in Pre-Industrial Society* (Cambridge: Cambridge University Press, 2002 edition), pp. 101–128

Chapman, Allan, 'Astrological Medicine' in Webster, Charles (ed.), *Health, Medicine and Mortality in the Sixteenth Century* (Cambridge: Cambridge University Press, 1979), pp. 275–300

Clarke, Simone, 'Visions of Community: Elizabeth Baker and Late Eighteenth-Century Merioneth' in Roberts, Michael and Clarke, Simone (eds), *Women and Gender in Early Modern Wales* (Cardiff: University of Wales Press, 2000), pp. 234–258

Davies, G.C., 'The Welsh Doctor as a Poet: Henry Vaughan the Silurist' in Cule, John (ed.), *Wales and Medicine* (Llandysul: Gomer Press, 1975), pp. 112–118

Fissell, Mary E., 'Making Meanings from the Margins: The New Cultural History of Medicine' in Huisman, Frank and Harley Warner, John (eds), *Locating Medical History: The Stories and Their Meanings* (Baltimore and London: Johns Hopkins University Press, 2004), pp. 364–389

Fissell, Mary E., 'The Marketplace of Print' in Jenner, Mark S.R and Wallis, Patrick (eds), *Medicine and the Market in England and its Colonies, c. 1450 – c. 1850* (Basingstoke: Palgrave Macmillan, 2007), pp. 108–132

Select bibliography

Gregory, Jeremy, 'Homo Religiosus: Masculinity and Religion in the Long Eighteenth Century' in Hitchcock, Tim and Cohen, Michele (eds), *English Masculinities 1660–1800* (London: Longman, 1999), pp. 85–110

Griffiths, Matthew, 'Land, Life and Belief: Wales, 1415–1642' in Jones, Gareth Elwyn and Smith, Dai (eds), *The People of Wales* (Llandysul: Gomer Press, 2000), pp. 49–82

Gruffydd, R. Geraint, 'The First Printed Books, 1546–1604' in Jones, Philip Henry and Rees, Eiluned (eds), *A Nation and its Books: A History of the Book in Wales* (Aberystwyth: National Library of Wales, 1998), pp. 55–65

Harley, David, 'The Theology of Affliction and the Experience of Sickness in the Godly Family, 1650–1714: The Henrys and the Newcomes' in Grell, Ole Peter and Cunningham, Andrew (eds), *Religio Medici: Medicine and Religion in Seventeenth-Century England* (Aldershot: Scolar Press, 1996), pp. 273–292

Harries, W. Gerallt, 'Bened Feddyg: A Welsh Medical Practitioner in the Late Medieval Period' in Cule, John (ed.), *Wales and Medicine* (Llandysul: Gomer Press, 1975), pp. 169–184

Hindle, Steve, 'Civility, Honesty and the Identification of the Deserving Poor in Seventeenth-Century England' in French, Henry and Barry, Jonathan (eds), *Identity and Agency in England, 1500–1800* (Basingstoke: Palgrave Macmillan, 2004), pp. 38–59

Huisman, Frank and Harley Warner, John, 'Medical Histories' in Huisman, Frank and Harley Warner, John (eds), *Locating Medical History: The Stories and Their Meanings* (Baltimore and London: Johns Hopkins University Press, 2004), pp. 1–32

Jenkins, Geraint H., '"The Sweating Astrologer": Thomas Jones the Almanacer' in Davies, R.R., Griffiths, Ralph A., Jones, Ieuan Gwynedd and Morgan, Kenneth O. (eds), *Welsh Society and Nationhood: Historical Essays Presented to Glanmor Williams* (Cardiff: University of Wales Press, 1984), pp. 161–177

Jones, Glyn Penrhyn, 'The Welsh Poet as a Medical Historian' in Cule, John (ed.), *Wales and Medicine* (Llandysul: Gomer Press, 1975), pp. 119–126

Jordanova, Ludmilla, 'The Social Construction of Medical Knowledge' in Huisman, Frank and Harley Warner, John (eds), *Locating Medical History: The Stories and Their Meanings* (Baltimore and London: Johns Hopkins University Press, 2006 edition), pp. 338–363

Kelly, James, 'The Emergence of Scientific and Institutional Medical Practice in Ireland, 1650–1800' in Jones, Greta and Malcolm, Elizabeth (eds), *Medicine, Disease and the State in Ireland, 1650–1940* (Cork: Cork University Press, 1999), pp. 21–39

Leong, Elaine and Pennell, Sara, 'Recipe Collections and the Currency of Medical Knowledge in the Early Modern "Medical Marketplace"' in Jenner, Mark S.R. and Wallis, Patrick (eds), *Medicine and the Market in England and its Colonies, c. 1450 – c. 1850* (Basingstoke: Palgrave Macmillan, 2007), pp. 133–152

Lloyd, Sarah, '"Agents in their own Concerns?" Charity and the Economy of Makeshifts in Eighteenth Century Britain', in King, Steven and Tomkins, Allanah (eds), *The Poor in England 1700–1850* (Manchester: Manchester University Press, 2003), pp. 100–136

Llwyd, Rheinallt, 'Printing and Publishing in the Seventeenth Century', in Jones, Philip Henry and Rees, Eiluned (eds), *A Nation and its Books: A History of the Book in Wales* (Aberystwyth: National Library of Wales, 1998), pp. 93–107

Select bibliography

Mortimer, Ian, 'The Rural Medical Marketplace in Southern England, c. 1570–1720' in Jenner, Mark S.R. and Wallis, Patrick (eds), *Medicine and the Market in England and its Colonies, c. 1450 – c. 1850* (Basingstoke: Palgrave Macmillan, 2007), pp. 69–87

Porter, Roy, 'Laymen, Doctors and Medical Knowledge in the Eighteenth Century: The Evidence of the *Gentleman's Magazine*' in Porter, Roy (ed.), *Patients and Practitioners: Lay Perceptions of Medicine in Pre-Industrial Society* (Cambridge: Cambridge University Press, 2002 edition), pp. 283–314

Porter, Roy, 'The Patient in England, c. 1660 – c. 1800' in Wear, Andrew (ed.), *Medicine in Society: Historical Essays* (Cambridge: Cambridge University Press, 1998 edition), pp. 91–118

Ralley, Robert, 'Medical Economies in Fifteenth-Century England' in Jenner, Mark S.R. and Wallis, Patrick (eds), *Medicine and the Market in England and its Colonies, c. 1450 – c. 1850* (Basingstoke: Palgrave Macmillan, 2007), pp. 24–46

Roberts, Michael, 'Gender, Work and Socialisation in Wales, c. 1450 – c. 1850' in Betts, Sandra (ed.), *Our Daughter's Land: Past and Present* (Cardiff: University of Wales Press, 1996), pp. 15–54

Roberts, Stephen, 'Religion, Politics and Welshness, 1649–1660' in Roots, Ivan (ed.), *'Into Another Mould': Aspects of the Interregnum* (Exeter: University of Exeter Press, 1998 edition), pp. 30–47

Sokoll, Thomas, 'Old Age in Poverty: The Record of Essex Pauper Letters, 1780–1834' in Hitchcock, Tim, King, Peter and Sharpe, Pamela (eds), *Chronicling Poverty: The Voices and Strategies of the English Poor, 1640–1840* (Basingstoke: Macmillan, 1997), pp. 127–154

Stoyle, Mark, 'Caricaturing Cymru: Images of the Welsh in the London Press 1642–46' in Dunn, Diana (ed.), *War and Society in Medieval and Early Modern Britain* (Liverpool: Liverpool University Press, 2000), pp. 162–179

Suggett, Richard, 'Pedlars and Mercers as Distributors of Print in Early Modern Wales' in Isaac, Peter and McKay, Barry (eds), *The Mighty Engine: The Printing Press and its Impact* (Winchester: St Paul's Bibliographies, 2000), pp. 23–32

Suggett, Richard, 'Vagabonds and Minstrels in Sixteenth-Century Wales' in Fox, Adam and Woolf, Daniel (eds), *The Spoken Word: Oral Culture in Britain, 1500–1850* (Manchester: Manchester University Press, 2002), pp. 138–172

Suggett, Richard and White, Eryn, 'Language, Literacy and Aspects of Identity in Early Modern Wales' in Fox, Adam and Woolf, Daniel (eds), *The Spoken Word: Oral Culture in Britain, 1500–1850* (Manchester: Manchester University Press, 2002), pp. 52–83

Thomas, Keith, 'The Meaning of Literacy in Early Modern England' in Baumann, Gerd (ed.), *The Written Word: Literacy in Transition* (Oxford: Clarendon Press, 1986), pp. 97–131

Walker, Garthine, '"Strange kind of Stealing": Abduction in Early Modern Wales' in Roberts, Michael and Clarke, Simone (eds), *Women and Gender in Early Modern Wales* (Cardiff: University of Wales Press, 2000), pp. 50–74

Walter, John and Schofield, Roger, 'Famine, Disease and Crisis Mortality in Early Modern Society' in Walter, John and Schofield, Roger (eds), *Famine, Disease and the Social Order in Early Modern Society* (Cambridge: Cambridge University Press, 1991 edition), pp. 1–74

Select bibliography

Wear, Andrew, 'Making Sense of Health and the Environment in Early Modern England' in Wear, Andrew (ed.), *Medicine in Society: Historical Essays* (Cambridge: Cambridge University Press, 1998 edition), pp. 119–147

Wear, Andrew, 'Puritan Perceptions of Illness in Seventeenth-Century England' in Porter, Roy (ed.), *Patients and Practitioners: Lay Perceptions of Medicine in Pre-Industrial Society* (Cambridge: Cambridge University Press, 2002 edition), pp. 55–100

White, Eryn M., 'Women, Religion and Education in Eighteenth-Century Wales' in Roberts, Michael and Clarke, Simone (eds), *Women and Gender in Early Modern Wales* (Cardiff: University of Wales Press, 2000), pp. 210–233

Williams, Glanmor, 'The Renaissance and Reformation' in Jones, Philip Henry and Rees, Eiluned (eds), *A Nation and its Books: A History of the Book in Wales* (Aberystwyth: National Library of Wales, 1998), pp. 41–54

Williams, Moelwyn, E., 'The Economic and Social History of Glamorgan, 1660–1760' in Williams, Glanmor (ed.), *Glamorgan County History, Vol. IV: Early Modern Glamorgan* (Cardiff: Glamorgan County History Trust, 1974), pp. 311–374

Journals

Allen, Richard C. 'Wizards or Charlatans? Doctors or Herbalists? An Appraisal of the "Cunning Men" of Cwrt-y-Cadno, Carmarthenshire', *North American Journal of Welsh Studies*, 1:2 (Summer 2001), pp. 68–85

Arkell, Tom, 'Multiplying Factors for Estimating Population Totals from the Hearth Tax', *Local Population Studies*, 28 (1982), pp. 51–57

Baker-Jones, D.L., 'Notes on the Social Life of Carmarthenshire During the Eighteenth Century', *Transactions of the Honourable Society of Cymmrodorion* 2 (1963), pp. 273–282

Barlow, Frank, 'The King's Evil', *English Historical Review*, 95:374 (1980), pp. 3–27

Borsay, Peter, Miskell, Louise and Roberts, Owen, 'Introduction: Wales, a New Agenda for Urban History', *Urban History*, 32:1 (2005), pp. 5–16

Bosanquet, Eustace F., 'English Seventeenth Century Almanacks', *Library*, 10:4 (March 1930), pp. 361–397

Boulton, Jeremy, 'London Widowhood Revisited: The Decline of Female Remarriage in the Seventeenth and Early Eighteenth Centuries', *Continuity and Change*, 5 (1990), pp. 323–355

Bowen, Lloyd, 'Representations of Wales and the Welsh during the Civil Wars and Interregnum', *Historical Research*, 77:197 (2004), pp. 358–376

Brockbank, William, 'Sovereign Remedies: A Critical Depreciation of the 17th Century London Pharmacopoeia', *Medical History*, 8:1 (1964), pp. 1–14

Burnby, Juanita, 'A Study of the English Apothecary From 1660 to 1760', *Medical History Supplement*, No. 3, 1983

Cerdeira, Christine, 'Early Modern Medical Wills, Book Ownership and Book Culture', *Canadian Bulletin of Medical History*, 12:2 (1995), pp. 427–439

Churchill, Wendy D., 'The Medical Practice of the Sexed Body: Women, Men and Disease in Britain *circa* 1600 to 1740', *Social History of Medicine*, 18:1 (2005), pp. 3–22

Claydon, 'Great Britain: Identities, Institutions and the Idea of Britishness', *Historical Journal*, 42:2 (1999), pp. 585–586

Corfield, Penelope J., 'From Poison Peddlers to Civic Worthies: The Reputation of the Apothecaries in Georgian England', *Social History of Medicine*, 22:1 (2009), pp. 1–22

Cule, John, 'The Court Mediciner and Medicine in the Laws of Wales', *Journal of the History of Medicine and Allied Sciences*, 22:3 (1966), pp. 213–236

Cule, John, 'Some Early Hospitals in Wales and the Border', *National Library of Wales Journal*, 20:2 (1977), pp. 97–130

Curth, Louise, 'The Commercialisation of Medicine in the Popular Press: English Almanacs, 1640–1700', *Seventeenth Century*, 17 (Spring, 2002), pp. 48–69

Curth, Louise, 'The Medical Content of English Almanacs', *Journal of the History of Medicine and Allied Sciences*, 60:3 (2005), pp. 255–282

Dacombe, Lucia, 'Noting the Mind: Commonplace Books and the Pursuit of the Self in Eighteenth Century Britain', *Journal of the History of Ideas*, 65:4 (2004), pp. 603–625

Davies, Edward, 'Llanrhaeadr-ym-Mochnant: Disease and Mortality in a Welsh Rural Parish in the Eighteenth Century', *Transactions of the Denbighshire Historical Society*, 55 (2007), pp. 66–95

Davies, Owen, 'Cunning-Folk in England and Wales during the Eighteenth and Nineteenth Centuries', *Rural History*, 8:1 (1997), pp. 91–107

Dingwall, Helen M., '"General Practice" in Seventeenth Century Edinburgh: Evidence from the Burgh Court', *Social History of Medicine*, 6:1 (1993), pp. 125–142

Dobson, Mary J., 'Disease, Mortality and the Environment in Early Modern England', *Health Transition Review*, 2 – Supplementary Issue (1992)

Dodd, A.H. 'The Old Poor Law in North Wales', *Archaeologia Cambrensis*, 81:6 (1926), pp. 111–132

Dunn, Peter M., 'Dr William Buchan (1729–1805) and his Domestic Medicine', *Archives of Disease in Childhood: Foetal and Neonatal Education and Practice*, 83 (2000), pp. 71–73

Durbach, Nadja, 'The Social History of British Medicine: An Essay Review', *Journal of the History of Medicine and Allied Sciences*, 57:4 (2002), pp. 487–489

Evans, Neil, 'Rethinking Urban Wales', *Urban History*, 32:1 (2005), pp. 114–131

Fissell, Mary E., 'Introduction: Women, Health and Healing in Early Modern Europe', *Bulletin of the History of Medicine*, 82:1 (2008), pp. 1–17

Hann, Andrew and Stobart, Jon, 'Sites of Consumption: The Display of Goods in Provincial Shops in Eighteenth-Century England', *Cultural and Social History*, 2 (2005), pp. 165–187

Harley, David, 'Rhetoric and the Social Construction of Sickness and Healing', *Social History of Medicine*, 12:3 (1999), pp. 407–435

Havens, Earle, '"Of Common Places or Memorial Books": An Anonymous Manuscript on Commonplace Books and the Art of Memory in Seventeenth Century England', *Yale University Library Gazette*, 76:3–4 (2002), pp. 136–153.

Haycock, David Boyd and Wallis, Patrick, 'Quackery and Commerce in Seventeenth-Century London: The Proprietary Medicine Business of Anthony Daffy', *Medical History Supplement No. 25*, 2005

Select bibliography

Hindle, Steve, 'Power, Poor Relief and Social Relations in Holland Fen c. 1600–1800', *Historical Journal*, 41:1 (1998), pp. 67–96

Hostick, Malvern, 'From the Parish Records for Misterton, Notts, 1730', *Lincolnshire Family History Society Journal*, 14:4 (November 2003), pp. 225–226

Ingman, John, 'The Early Days of the Caernarvonshire and Anglesey Hospital, with Notes on Some of Bangor's Medical Practitioners 1772–1856', *Caernarvonshire Historical Society Transactions*, 2 (1950), pp. 61–72

Jenkins, David, 'A Late Seventeenth Century Llanfyllin Shopkeeper: The Will and Inventory of Cadwalader Jones', *Montgomeryshire Collections*, 69 (1981), pp. 45–56

Jenkins, Geraint H., 'Popular Beliefs in Wales from Restoration to Methodism', *Bulletin of the Board of Celtic Studies*, 27:3 (1977), pp. 440–462

Jenkins, Geraint H., '"A Rank Republican [And] a Leveller": William Jones, Llangadfan', *Welsh History Review*, 17:3 (1995), pp. 365–386

Jenkins, Philip, 'A New History of Wales', *Historical Journal*, 32:2 (1989), pp. 387–393

Jones, Brinley J., 'The Population of Eighteenth Century West Glamorgan: The Evidence of the Parish Registers', *Glamorgan Historian*, 12, pp. 177–198

Jones, Evan D., 'Gleanings from the Radnorshire Files of Great Sessions Papers, 1691–1699', *Radnorshire Society Transactions*, 13 (1943), pp. 7–34

Jones, Glyn Penrhyn, 'Some Aspects of the Medical History of Caernarvonshire', *Caernarvonshire Historical Society Transactions*, 23 (1962), pp. 67–91

Jones, Glyn Penrhyn, 'Some Aspects of the Medical History of Denbighshire', *Denbighshire Historical Society Transactions*, 8 (1959), pp. 40–66

Jones, Ida B., 'Hafod 16: A Mediaeval Welsh Medical Treatise', *Études Celtiques*, 8 (1958–59), pp. 346–393

Jordanova, Ludmilla 'Has the Social History of Medicine Come of Age?', *Historical Journal*, 36:2 (1993), pp. 437–449

Kent, Joan and King, Steve, 'Changing Patterns of Poor Relief in Some English Rural Parishes', *Rural History*, 14:2 (2003), pp. 119–156

King, Steve, 'Dying with Style: Infant Death and its Context in a Rural Industrial Township c. 1650–1830', *Social History of Medicine*, 10:1 (1997), pp. 3–24

Lawton, Julia, 'Lay Experiences of Health and Illness: Past Research and Future Agendas', *Sociology of Health and Illness*, 25 (2003), pp. 23–40

Leong, Elaine, 'Making Medicines in the Early Modern Household', *Bulletin of the History of Medicine*, 82:1 (2008), pp. 145–168

Lovering, G.W.J., 'Some Glimpses of Seventeenth Century Monmouthshire', *Gwent Local History*, 73 (1992), pp. 9–34

Lyman Dixon, Anthony, 'The Physicians of Myddfai', *Herbs*, 24:2 (1999), pp. 18–23

McKay, Elaine, 'English Diarists: Gender, Geography and Occupation, 1500–1700', *History*, 90:298 (2005), pp. 191–212

Manley, G., 'Central England Temperatures: Monthly Means 1659 to 1973', *Quarterly Journal of the Royal Meteorological Society*, 100 (1974), pp. 389–405

Matthews, Leslie A., 'Day Book of the Court Apothecary in the Time of William and Mary, 1691', *Medical History*, 22 (1978), pp. 161–173

Select bibliography

Morgan, Gerald, 'Bottom of the Heap: Identifying the Poor in West Wales Records', *Llafur*, 7:1 (1996), pp. 13–28

Morgan, Prys, 'A Welsh Snakestone: Its Tradition and Folklore', *Folklore*, 94:2 (1983), pp. 184–191

Morris, T.E., 'The Parish Book of Cefnllys, Radnorshire', *Archaeologia Cambrensis*, 19:1 (1919), pp. 35–94

Mortimer, Ian, 'Diocesan Licensing and Medical Practitioners in South-West England, 1660–1780', *Medical History*, 48:1 (2004), pp. 49–68

Owen, Hugh, 'The Corporation of Beaumaris Minute Book (1694–1723)', *Transactions of the Anglesey Antiquarian Society* (1932), pp. 75–91

Owen, Hugh, 'The Diary of Bulkeley of Dronwy, Anglesey 1630–1636', *Transactions of the Anglesey Antiquarian Society* (1937), pp. 26–169

Owen, Leonard, 'The Letters of an Anglesey Parson, 1712–1732', *Transactions of the Honourable Society of Cymmrodorion*, 1 (1961), pp. 72–100

Owen, Leonard, 'The Population of Wales in the Sixteenth and Seventeenth Centuries', *Transactions of the Honourable Society of Cymmrodorion* (1959), pp. 99–113

Owen, Morfydd E., 'The Medical Books of Medieval Wales and the Physicians of Myddfai', *Carmarthenshire Antiquary*, 31 (1995), pp. 34–45

Owen, T.J., 'The Records of the Parish of Aber', *Caernarvonshire Historical Society Transactions*, 14 (1953), pp. 74–93

Pelling, Margaret, 'The Women of the Family? Speculation around Early Modern British Physicians', *Social History of Medicine*, 7:3 (1995), pp. 383–401

Pettegree, Andrew, 'Centre and Periphery in the Early Modern Book World', *Transactions of the Royal Historical Society*, 18 (2008), pp. 101–128

Porter, Roy, 'Lay Medical Knowledge in the Eighteenth Century: The Evidence of the *Gentleman's Magazine*', *Medical History*, 29:2 (1985), pp. 138–168

Powell, Nia, 'Do Numbers Count? Towns in Early Modern Wales', *Urban History*, 32:1 (2005), pp. 46–67

Powell, Nia, 'Urban Population in Early Modern Wales Revisited', *Welsh History Review*, 23:3 (June 2007), pp. 1–31

Raven, James, 'New Reading Histories, Print Culture and the Identification of Change: The Case of Eighteenth-century England', *Social History*, 23:3 (1998), pp. 268–287

Rogers, Shannon, L. 'From Wasteland to Wonderland: Wales in the Imagination of the English Traveller, 1720–1895', *North American Journal of Welsh Studies*, 2:2 (Summer 2002), pp. 15–26

Rublack, Ulinka (translated by Pamela Selwyn), 'Fluxes: The Early Modern Body and the Emotions', *History Workshop Journal*, 53 (2002), pp. 1–16

Seguin, Colleen M. 'Cures and Controversy in Early Modern Wales: The Struggle to Control St Winifred's Well', *North American Journal of Welsh Studies*, 3:2 (Summer 2003), pp. 1–17

Shammas, Carol, 'Food Expenditure and Economic Well-Being in Early Modern England', *Journal of Economic History*, 43:1 (March 1983), pp. 89–100

Select bibliography

Sharpe, J.A., '"Last Dying Speeches": Religion, Ideology and Public Execution in Seventeenth Century England', *Past and Present*, 107:1 (1985), pp. 144–167

Shepard, Alexandra, 'Poverty, Labour and the Language of Self-Description in Early Modern England', *Past and Present*, 201:1 (2008), pp. 51–95

Skeel, Caroline, 'Social and Economic Conditions in Wales and the Marches in the Early Seventeenth Century, as Illustrated by Harl. MS 4220', *Transactions of the Honourable Society of Cymmrodorion* (1916–17), pp. 119–144

Stedman Davies, Rev. D. and Mason, Rev. A., 'Llangynllo', *Radnorshire Society Transactions*, 12 (1942), pp. 64–73

Stobart, Jon, 'Shopping Streets as Social Spaces: Leisure, Consumerism and Improvement in an Early Eighteenth Century Town', *Urban History*, 25:1 (1998), pp. 3–21

Stoyle, Mark, 'English "Nationalism", Celtic Particularism and the English Civil War', *Historical Journal*, 43:4 (2000), pp. 1,113–1,128

Sugg, Richard, '"Good Physic but Bad Food": Early Modern Attitudes to Medicinal Cannibalism and its Providers', *Social History of Medicine*, 19:2 (2006), pp. 225–240

Tallis, Lisa, 'The "Doctor Faustus" of Cwrt-Y-Cadno: A New Perspective on John Harries and Popular Medicine in Wales', *Welsh History Review*, 24:3 (2009), pp. 1–28

Teale, Adrian, 'The Battle against Poverty in North Flintshire, c. 1660–1714', *Flintshire Historical Society Journal*, 31 (1983/84), pp. 71–108

Thomas, G.B., 'Llanaber Vestry Records, 1726–54', *Journal of the Merioneth Historical and Record Society*, 2 (1953–56), pp. 271–284

Thomas, Henry, 'An Old Vestry Book', *Journal of the Merioneth Historical and Record Society*, 2 (1953–56), pp. 39–44

Turner, I. and Turner, D.T., 'The Pharmacy of the Physicians of Myddfai', *Pharmaceutical History*, 13:2 (1983), pp. 1–27

Vaughan, Mary, 'An Old Receipt Book', *Journal of the Merioneth Historical and Record Society*, 4 (1964), pp. 318–323

Wallis, Patrick, 'Consumption, Retailing and Medicine in Early Modern London', *Economic History Review*, 61:1 (February 2008), pp. 26–53

Walsham, '"Frantick Hacket": Prophecy, Sorcery, Insanity and the Elizabethan Puritan Movement', *Historical Journal*, 41:1 (1998), pp. 27–66

Weber, A.S., 'Women's Early Modern Medical Almanacs in Historical Context', *English Literary Renaissance*, 33:3 (2003), pp. 358–402

Whittet, T. Douglas, 'Welsh Apothecaries' and Barber-Surgeons' Tokens and their Issuers', *Archaeologia Cambrensis*, 138 (1990), pp. 99–109

Whyte, Nicola, 'Landscape, Memory and Custom: Parish Identities c. 1550–1700', *Social History*, 32:2 (2007), pp. 166–186

Willen, Diane, 'Women in the Public Sphere in Early Modern England: The Case of the Urban Working Poor', *Sixteenth Century Journal*, 19:4 (1988), pp. 559–575

Williams, Moelwyn E., 'A General View of Glamorgan Houses and their Interiors in the Seventeenth and Eighteenth Centuries', *Glamorgan Historian*, 10 (1974), pp. 157–176

Withey, Alun, 'Medicine and Mortality in Early Modern Monmouthshire: The

Select bibliography

Commonplace Book of John Gwin of Llangwm', *Welsh History Review*, 23:1 (June 2006), pp. 48–73

Withey, Alun, 'Unhealthy Neglect? The Medicine and Medical Historiography of Early Modern Wales, *Social History of Medicine*, 21:1 (2008), pp. 163–174

Woodward, Nick, 'Crisis Mortality in a Welsh Market Town: Carmarthen, 1675–1799', *Welsh History Review*, 22:3 (June 2005), pp. 432–462

Woodward, Nick, 'Infanticide in Wales, 1730–1830', *Welsh History Review*, 23:3 (June 2007), pp. 94–125

Wunderli, Richard and Broce, Gerald, 'The Final Moment before Death in Early Modern England', *Sixteenth Century Journal*, 20:2 (1989), pp. 259–275

Young, J.T., 'Illness Behaviour: A Selective Review and Synbook', *Sociology of Health and Illness*, 26:1 (2004), pp. 1–31

Theses

Jones, Glyn Penrhyn, 'A History of Medicine in Wales in the Eighteenth Century' (Liverpool University: Unpublished MA Thesis, 1957)

Leong, Elaine, 'Medical Recipe Collections in Seventeenth Century England: Knowledge, Text and Gender' (University of Oxford: Unpublished DPhil Thesis, 2006)

Stine, Jennifer K., 'Opening the Closets: The Discovery of Household Medicine in Early Modern England' (Stanford University: Unpublished PhD Thesis, 1996)

Stobart, Anne, 'The Making of Domestic Medicine: Gender, Self-Help and Therapeutic Determination in Household Healthcare in South-West England in the Seventeenth Century' (Middlesex University: Unpublished PhD Thesis, 2008)

Tallis, Lisa M., 'The Conjuror, the Fairy, the Devil and the Preacher: Witchcraft, Popular Magic and Religion in Wales, 1700–1905' (University of Wales, Swansea: Unpublished PhD Thesis, 2007)

Williams, Gareth Haulfryn, 'A Study of Caernarfonshire Probates, 1630–1690' (University of Wales: Unpublished MA Thesis, 1972)

Index

Index

Index

Lightning Source UK Ltd.
Milton Keynes UK
UKOW05f1539101013

218809UK00002B/12/P